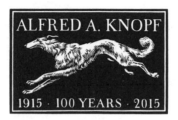

ALSO BY CHRISTOPHER MCDOUGALL

Born to Run

NATURAL BORN HEROES

NATURAL BORN HEROES

How a Daring Band of Misfits Mastered the

Lost Secrets of Strength and Endurance

Christopher McDougall

ALFRED A. KNOPF · NEW YORK · 2015

THIS IS A BORZOI BOOK
PUBLISHED BY ALFRED A. KNOPF

www.aaknopf.com

Library of Congress Cataloging-in-Publication Data
McDougall, Christopher, 1962–
Natural born heroes : how a daring band of misfits mastered the lost secrets of strength and
endurance / by Christopher McDougall. — First edition.
pages   cm
"This is a Borzoi book"—Title page verso.
ISBN 978-0-307-59496-9   (hardback) ISBN 978-0-307-96228-7
1. World War, 1939–1945—Underground movements—Greece—Crete.   2. Kreipe, Karl—
Kidnapping, 1944.   3. Soldiers—Greece—Crete—History—20th century.   4. Heroes—
Greece—Crete—History—20th century.   5. Long-distance running—Greece—History.
6. Physical fitness—Greece—History.   7. Heroes—History.   8. Physical fitness—
Philosophy.   9. Athletics—Philosophy.   I. Title.
D766.7.C7M535 2015
940.53'4959—dc23
2014047459

Map illustration by Robert Bull

Jacket composite image by Terry Sanders:
(man) Larry Lilac/Alamy; (hill) 24BY36/Alamy
Jacket design by Chip Kidd

Manufactured in the United States of America

First Edition

To my parents, John and Jean McDougall.
"Anything which I have done
which you may consider worthwhile,"
as Howard Hughes once said,
"has been made possible
by the genius of my father."

Tradition carries a nasty wallop.

—JOURNALIST HEYWOOD BROUN,
as he watched an old boxer destroy a young challenger in 1922

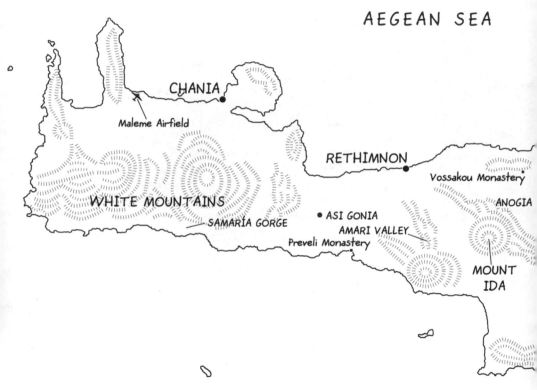

AEGEAN SEA

CHANIA

Maleme Airfield

RETHIMNON

Vossakou Monastery

ANOGIA

WHITE MOUNTAINS

SAMARIA GORGE

ASI GONIA

AMARI VALLEY

Preveli Monastery

MOUNT
IDA

MEDITERRANEAN SEA

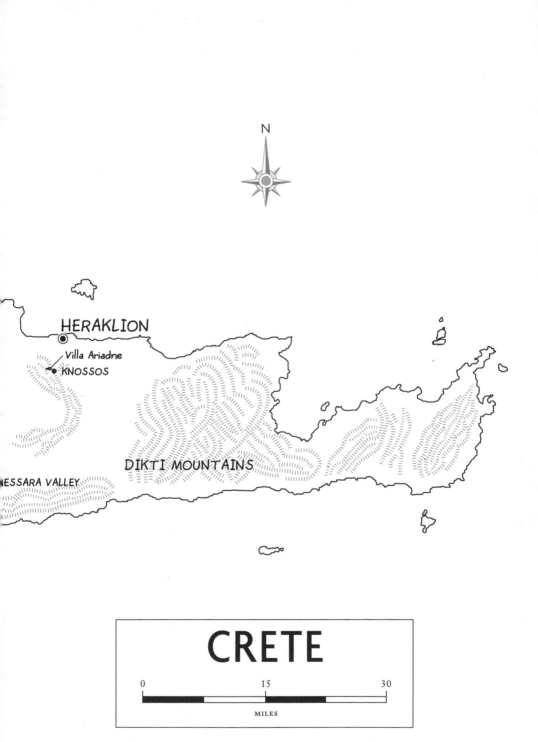

N

HERAKLION

Villa Ariadne

KNOSSOS

DIKTI MOUNTAINS

MESSARA VALLEY

CRETE

0   15   30

MILES

NATURAL BORN HEROES

CHAPTER 1

YOU'VE GOT TO PUT YOURSELF in the Butcher's shoes.

You're General Friedrich-Wilhelm Müller, one of two German commanders on the Greek island of Crete. Hitler is worried that something terrible is about to happen right under your nose, something that could severely damage the German offensive, but you've got it all under control. The island is small and your manpower is huge. You've got 100,000 seasoned troops, with search planes prowling the mountains and patrol boats monitoring the beaches. You've got the Gestapo at your service, and you're scary enough to be called the Butcher. No one is going to mess with you.

And then you wake up on the morning of April 24, 1944, to discover the other you is gone. Your fellow commander, General Heinrich Kreipe, has disappeared. There's no hint of foul play: no shots fired, no bloodshed, no signs of a scuffle. Stranger yet, the general vanished from somewhere around the capital, the most heavily guarded corner of the island. Whatever happened, it happened right in front of the general's own men. Kreipe was no toy soldier, either; he was a serious hard case, a Great War survivor with an Iron Cross who'd battled his way up through the ranks and just transferred in from the Russian front. He had a personal security force and an armed driver and a villa surrounded by attack dogs, razor wire, and machine-gun posts.

So where was he?

All the Butcher knew was this: shortly after 9 P.M., General Kreipe left his command base and drove into the center of town. It was Saturday, so foot traffic was thicker than usual. Troops from outlying garrisons had been bused in for a movie, and the streets were jammed with strolling soldiers. The movie had just let out; the Butcher knew this because hundreds of soldiers had seen the black sedan with the general's flags on the bumper inching its way through the streets. General Kreipe's driver had to honk them out of the way, even rolling down his window at one point to holler, *"GENERALS WAGEN!"* Kreipe was right there in the front passenger seat, nodding his head and returning salutes. Every road in every direction at every half-mile was guarded by checkpoints. The general's car passed Gestapo headquarters and funneled through the last checkpoint, the narrow opening at the Canae Gate. *"Gute Nacht,"* the general's driver called. The sedan slid beneath the crossbar and exited the city.

Early the next morning, the general's car was discovered on a scruff of beach just outside the city. The general and his driver were gone, as were the eagle flags from the front bumper. Around the car was a weird scattering of rubbish: an Agatha Christie novel, Cadbury milk chocolate wrappers, a bunch of English "Player's" cigarette butts, and a green British commando beret. On the dashboard was a letter. It was addressed to "The German authorities on Crete" and said that Kreipe had been captured by a British raiding force and taken off the island. The letter was ceremonially sealed with red wax and signet rings, and included a jaunty postscript:

> **We are very sorry to have to leave this beautiful motor car behind.**

Something didn't add up. The general must have been grabbed after he left the city, but his car was found only a twenty-minute drive away. So within that brief window, these mystery men had executed an ambush, disarmed and subdued two prisoners, smoked a pack of cigarettes, shared some snacks, lost a hat, melted wax, and what else— browsed a paperback? Was this an abduction or a family vacation? Plus that stretch of coast was floodlit by klieg lights and patrolled by planes. Why would seasoned commandos choose the most exposed part of the island as their extraction point? From that beach, their escape boat would have to head north into hundreds of miles of German-occupied waters, making them sitting ducks as soon as the sun came up.

Whoever did this was trying very hard to look very British, very cool and under control. But the Butcher wasn't buying it. He was in the midst of his second World War and to his knowledge, no general had ever been kidnapped before. There was no precedent for this sort of thing, no tactics, so they had to be making it up as they went along. Which meant that sooner or later, they'd make a blunder and fall right into his hands. Already, they'd made a big mistake: they'd badly underestimated their opponent. Because the Butcher had seen through their feints and realized two things:

They were still on his island, and they were running for their lives.

CHAPTER 2

Those brave in killing will be killed.
Those brave in not killing will live.

—LAO-TZU

ON A SPRING MORNING IN 2012, I stood where the general's car was found, wondering the same thing as the Butcher: where could they possibly go?

At my back is the Aegean Sea. In front, there's nothing but a snarl of chest-high brambles leading to a sheer cliff. In the far distance and cutting the island in half like a giant border fence is the craggy range of snowy Mount Ida, the highest climb in Greece. The only possible escape is the southern coast, but the only way to get there is up and over that eight-thousand-foot peak. The trek alone would be a challenge, but pulling it off with a belligerent prisoner in tow and a massive manhunt hot on your heels? Impossible.

"Ah!" There's a shout from somewhere inside the brambles, then a hand jerks up like it's hailing a cab. "Come toward me."

Chris White remains rooted in place, his arm high so I can find him and his eyes pinned on whatever he's spotted. I heave my backpack over my shoulders and begin fighting my way toward him, thorns tearing at my clothes. No one alive knows more about what happened to General Kreipe than Chris White, which is odd, because there's no reason Chris White should know anything about what happened to General Kreipe. Chris isn't a scholar or a military historian. He doesn't speak Greek or German, and as a lifelong pacifist he has no real taste for war stories. By day, Chris is a social worker who manages care for the elderly and the mentally disabled in the quiet English city of Oxford. But at night and on weekends, he's buried in a stack of topographical maps and out-of-print books in a little wooden shack behind his country cottage. In the great tradition of British amateur obsessives, Chris has spent the past ten years piecing together the mystery the Butcher faced on the morning of April 24, 1944: how do you make a German general disappear on an island swarming with German troops?

It was a magical idea. That's what Chris White loved about it. The scheme was so perfectly, defiantly *un*-Nazi: instead of force and brutality, the plan was to trip Hitler up with ingenuity and finesse. There would be no bullets, no blood, no civilians in the middle. Killing the general would have made him just another casualty of war, but *not* killing him would flip the tables and inflict a touch of fear in the men who were terrorizing Europe. The sheer mystery would make the Nazis crazy and plant an itch of doubt in every soldier's mind: if these phantoms could get the most protected man on a fortified island, then who was safe?

But getting him was only the beginning. The Butcher would throw everything he had into the manhunt, and what he had was a lot. He'd have troops combing the woods, attack dogs searching for scent, recon planes buzzing the mountains and clicking photos of goat trails for ground scouts to later follow on foot. The Gestapo would offer bribes and rewards and activate its network of local traitors. The Butcher had more than one soldier for every four civilians, giving him a tighter security ratio than you'd find in a maximum-security prison. And that's what Crete had become: a prison fenced in by the sea. Crete had never been an ordinary island in the first place, at least not in Hitler's eyes. The Führer counted on Crete as a crucial transit point for German troops and supplies heading to the Russian front, and he intended to keep it safe as a bank vault. The slightest hint of any Cretan resistance, Hitler had ordered, should be crushed with *eine gewisse brutalität*—"a good bit of brutality."

And to make it clear what he meant by *brutalität*, Hitler put the island in the hands of his dream warrior: General Müller, a seventeen-year veteran with a Knight's Cross for extreme bravery whose ruthlessness soon earned him the nickname "the Butcher of Crete." The Butcher's chief henchman was a Gestapo sergeant named Fritz Schubert, a Middle East–born German better known as "the Turk." With his walnut skin and fluency in Greek and English, the Turk was able to disguise himself as a shepherd and sniff out information by hanging around cafés and village squares. His favorite trick was putting on a British uniform, then pulling a Cretan with a death sentence from the dungeon and offering him freedom if he introduced the Turk around his village as a British commando who'd come to help the Resistance. "They were very skillful, well used to deceiving guileless people," one Cretan survivor would recall.

But maybe the Butcher was the sucker this time. Maybe the kidnappers deliberately overdid it with the rubbish around the general's car because they wanted to toy with the Butcher and make him wonder if the general was still on the island. Then he'd fan out his troops all across those mountains . . . only to wheel around and discover Allied troops were storming the beaches. If so, then bravo—the Butcher had to applaud their cunning.

Crete, that remote little island, was secretly one of Hitler's constant anxieties. "A fear that Greece and Crete would be invaded arose in January 1943," explained Antony Beevor, the British military historian whose father served with wartime intelligence. "The innermost German terror was of a Cretan uprising in the rear." Hitler's forces were already stretched dangerously thin, occupying more than a dozen countries while locked in vicious fighting across Russia and North Africa. A stab in the back in Crete could be a disaster. Either way, the Butcher had to wrap this mess up fast. The longer the general was missing, the more the Butcher looked weak and vulnerable—both to his enemies and to his own men.

So by noon of that first morning, the Butcher came up with a plan to trap the rats. His planes were soon in the air and snowing down leaflets over Heraklion, the coastal city that would become Crete's capital:

> IF THE GENERAL IS NOT RETURNED WITHIN THREE DAYS,
> ALL VILLAGES IN THE HERAKLION DISTRICT WILL BE BURNED
> TO THE GROUND. THE SEVEREST MEASURES OF REPRISAL
> WILL BE BROUGHT TO BEAR ON THE CIVILIAN POPULATION.

The clock was ticking. The Butcher had plenty of brave soldiers; what he needed was frightened civilians. *Let's see how far those bandits get once everyone on the island turns against them.*

Chris White parted the brambles and pointed. In the dirt, a thin scuff led to a low tunnel through the brush. It wasn't much of a scuff, but it was the best we'd seen all morning.

"They went this way," Chris said. "Let's go."

CHRIS TOOK POINT. Brambles twined across the trail like netting and the footing was a loose jumble of scrabbly stone. The scuff kept twisting places it shouldn't—veering back on itself, disappearing into overgrown gullies—but Chris was unstoppable. Whenever the trail seemed to die for good, Chris would disappear in the mess until eventually, his hand shot back up:

"AH!"

No, my gut kept telling me. *This is all wrong.* Why would anyone blaze a trail that runs smack into a boulder? Or in and out of a gully instead of alongside it? I had to remind myself we were steering by goat logic; on Crete, goats break the trail and goatherds follow, adapting themselves to the animals' feel for the landscape. And once I stopped doubting the goat logic, I noticed the slickness of the stones and remembered something else: water only travels in one direction. No matter how weirdly these washouts twisted us around, we had to be gaining altitude. Imperceptibly, we were wormholing our way up the cliff.

"Doesn't it take your breath away?" said Chris. "Before we came, it's possible no one had walked through here since the German occupation. It's like going into an ancient tomb."

Soon Chris and I were beetling along at a steady clip. Well, Chris beetled and I followed. He broke the trail and ranged ahead while I focused on just keeping pace. I'm ten years younger than Chris and I *thought* in much better shape, so it was humbling to face the fact that this sixty-year-old social-services administrator who never works out and looks like he's best suited for a comfy chair and a Sunday paper could shame me with his endurance and uphill agility.

"It must come naturally." Chris shrugged.

Did it? That's what I was on Crete to find out.

The ancients called Crete "the Sliver," and when your plane is coming in for a landing with no hint of land below, you'll know why. Right when you think you're about to plunge into the sea, the pilot banks and the island bursts into view, frothy around the edges as if it just popped up from the deep. Looming in the harbor behind the airport is a gloomy stone fortress, a sixteenth-century Venetian relic that only adds to the sensation that you're punching through a portal in time and about to enter a world summoned back from the past.

Crete has another nickname—"the Island of Heroes"—which I'd only discovered by accident. I was researching Pheidippides, the ancient Greek messenger who inspired the modern marathon, when I came across an odd reference to a modern-day Pheidippides named George Psychoundakis, better known as "the Clown." The Clown was awe-inspiring. When Hitler's forces invaded Crete, he transformed himself overnight from a sheep farmer into a mountain-running messenger for the Resistance. Somehow, George was able to master challenges that would stagger an Olympic athlete: he could scramble snowy cliffs with a sixty-pound pack on his back, run fifty-plus miles through the night on a starvation diet of boiled hay, and outfox a Gestapo death squad that had him cornered. George wasn't even a trained soldier; he was a shepherd living a sleepy, peaceful life until the day German parachutes popped open over his home.

Until then, I'd thought the secrets of ancient heroes like Pheidippides were either half myth or lost to antiquity, but here was a normal man pulling off the same feats 2,500 years later. And he wasn't alone: George himself told the story of a fellow shepherd who singlehandedly saved a villageful of women and children from a German massacre. The Germans had come to search for weapons and became suspicious when they realized all the men were missing and none of the women were talking. The German commander had the women lined up for execution. Just as he was about to say "Fire!" his skull exploded. A shepherd named Costi Paterakis had raced to the rescue through the woods, arriving just in time to take aim from a quarter-mile away. The rest of the Germans scattered for cover—and fell right into the crosshairs of Resistance fighters who arrived on Costi's heels.

"It still seems to me one of the most spectacular moments of the war," said a British Resistance operative whose own life was saved by the silence of those brave women. The story is so stirring, it's easy to forget what it really required. Costi had to ignore self-preservation and propel his body toward danger; he had to cover miles of cross-country terrain at top speed without a stumble; he had to quickly master rage, panic, and exhaustion as he slowed his pounding heart to steady his gun. It wasn't just an act of courage—it was a triumph of natural heroism and physical self-mastery.

The more I looked into Crete during the Resistance, the more stories like that I found. Was there really an American high school student fighting alongside the rebels behind German lines? Who was the starving prisoner who escaped a POW camp and turned himself into a master of retaliation known as "the Lion"? And most of all: what really happened when a band of misfits tried to sneak the German commander off the island? Even the Nazis realized that when they landed on Crete, they'd entered an entirely different kind of fight. On the day he was sentenced to death for war crimes, Hitler's chief of staff didn't blame the Nuremberg judges for his fate. He didn't blame his troops for losing, or even the Führer for letting him down. He blamed the Island of Heroes.

"The unbelievably strong resistance of the Greeks delayed by two or more vital months the German attack against Russia," General Wilhelm Keitel lamented shortly before he was led out to be hanged. "If we did not have this long delay, the outcome of the war would have been different . . . and others would be sitting here today."

And nowhere in Greece was the Resistance more ingenious, immediate, and enduring than on Crete. So what exactly were they tapping into?

There was a time when that question wouldn't be a mystery. For much of human history, the art of the hero wasn't left up to chance; it was a multidisciplinary endeavor devoted to optimal nutrition, physical self-mastery, and mental conditioning. The hero's skills were studied, practiced, and perfected, then passed along from parent to child and teacher to student. The art of the hero wasn't about being brave; it was about being so competent that bravery wasn't an issue. You weren't supposed to go down for a good cause; the goal was to figure out a way not to go down at all. Achilles and Odysseus and the rest of the classical heroes hated the thought of dying and scratched for every second of life. A hero's one crack at immortality was to be remembered as a champion, and champions don't die dumb. It all hinged on the ability to unleash the tremendous resources of strength, endurance, and agility that many people don't realize they already have.

Heroes learned how to use their own body fat for fuel instead of relying on bursts of sugar, the way nearly all of us do today. Roughly one-fifth of your body is stored fat; that's all premium caloric energy, ready for ignition and plentiful enough to power you up and down a mountain without a bite of food—*if* you know how to tap into it. Fat as fuel is an all-but-forgotten secret of endurance athletes, but when it's revived, the results are astonishing. Mark Allen, the greatest triathlete in history, made his breakthrough when he discovered a way to burn body fat in place of carbs. It revolutionized his approach to the sport and led to six Ironman titles, a top-three finish in nearly every race of his career, and recognition in 1997 as the "World's Fittest Man."

Heroes also didn't bulk up on muscle; instead they relied on the lean, efficient force of their fascia, the powerful connective tissue that is like your body's rubber band. Bruce Lee was a so-so martial artist until he became fascinated by Wing Chun, the only fighting art created by a woman. Wing Chun relies on fascial *snap* instead of muscular force. Lee became so adept at harnessing the power of his fascia that he perfected a one-inch punch, a blow from a barely moving fist that could send a man twice his size sailing across the room. Fascia power is an egalitarian and almost undepletable resource. It's the reason Masai warriors, in their jumping rituals, can bounce along as high as a man's head, and it's the essence of both Greek pankration and Brazilian jiu-jitsu, two of the most lethal self-defense styles ever created.

Heroes had to be masters of the unpredictable. They trained their amygdalae by practicing "natural movement," which used to be the only kind of movement we knew. Just to survive, humans had to be able to flow across the landscape, bending their bodies over and around any obstacle in their path, leaping without fear and landing with precision. Back in the early 1900s, a French naval officer named Georges Hébert dedicated himself to the study of natural movement; he watched the way children play—running and climbing and tussling around—and began to appreciate the importance of spontaneity and improvisation. When Hébert's natural movement disciples were later tested for strength, speed, agility, and endurance, they scored on par with world-class decathletes.

That's why the Greeks didn't wait for heroes to appear; they built their own instead. They perfected a hero's diet, which curbs hunger, boosts power, and converts body fat into performance fuel. They developed techniques for controlling fear and adrenaline surges, and they learned to tap into the remarkable hidden strength of the body's elastic tissue, which is far more powerful and effective than muscle. More than two thousand years ago, they got serious about the business of releasing the hero inside us all. And then they were gone.

Or maybe not. When a middle school teacher in San Antonio, Texas, named Rick Riordan began thinking about the troublesome kids in his class, he was struck by a topsy-turvy idea. Maybe the wild ones weren't hyperactive; maybe they were misplaced heroes. After all, in another era the same behavior that is now throttled with Ritalin and disciplinary rap sheets would have been the mark of greatness, the early blooming of a true champion. Riordan played with the idea, imagining the what-ifs. What if strong, assertive children were redirected rather than discouraged? What if there were a place for them, an outdoor training camp that felt like a playground, where they could cut loose with all those natural instincts to run, wrestle, climb, swim, and explore? You'd call it Camp Half-Blood, Riordan decided, because that's what we really are—half animal and half higher-being, halfway between each and unsure how to keep them in balance. Riordan began writing, creating a troubled kid from a broken home named Percy Jackson who arrives at a camp in the woods and is transformed when the Olympian he has inside is revealed, honed, and guided.

Riordan's fantasy of a hero school actually does exist—in bits and pieces, scattered across the globe. The skills have been fragmented, but with a little hunting, you can find them all. In a public park in Brooklyn, a former ballerina darts into the bushes and returns with a shopping bag full of the same superfoods the ancient Greeks once relied on. In Brazil, a onetime beach huckster is reviving the lost art of natural movement. And in a lonely Arizona dust bowl called Oracle, a quiet genius disappeared into the desert after teaching a few great athletes—and, oddly, Johnny Cash and the Red Hot Chili Peppers— the ancient secret of using body fat as fuel.

But the best learning lab of all was a cave on a mountain behind enemy lines—where, during World War II, a band of Greek shepherds and young British amateurs plotted to take on 100,000 German soldiers. They weren't naturally strong, or professionally trained, or known for their courage. They were wanted men, marked for immediate execution. But on a starvation diet, they thrived. Hunted and hounded, they got stronger. They became such natural born heroes, they decided to follow the lead of the greatest hero of all, Odysseus, and attempt their own version of the Trojan horse.

It was a suicide mission—for anyone, that is, who hadn't mastered a certain ancient art.

CHAPTER 4

When Hitler came to power Churchill didn't use judgement
but one of his deep insights. . . . *That* was what we needed.

—C. P. SNOW,
scientist and wartime spymaster, in his 1961 Harvard lecture
"Science and Government"

FOUR YEARS EARLIER, England was doomed. That's the reality Winston Churchill faced when he took over as prime minister in 1940.

"We are told that Herr Hitler has a plan for invading the British
Isles," Churchill announced. At that very moment, in fact, tank commander Erwin Rommel was bearing down on the Channel with his
fabled "Ghost Division," so known because it blasted through enemy
territory with such supernatural speed—once thrusting nearly two
hundred miles in a single day—that Rommel could be storming into
London within twenty-four hours of rumbling up on British shores.

Clearly, surrender was England's only hope. For every British plane,
Hitler had three; for every British soldier, Hitler had two. U-boat
wolf packs and magnetic mines had turned the Channel into a death
trap, crippling all but eleven of the Royal Navy's forty destroyers.
British soldiers were bloodied and barely armed; tens of thousands
had been captured or killed, and the survivors had ditched their guns
and gear in the rush to escape. German troops, by contrast, were so

disciplined, ferocious, and euphoric, Hitler actually wanted them to ease up and not overextend themselves by advancing so fast.

"Gentlemen, you have seen for yourself what criminal folly it was to try to defend this city," Hitler said while touring the smoking remains of Warsaw, which had been bombed into a nightmare landscape of rubble and rotting corpses as its mayor was dragged off to Dachau. "I only wish that certain statesmen in other countries who seem to want to turn all of Europe into a second Warsaw could have the opportunity to see, as you have, the real meaning of war."

But Churchill knew the real meaning of Hitler. During the chaotic early months of the Nazi onslaught, few were as quick as Churchill to pierce the Third Reich's gun smoke and pageantry and see into the heart of the man behind it all. *If you think you're dealing with a fellow statesman,* Churchill warned Parliament, *or an empire builder, or even a run-of-the-mill megalomaniac, you're making a terrible mistake.* War wasn't Hitler's means to something greater; it was the greatest thing he knew.

"Nazi power," Churchill said, "derives strength and perverted pleasure from persecution." Fear and pain were an erotic thrill for "these most sinister men." By Hitler's own telling, the most wonderful day of his young life was one of the darkest in history: he was "overcome with rapturous enthusiasm" when he heard that World War I had broken out. "I fell to my knees and thanked Heaven from an overflowing heart." As a soldier, Corporal Hitler adored the ghoulish world of frontline fighting; he resisted evacuation from the trenches when his thigh was torn up with shrapnel, and on his first night back after recovering, he was too excited to sleep and stalked around with a flashlight, spearing rats with his bayonet, until someone hit him with a boot and told him to knock it off.

"When we see the originality of malice, the ingenuity of aggression, which our enemy displays," Churchill warned, "we may certainly prepare ourselves for every kind of novel stratagem and every kind of brutal and treacherous maneuver."

So Churchill came up with a novel maneuver of his own. This was a new kind of fight, so Churchill wanted a new kind of fighter: lone phantoms with the inventiveness and self-reliance to test "the unwritten laws of war," as Churchill put it, and execute whatever havoc they could dream up. The British Army was outgunned and outnumbered, but maybe this way they could even the odds by tying up entire German regiments in pursuit of a single man. Or a single woman. Or a single woman who, in one recruit's case, was actually a man. Anytime a German soldier tried to close his eyes and sleep, Churchill wanted him plagued—and trailed—by lethal shadows.

He couldn't use seasoned soldiers for an operation like that; anyone fit enough to fight was needed on the battlefield. Instead, Churchill's new operation began recruiting poets, professors, archeologists—anyone who'd traveled a bit and knew his or her way around foreign countries. Two middle-aged professors were so electrified when they got wind of Churchill's scheme that they reversed their conscientious objector status and decided to fight instead. For British academics, this was their fantasy world come to life. The classics were their comic books; they'd grown up on Plutarch's *Lives*—"the bible for heroes," as Emerson declared—and came of age with their heads buried in the adventures of Odysseus and Richard the Lionheart and Sigurd the Dragonslayer. They understood that in ancient Greece, entire wars could pivot on the performance of one or two extraordinary individuals.

Hold on. British high command was appalled. Was Churchill really going to pit these oddballs against the most ruthless killers on the planet? The Nazis had just ripped apart the armies of nine European nations, and Churchill's counterpunch was . . . *this?* They're not commandos, Churchill's general argued; they're calamities. If their fake passports and ludicrous accents don't betray them, the villagers will; as soon as these misfits are dropped behind enemy lines, they'll have to depend for food and hideouts on the very people most likely to give them away. Why *wouldn't* a farmer with a storm trooper's gun in his face trade a British life for his own? Churchill's adventurers will have no escape if pursued and no hope if they're caught: by the code of combat, no uniform means no mercy. They won't be marched into camps and visited by the Red Cross, like other prisoners of war; they'll be beaten and tortured till they scream out every secret they know, then executed on the spot.

But Churchill was undeterred. Few knew that in his early life, Churchill had been one of those calamities himself. He was "hardly the stuff of which gladiators are made," *The Last Lion* biographer William Manchester would note. "Sickly, an uncoordinated weakling with the pale fragile hands of a girl, speaking with a lisp and a slight stutter, he had been at the mercy of bullies. They beat him, ridiculed him, and pelted him with cricket balls. Trembling and humiliated, he hid in a nearby woods." Young Winston was so far from rugged, he could only tolerate silk underwear and even in winter had to sleep naked beneath silk sheets. "I am cursed with so feeble a body," he'd complain, "that I can hardly support the fatigues of the day." But over time, Churchill managed to transform himself from that bullied wisp into the dashing war correspondent and army officer who'd become Great Britain's cigar-chomping, bulldog-tough defender of freedom. If he could do it, Churchill was certain, so could his fellow misfits.

And his misfits believed him—because some of them had already seen a real superhero in the flesh. All they had to do was look out the window and wait for Thomas Edward Lawrence—winner of dagger fights, conqueror of evildoers, chieftain of desert bandits— to come roaring across the Dorset countryside on his big Brough Superior motorcycle. Lawrence of Arabia was more than their idol; he was their evolutionary road map, a guide to the transformation he'd followed from *them* into *him*. Back at the start of World War I, T. E. Lawrence had been just as bookish and inept as they were now; as an Oxford scholar with the build of a preteen girl and an aversion to rough sports, let alone brawls, Lawrence was originally assigned to draw maps and military postage stamps and was so out of place on the battlefield that one superior dismissed him as "a bumptious young ass" who "wants a kicking and kicking hard."

Then something happened. Lawrence rode into the desert, and someone else rode back out. Gone was the "little silk-shirted man," as Lawrence described himself; in his place was a turbaned warrior with a scimitar on his hip, bullet scars on his chest, and a battered infantry rifle notched with kills slung across his back. No one expected him to still be alive, let alone commanding a band of Arab raiders. Lawrence had managed to marshal these nomadic tribesmen into a camel-mounted attack squad, leading them on hit-and-run raids against the forces of the Ottoman Empire. The Oxford graduate student could now leap astride a fleeing camel, throw burning sticks of dynamite at pursuers, and vanish into a sandstorm, only to reappear a thousand miles away as he galloped from the twisted wreckage of another sabotaged train. The same colonel who'd wanted to boot Lawrence's bumptious behind was now amazed by his "gallantry and grit," while Lawrence's enemies paid him an even greater compliment: the Turks put a dead-or-alive bounty on his head of fifteen thousand pounds, the equivalent today of more than half a million dollars.

Out there in the wilderness, Lawrence had learned a secret. He'd gone back in time, to a place where heroes weren't a different breed— they just had different breeding. They were ordinary people who'd mastered extraordinary skills, who'd found that by tapping into a certain body of primal knowledge, they could perform with remarkable amounts of stamina, strength, nerve, and cunning. The ancient Greeks knew this; their entire culture was built on the premise that everyone is tinged with a touch of the godly. To be a hero, you had to learn how to think, run, fight, and talk—even eat, sleep, and crawl— like a hero.

Which was excellent news if you were a one-eyed archeologist like John Pendlebury, or a penniless young artist like Xan Fielding, or a wandering playboy-poet like Patrick Leigh Fermor—three men whose fates would become intertwined on Crete. Churchill might have been offering misfits like them a death sentence—and to many, he was—but he was also offering a new way to live. If Lawrence of Arabia could learn the art of the hero, so could they.

This was their chance.

CHAPTER 5

The right man in the right place is a devastating weapon.

—MOTTO OF U.S. SPECIAL FORCES

MY LAWRENCE OF ARABIA—the person who first made me realize
heroism was a skill, not a virtue—was a middle-aged woman with big
round glasses who ran a small elementary school in the Pennsylvania
countryside. On February 2, 2001, Norina Bentzel was in her office
when a man with a machete went after her kindergartners. It's been
ten years since I heard what happened next, and only now am I beginning to understand the answer to one question:

Why didn't she quit?

How does a forty-two-year-old grade school principal who's never
been in a fight take on a frenzied Army vet and keep battling him—
relentlessly, with her bare hands, at only five foot three—as he's
slashing at her with a blade that can cut through a tree branch? It's
remarkable that she had the tenacity to confront him, but the real
mystery is how she persisted when, very quickly, she must have realized she was doomed to lose. Because that's the ugly truth about heroism: the tests don't start when you're ready or stop when you're tired.
You don't get time-outs, warm-ups, or bathroom breaks. You may
have a headache or be wearing the wrong pants or find yourself—the

way Norina did—in a skirt and low heels in a school hallway becoming slick with your own blood.

Michael Stankewicz was a social studies teacher at a Baltimore high school who began simmering with rage and paranoia after his third wife left him. His violent threats got him fired, hospitalized, and eventually jailed. After he was released, he picked up a machete and drove to the school his stepchildren once attended—North Hopewell–Winterstown Elementary, in sleepy, rural York County, Pennsylvania. Just before lunch, Norina Bentzel happened to glance out her window and see someone slip through the front door behind a mother with two children. She went to find out who he was and discovered a stranger peering into the kindergarten.

"Excuse me, sir," Norina said. "Is there someone I can help you find?"

Stankewicz wheeled, yanking the machete out of his left pant leg. He slashed at Norina's throat, missing by a hair and slicing off the plastic ID tag hanging around her neck. A sad and strangely articulate thought ran through her mind: *There is no one in my environment who can help.* She was alone in this. Whatever she did in the next few seconds would determine who made it out of that school alive.

Norina could have screamed and fled. She could have curled up in a ball and begged for mercy, or lunged for Stankewicz's wrist. Instead she crossed her arms in front of her face in an X and backed away. Stankewicz kept chopping and slashing, but Norina rolled with the blows, never taking her eyes off him or allowing him to close the gap and get her on the floor. Norina led Stankewicz away from the classrooms and down the hall toward her office. She managed to slip inside, bolt the door, and hit the lockdown alarm with her gashed and blood-soaked hand.

She was a second too late. Some of the kindergartners were just exiting their classroom as the alarm sounded. Stankewicz went after them. He gashed the teacher's arm, sliced off a girl's ponytail, broke a boy's arm. The children fled toward the office, where Norina once again faced Stankewicz. The machete slashed deep into her hands, severing two of her fingers. Norina looked done for, so Stankewicz turned to seek fresh victims—and that's when Norina leaped. She wrapped him in a bear hug, hanging on with the last of her strength as he thrashed and lunged and—

Clink.

He dropped the machete. The school nurse grabbed it and ran out to hide it in the hall. Stankewicz staggered to the desk, Norina still clinging to his back. Soon sirens and thundering footsteps were approaching. Norina had lost nearly half her blood but was rushed to the hospital in time to save her life. Stankewicz surrendered.

"Luck" and "courage" were mentioned often in the days following the attack, but of all the factors involved, luck and courage were the least significant. Courage gets you into predicaments; it doesn't necessarily get you back out. And unless he slips and falls, there's nothing lucky about outfighting a man coming at you with a machete. Norina Bentzel survived because she made a series of decisions, instantly and under extraordinary pressure, and her success rate was the difference between life and death.

When she crossed her arms and retreated, she instinctively seized on exactly the posture recommended in pankration, the ancient Greek art of no-rules fighting, later adopted in World War II by the "Heavenly Twins"—Bill Sykes and William Fairbairn—whose close-combat technique is still used by Special Forces today. Norina didn't stumble frantically or bolt into a dead end, but maneuvered backwards with purpose. If she'd allowed her adrenaline to redline, she'd have burned through her energy and been left helpless. Instead it was Stankewicz who ran out of gas, allowing Norina to wait for her opportunity and seize it.

When it came to strength, bulk, and savagery, Norina was hopelessly outmatched. So instead of going muscle-to-muscle, she found a better solution. She relied on her fascia, the fibrous connective tissue that encases our bodies beneath the skin. Your upper body has a belt of fascia running across your chest from one hand to the other. By wrapping her arms around Stankewicz, Norina closed the fascia loop; she turned herself into a human lasso, essentially banding Stankewicz's arms with a thick rubber cable and neutralizing his force.

But for any of that to happen, Norina first had to master her amygdala: the fear-conditioning portion of the brain. The amygdala accesses your long-term memory, scanning whether anything you've done in the past resembles something you're about to attempt in the present. If it hits a match, you're good to go: your muscles will relax, your heart rate will stabilize, your doubts will vanish. But if the amygdala finds no evidence that you've ever, say, climbed down a tall tree, it will lobby your nervous system to shut down the operation. The amygdala is what causes people to burn to death instead of stepping onto a firefighter's ladder, or drown by refusing to release their grip on a lifeguard's neck. It's also what makes riding a bike so hard when you're five, yet so easy after a five-year break; once learned, your amygdala recognizes the behavior and gives the go-ahead. Your amygdala doesn't reason; it only responds. It can't be tricked, only trained.

For most of us, no matter how strong or brave, the bizarreness of a machete attack would overwhelm our amygdala and freeze us in our tracks. Norina's genius was finding a strategy that suited her skills: she wasn't a fighter, but she was a hugger. Wrapping her arms around someone was a movement so familiar, her sensory system didn't object. Norina managed that hug because she'd had a flash of insight: she couldn't conquer Stankewicz's rage, but maybe she could calm it.

"I put my arms around you," she would tell Michael Stankewicz from the witness stand on the day he was sentenced. "To *comfort* you."

Stankewicz stared at her. Then he silently mouthed "Thank you" and was led off to serve a 264-year term in prison.

So how do you prepare for an attack by a maniac with a machete?

The question feels stupid coming out of my mouth and almost indecent, given the circumstances. I'm at Norina's school, and it's been barely a year since the attack. But privately, Norina has been wondering the same thing herself.

"Let's talk outside," she suggests. She's gracious and good-humored, and so charmed by children that after seventeen years as an educator she still likes spending her breaks watching the kids tear around at recess. Her arms are now covered with lightning-bolt scars. After four reconstructive surgeries, her hands have recovered a good bit of function, but they don't feel like her hands anymore; they're so cold and numb all the time that even on this warm autumn afternoon, she's clutching heat packs. But she can hold hands with her husband and children again and play her alto sax at Penn State Blue Band reunions and tousle the hair of the schoolkids who come charging up as soon as they see us on the playground.

Strange as it sounds, Norina says, she was ready that day. She must have been. She was calm, rational, strong. She wasn't panicking or preparing to die; she was running through her options and planning her next move. Her reactions weren't random; they were natural and deliberate. So deliberate, in fact, she felt "guided from above." But for practical purposes, she was guided from within: she knew what to do, and her body knew how to do it.

"If you want to call me a hero because I treasure these children, that's fine, but I do that every day in my job," Norina says. It's an interesting clue. Was she poised because she's a lifelong teacher who's trained herself to stay cool when things get hot? Did she hold eye contact because she deals with tantrumy children and agitated parents that way every day? Was it a coincidence that her hands came up in the same position she'd practiced for decades as a saxophonist, and she likewise had the ambidexterity to deflect and defend with both arms?

All it takes is a few minutes with her on the playground to understand why she'd fight to the death for these kids. What's still baffling—to Norina most of all—is why she won.

"What I find fascinating is how rare it is today for even a hero to understand his own heroism," says Earl Babbie, Ph.D., a professor emeritus in behavioral sciences at Orange County's Chapman University whose research focuses on heroics. "I'll bet you won't find a single example of a person who says, 'Yes, I'm a hero.' A few years back, a hijacker on a plane pointed a gun at a passenger. The flight attendant got between the gun and the passenger and said, 'You'll have to kill me first.' Afterward, the flight attendant said, 'No, no, I'm no hero.'

"And I thought, *For Christ's sake!* If that doesn't qualify, what does?" Babbie continues. "I don't think it's modesty. I think it's bewilderment."

Babbie has a dream experiment he'd love to perform. "I wish it were possible to interview heroes the day before they risk their lives for someone else," he says. "I bet you won't find anyone who can tell you with assurance what he or she would do in a life-threatening situation." Just the opposite, in fact: Babbie has found that the art of the hero has been neglected for so long, most people are uncomfortable even discussing it. He likes to read the Boy Scout Oath and Law out loud in class and watch his students squirm when he comes to the parts about being *trustworthy, loyal, helpful,* and *friendly.*

"Virtue isn't respectable these days, and we've certainly seen enough hypocrisy among so-called moral leaders to question what they tell us to do," Babbie says. "But at some deeper level, we still instinctively idolize the kind of heroic behavior we claim is foreign to us, and keep acting on the heroic urges we claim we don't have."

Even Charles Darwin found heroes bewildering. Darwin's great gift to science was simplifying all life to pure mathematics: your one and only goal on earth is multiplication. Everything you do, every instinct you have, is an evolutionary urge to make babies and leave behind as many copies of yourself as possible. From that perspective, heroism makes no sense. Why risk the grave for someone else if there's no guarantee of a biological payoff? Dying for your own kids: smart. Dying for a rival's? Genetic suicide.

Because no matter how many virile, healthy heroes you raised, it would take just one selfish bastard with a hearty sex drive to wipe out your entire bloodline. Selfish Bastard's kids would thrive and multiply, while Hero Dad's kids would eventually follow their father's example and sacrifice themselves into extinction. "He who was ready to sacrifice his life, as many a savage has been, rather than betray his comrades," Darwin concluded, "would often leave no offspring to inherit his noble nature."

So if natural selection eliminates natural heroism, why does it still exist?

Andrew Carnegie was just as stumped as Darwin. The nineteenth-century steel baron built his fortune on his ability to read human nature, but heroism was one personality quirk he couldn't crack. When he arrived in the United States from Scotland at age thirteen, Carnegie was a penniless, barely educated immigrant who was lucky to land work in a railroad yard, but his skill at outmaneuvering the most ruthless sharks of his time—including that notorious man-eater J. P. Morgan—helped speed his rise to the top of the steel industry. He wanted money, so he worked hard and gambled well. No voodoo there. But how do you explain someone who strives harder and risks more for free?

Carnegie was so intrigued by heroes, he began hunting them. In 1904, he set up the Carnegie Hero Fund, as much a research tool as a reward. Only pure altruists are eligible, not firemen or police officers or parents rescuing their own children. Every year, the fund collects tales of heroics from across the country, cataloguing them by gender, region, age, and incident and awarding a cash prize to the heroes or their surviving families. Carnegie was soon hearing about Thelma McNee, the teenage girl who leaped from her apartment roof onto the burning building next door to rescue two children trapped inside by the flames. A submission came in for Wava Campredon, a seventy-year-old New Mexico woman who was mauled but kept battling two savage dogs with her garden hoe to save her neighbor. Mary Black, a twenty-five-year-old Oregon housewife, was "encumbered by four skirts" but still swam twice into a flood-engorged river to save a pair of drowning sisters.

Was there some kind of pattern at work? Carnegie couldn't figure out if he was looking at a performance model that could be reproduced or just a happy string of accidents in which the right person turned up at the right time, sometimes with a hoe. Because if he could boil heroism down to a formula—to an art—then good God! He'd go down as one of the world's great peacemakers, a name spoken in the same breath as Christ. Once everyone became protectors, who'd be left undefended? Every classroom would have a hero like Norina Bentzel, every home a Thelma McNee, every riverbank a Mary Black. Carnegie had a reputation as a brass-knuckled fighter, but he was actually a pacifist who believed that violence was a disease that someone—maybe even Carnegie himself—could cure.

But in the end, he gave up. Carnegie would continue rewarding heroes, although he'd never understand them. "I do not expect to stimulate or create heroism by this fund," he conceded, "knowing well that heroic action is impulsive."

Impulsive. That was Carnegie's mistake.

Carnegie and Darwin were men of science, but they were approaching the problem like poets. *Sacrifice . . . betray . . . noble . . . impulsive . . .*

Those are judgments of intent, not descriptions of behavior. Carnegie and Darwin were wondering about thoughts and feelings—the *why?*—when they should have been focusing on action, on the cold, hard facts of *how?* Detectives don't begin a case by worrying about motive, an infinite onion you can peel forever and still end up with nothing. First pin down what someone did, and maybe then you'll discover why they did it.

That's how the Ancient Greeks went about it. They put heroes at the center of their theology, which for all its tales of godly feuds and magical transformations still stands alone as the most pragmatic of world religions. Instead of bowing down to saints and miracles, the Greeks worshipped problem solvers and hard how-to. They understood the difference between heroism and impulse, and they devised an easy, two-step test for telling them apart:

1. Would you do it again?
2. And could you?

Hercules didn't have one Labor; he had twelve, plus plenty of mini-labors on the side. Odysseus's to-do list was relentless: he not only came up with a way to win the Trojan War, but he battled his way home afterwards by outsmarting, outfighting, and outrunning typhoons, warriors, enchantresses, a Cyclops, the powers of the underworld, and the charms of a sex goddess. Atalanta, one of the Greeks' rare female heroes, showed the boys she could beat up a pair of degenerate Centaurs, defeat a legendary wrestler, help Jason recover the Golden Fleece, and hunt down the monstrous Calydonian Boar. Perseus, who was "skilled in all manner of things, from the craft of the fisherman to the use of the sword," had to brainstorm a plan for cutting off Medusa's head without being turned to stone, then rescue a chained and naked princess from a sea monster.

Luckily, one man appeared who could turn all that crazy drama into a hard, clear code of conduct: Plutarch, the great Greek umpire of all things heroic. Plutarch was fascinated by heroism the way nuclear scientists are fascinated by uranium: he saw it as a fantastic natural superfuel, powerful and abundant and just waiting to be harnessed. Plutarch spent his life analyzing heroes and threw his net wide: he believed even fantasy has its roots in real-life experiences, so he studied true stories and tall tales, Roman history and Greek myths. By the time he was ready to write his epic work, *Parallel Lives*, he'd heard it all, so you couldn't dazzle him; even the most beloved heroes got a blasting from Plutarch if they stepped out of line.

He reconstructed the lives of Alexander the Great and Julius Caesar; he exposed the shortcomings of Pericles—a brilliant tactician who nonetheless blundered Athens into the Peloponnesian War—and the fatal flaw of Pyrrhus, "the fool of hope" who took awful losses whenever his imagination outstripped his might. Plutarch admired Romulus, the wolf-suckled founder of Rome, for remaining true to his humble birth and kind to his eight hundred mistresses. But he blistered Theseus, who defeated the Minotaur in the Labyrinth; just because you kill monsters and thwart tyrants, you don't get a free pass for sex crimes. "The faults committed in the rapes of women admit of no plausible excuse in Theseus," Plutarch scolded. "It is to be suspected these things were done out of wantonness and lust."

Plutarch did such a remarkable job, *Parallel Lives* became the handbook for modern history's heroes. "It has been like my conscience," Henry IV of France commented, "and has whispered in my ear many good suggestions and maxims for my conduct and the government of my affairs." Abraham Lincoln was a devoted reader, as were Teddy Roosevelt, George Patton, and John Quincy Adams. When England was rebuilding after the Great War, the hero's bible was its guide. "Plutarch's *Lives* built the heroic ideal of the Elizabethan age," C. S. Lewis acknowledged.

And what Plutarch taught them is this: Heroes care. True heroism, as the ancients understood, isn't about strength, or boldness, or even courage. It's about compassion.

When the Greeks created the heroic ideal, they didn't choose a word that meant "Dies Trying" or "Massacres Bad Guys." They went with ἥρως (or *hērōs*)—"protector." Heroes aren't perfect; with a god as one parent and a mortal as the other, they're perpetually teetering between two destinies. What tips them toward greatness is a sidekick, a human connection who helps turn the spigot on the power of compassion. Empathy, the Greeks believed, was a source of strength, not softness; the more you recognized yourself in others and connected with their distress, the more endurance, wisdom, cunning, and determination you could tap into.

The nearly indestructible Achilles had his loyal friend Patroclus. Odysseus fought his greatest battle with two loyal herdsmen by his side. Even Superman, who wasn't human at all, kept Jimmy Olsen hanging around. Hercules had his twin brother and adoring nephew, and when things were darkest, his best bud, Theseus, was always there. And of course, brainy boy detective Encyclopedia Brown had two-fisted Sally Kimball. A sidekick is a hero's way of looking into his soul, of drawing strength from his *weakest* side, not his strongest. He has to remember that even though he shares the blood of a god, he's still human at heart. He's not a Titan who will swallow a baby to get out of a jam, or a god who will never die. He has one shot at immortality, and it's in the memories and stories of the grateful and inspired.

He has to care so much for what's human, it brings out what's godly.

You can hope an impulse or "noble nature" will spontaneously create those kinds of heroic skills. Or you can follow the lead of the Spartans, who went right to the source: Crete. Sparta's founding father, Lycurgus, traveled to the island to soak up ideas and was so impressed he smuggled a Cretan back with him in disguise, pretending he was a poet while secretly relying on him as Sparta's most influential lawmaker. Sparta's social code "is, in a very great measure, a copy of the Cretan," Aristotle points out in *Politics*, and its defining spirit would become the foundation of both Greek theology and Western democracy: the notion that ordinary citizens should always be ready for extraordinary action.

The Greek myths are really the same performance parable, over and over; they're showcases for underdogs using the art of the hero to deal with danger. Need to tame a savage bull? Wait for it to take a drink, then wrestle it down by the horns. Ordered to clean a toxic stable? Flood it. Up against a giant man-bull, a three-headed hellhound, or a lion with an impenetrable pelt? Get behind them and choke 'em out. These techniques weren't just mythical make-believe; some were so spot-on, they're still used today in the Greek fighting art of pankration. If you're ever up against a guy who can tear your head off, take a lesson from Odysseus: "Odysseus knew a trick or two," Homer notes in the *Iliad*. "He kicked Ajax hard in the back of his knee and toppled him backwards, falling on his chest."

Because the way the Greeks looked at it, you have a choice: you can either hope a Norina Bentzel comes to the rescue when your kids are in danger, or you can guarantee it. Daredevils aren't the answer; spinal rehab wards are full of daredevils. Fearlessness doesn't really help, either: when your car breaks down, you don't want the mechanic to say, "I've never done this before, but I'm willing to die trying." What you want to hear is "Don't worry. This is right up my alley." Heroism isn't some mysterious inner virtue, the Greeks believed; it's a collection of skills that every man and woman can master so that in a pinch, they can become a Protector.

And for a long time, they were great at it. For centuries, the art of the hero thrived. But as the Greek empire faded, so did its influence, closing in on itself and disappearing. . . .

Until the last place the art of the hero remained intact was the wild mountains of Crete, where a band of British Army rejects arrived during World War II for a crash course in wisdom from the past.

CHAPTER 6

Until now, we would say that the Greeks fight like heroes.
From now on, we will say that heroes fight like Greeks.

—WINSTON CHURCHILL, 1941

SECRETLY, HITLER was dealing with a problem of his own. He was about to risk everything on Operation Barbarossa, his master plan to conquer the Soviet Union. If he miscalculated, Germany was doomed. But if Hitler played it right and brought the Russian Bear to its knees, no power on earth could defy him.

Once Germany grabbed control of Russia's oil fields, plus all those Soviet farms, tanks, and Red Army soldiers, the Third Reich would have the biggest, fastest, best-equipped fighting force the world had ever seen. Ponder *that*, America. Franklin D. Roosevelt would have to gulp hard before coming to Britain's aid. Hitler didn't necessarily intend to invade the United States—he'd be content for the present with all of continental Europe—but if pushed, he could make life in the United States very ugly, very fast. South American friends were standing by; Brazil and Argentina were already pro-fascist, and bringing Mexico on board was just a matter of promising the return of California, New Mexico, and Arizona and the easing of America's economic bootheel. The Imperial Japanese Navy and German

U-boats would strangle American shipping, while Germany's long-range Amerika Bombers, still in demo but coming along nicely, could unload a firestorm on Washington, D.C., and make it all the way back to Munich without refueling.

But Hitler had to move fast. Russia, as Napoleon learned the hard way, is a mousetrap that opens only briefly each summer before snapping shut on your neck. In 1812, Napoleon marched into Russia with nearly a half-million soldiers and most of Europe under his command; he came home with ten thousand skeletal survivors and soon lost his own country. Russia is too vast, too cold, and too populated with fighting men to risk the slightest miscalculation. If you're lucky, you have a four-month window: you have to get in as soon as the snows thaw in early spring, and be in control before *rasputitsa*, autumn's quagmire season. Once the *rasputitsa* rains start falling, Russian roads dissolve into wheel-sucking mud swamps. Bullets didn't defeat Napoleon; he was doomed the moment the mousetrap snapped and his foundering soldiers began dying from frostbite, exhaustion, and starvation.

Hitler knew the risks but liked his odds. Germany had the best army in Europe, while Stalin had done a spectacular job of turning the Red Army into possibly the worst. Stalin was always fretting that any general good enough to defend the country was also good enough to seize it, so he kept executing the best Russian officers and replacing them with lackeys. The troops under their command were often poor peasants who'd never touched a rifle in their lives. Field weapons were scarce and outdated, and the units lucky enough to have functioning artillery lacked enough shells for target practice.

So on November 13, late at night and all alone, Hitler made his decision. It was time to become invincible. It stung him that England was still standing after four months of hellacious bombing, but no matter; he could circle back later for the kill. "The German armed forces must be prepared, even before the end of the war against England, to overthrow the Soviet Union in a rapid campaign," Hitler told his generals. He chose the name Barbarossa—"Red Beard"—after the swashbuckling German emperor of the twelfth century who, legend had it, was still asleep in a Bavarian cave, attended by ravens and awaiting the call to restore Germany to its ancestral glory.

Barbarossa would be unleashed, Hitler decided, on May 15, 1941. By Christmas, swastikas would be flying over London and Moscow.

America wouldn't even have a chance to react. The war would be over. It was foolproof.

STEP #1: CONQUER CRETE

"Mastery of the eastern Mediterranean was dependent upon Crete," said General Franz Halder, one of Hitler's top strategists. As Greece's largest island, Crete was the perfect staging area for Germany's eastern push. But that left Hitler in a jam, because Mussolini had already gone behind the Führer's back and tried grabbing Greece on his own. "If there's any trouble beating the Greeks," Mussolini had boasted, "I'll resign from being an Italian." *Greece will be ours by December,* Mussolini assured Hitler. *Consider it a Christmas present.*

Instead, it turned into a bloodbath.

Greek civilians raced into the mountains to join frontline troops, and together they managed to bottle up the Italians in the narrow passes. From across the sea, Crete sent the mountain men of its 5th Division. The Cretans could live off the land, skitter by night across cliff fronts, and kill as easily with a knife as they could with a gun. Instead of steamrolling to victory, the Italians found themselves struggling to hold their ground as Cretan phantoms picked them off from the crags. Dressed in rags, carrying their rifles across their shoulders like shepherd's crooks, joking and cheerful despite the snow and deadly cold, the Cretans were soon spearheading the Greek attack. In one battle, a Cretan regiment was outnumbered ten to one and still chased back an entire Italian division.

Watching this unfold from afar, Hitler was aghast. Attacking Greece through the mountains, *in the middle of the rainy season?* With winter on the way? If mud didn't stop the Italians, just wait for the snow. Right when the Third Reich was awing the world with its might, Hitler fumed, Mussolini's bungling "struck a blow at the belief in our invincibility." Christmas came and went, and instead of marching into Athens, the Italians were retreating into Albania. Germany would now have to step in and clean up this mess, if only to save face and avenge the disgrace.

Hitler took his time. He wasn't going to repeat Mussolini's mistake and monkey around with the weather. He left the Greeks and Italians snowbound in the mountains through the worst winter in a half-century. He didn't even bother trying to stop British troops from coming to Greece's aid. He waited till the weather warmed, on April 6, and then he gave Russia a look at its future.

"When it comes to hundreds of dive bombers at you and you can't hit back at the swine, by god it's nerving dear," one Australian corporal wrote from Greece to his wife after the German invasion. "It makes the strongest man feel helpless as a baby." German armored vehicles smashed through the mountain passes, while Luftwaffe planes machine-gunned and carpet-bombed anything that moved. The Greeks dug in courageously—so courageously, in fact, that after one garrison finally ran out of ammunition, the Germans spontaneously stood and saluted—but the long winter's war had left them exhausted. The Greeks were soon forced to surrender, while some fifty thousand British Commonwealth troops scrambled aboard ships to escape to Crete, throwing aside their heavy weapons as they had at Dunkirk.

In just twenty-four days, Hitler mopped up Greece and captured Yugoslavia at the same time. Now for the finale: Crete.

This would take some finesse. Thanks to Mussolini's bungling, the whole Greek adventure had put Operation Barbarossa behind schedule, but storming straight into Crete could be trouble. If Hitler invaded with a big ground force, he'd tie up troops that were already supposed to be on their way to Russia. But if he went in shorthanded, those mountain men could cause him the same headaches they'd just given Mussolini. Hitler assembled his generals and spelled out his dilemma.

That's no dilemma, argued General Kurt Student, commander of the elite XI Air Corps. *That's the opportunity of a lifetime.*

Of *Student's* lifetime, at least. Student had grown up poor and clawed his way up through the ranks by taking jobs that were supposed to kill him. He started as a trench fighter in World War I, then was trained to fly and volunteered for dead man's duty as a dogfight pilot over the Russian front. He became a legend for shooting down a notoriously elusive French plane, then bolting a German machine gun to its nose and taking it right back into combat. As one of the few German fliers to survive the war, he was recruited into an underground brotherhood that, in violation of the Treaty of Versailles, was secretly rebuilding the German air force. Airborne shock and awe was Germany's greatest weapon, Student was convinced, and he was willing to prove it with his own battered body; even though he was a fifty-year-old senior officer at the start of World War II and never learned to skydive, he personally commanded the invasion of Holland by slicing through shrapnel fire to arrive by seaplane. He was accidentally shot in the forehead by one of his own soldiers, but not even that stopped him; when Hitler was vexed by Crete, Student had recovered and was strong enough to step forward with a spectacular solution.

Crete was Hitler's opportunity to launch the biggest airborne invasion in history. He could awe the world with the Third Reich's newest and most terrifying innovation: a flying army. No military had ever attempted to swarm a major target by dropping in entirely from above, arriving from the clouds without the support of ground troops or sea reinforcements. Germany's big Junkers were powerful enough to tow gliders holding a force of ten Storm Regiment commandos. Cut the gliders loose and they're silent; steer them out of the blinding sunrise and they're invisible. It was the ultimate sneak attack: a fighting force that could suddenly appear right over your head—anywhere, anytime—without a moment's warning.

Hitler heard him out . . . then said no. Dangling that many men over the enemy's guns? Far too risky.

But they weren't talking about men, Student insisted; they were talking about the *Fallschirmjäger*, an elite corps of paratroopers known as "Hunters from the Sky." You had to be extraordinarily ferocious, tough, ingenious, and athletic to even apply to be a Hunter, and even then, two of every three candidates flunked out. To earn the badge of the attacking eagle, you had to run an obstacle course under live fire; jump by night into forests; fire a submachine gun with accuracy while falling through the air at thirty-five miles per hour; survive for days on only the gear in the forty-seven pockets of your jumpsuit; and be able to disarm an enemy with your bare hands and use his own weapon against him. The Hunters could hit the ground, by day or by darkness, and come up fighting before a stunned enemy could react. A force of only eighty *Fallschirmjäger* had forced the surrender of fifteen hundred Belgian soldiers. Plus the Hunters relied on one of the Nazis' secret weapons: before jumping, they were issued tablets of Pervitin, an early version of crystal meth.

Hitler started coming around. Despite his misgivings, he loved the Wagnerian overkill of Student's plan: no clanking tanks or common foot soldiers, just wave after wave of Germany's fiercest commandos raining down from the sky like apocalyptic demons. It was more than warfare; it was biblical doom. Hitler found the theatrics so tantalizing, he insisted they feature Germany's greatest star, Max Schmeling, the world heavyweight boxing champion who'd knocked out Joe Louis. Having a celebrity like Max Schmeling leap out of a plane behind enemy lines was an astonishing command, but it neatly served two purposes.

Privately, it settled a personal grudge between the Führer and the famous fighter, who refused to join the Nazi Party and, it was rumored, had saved the lives of his Jewish trainer's two sons by hiding them in his hotel room and smuggling them to safety in the United States. Publicly, it added another chilling image to the Nazis' gallery of terror. A photo of the muscular German colossus as his big boots thumped down on the dust of Crete would send an unmistakable message: *Our giants are coming, and they can't be stopped.* For a Third Reich so enraptured by death's-head skulls, blood-red flags, and the raw rape symbolism of the swastika, with its two interlocked bodies representing, as Hitler put it, "the struggle for the victory of the Aryan man," the sight of Germany's two-fisted champion striding across the ancient world was irresistible. Crete was the birthplace of the modern world, the origin of every great achievement in civilization, and Hitler would show he could snatch it up in a matter of hours.

Besides, wasn't it time the Nazis were greeted as heroes for a change? German troops weren't really invading Crete, General Student pointed out; they were *liberating* it. The Cretan islanders were so sick of being ruled by the Greek king, Hitler would become their idol as soon as they realized the arrival of the Germans meant the end of the monarchy. In fact, Student had it on good authority that a supersecret underground of Cretan rebels was eager to greet its new German friends and had already worked out a pass code. "Top Dog!" the Germans were supposed to call out. "Big Buck!" the Cretan underground would reply, and the celebration would begin.

Hitler relented. He dubbed Student's plan Operation Mercury, after the Roman god of thievery and lightning speed, and set the go date for May 20. It took twenty-four days to capture the mainland; Hitler would allow twenty-four hours for Crete.

One day. Then it was on to Russia.

• • •

May 20, 1941, dawned beautifully, so Colonel Howard Kippenberger of the New Zealand 10th Brigade grabbed a plate of porridge and went outside to enjoy the sun rising over the Aegean. *Weird*, he thought as he settled in under a plane tree. *What happened to the sun?* A minute earlier, there wasn't a cloud in the sky, but now all of a sudden he's sitting in shadows. *Wait . . .* He jerked his head up, stunned.

Overhead, German gliders were silently soaring in, so many they darkened the sky. Kippenberger grabbed for his rifle, but he'd left it in his room. Kippenberger had never seen anything like it. There had to be hundreds of commandos inside those gliders. Hard behind was a sea of transport planes, with wave after wave of elite *Fallschirmjäger* paratroopers pouring out the jump doors.

"STAND TO YOUR ARMS!" Kippenberger shouted, praying that not too many of his troops were splashing naked in the sea at that moment. By the time he got his rifle, Germans were on the ground and scrambling for position. Bullets splintered the olive trees; snipers had already nested, with sight lines toward the little house serving as Kippenberger's headquarters. Above, the sky was so hectic with men and machines that one stunned soldier felt he was witnessing the Martian occupation of Earth from H. G. Wells's *War of the Worlds*.

Many of Kippenberger's men were mechanics and drivers, not frontline soldiers. They backed up, firing desperately and uncertainly, while Kippenberger hurried to the top of a hill to get a clear view of how much trouble they were in.

Lots, it turned out.

When it came to troops, Crete was an island of castaways. Nearly every soldier there was a refugee from the fighting on the Greek mainland—a hodgepodge of Australians, New Zealanders, Brits, and Greeks. As ordered, they'd chucked their heavy weapons when they were ferried to Crete, where they'd hunkered down to await one of two things: either massive reinforcement or a speedy retreat. Anything else would be a massacre. One battalion didn't even have boots; their ship had been torpedoed on the way to Crete, so they'd dumped their rifles and shoes to swim for it.

"Forces at my disposal are totally inadequate to meet the attack envisaged," concluded Major General Bernard Freyberg of New Zealand after he arrived on Crete to take command. Was Freyberg seriously expected to defend one of the most strategically important islands in the Mediterranean with, as he put it, "gunners who had lost their guns, sappers who had lost their tools, and R.S.A.C. drivers who had lost their cars"? He wasn't sure what Hitler had in mind, but if it was even a fraction of the firepower unleashed on the mainland, the Brits were doomed.

Coming from a wild man like Freyberg, gloom like that had to be taken seriously. Churchill loved Freyberg and had nicknamed him the Salamander, after the myth that salamanders are created by fire. Freyberg had left New Zealand as a young man to join Pancho Villa's rebels in Mexico, so hungry for action that he'd traveled across the globe to plunge into a war he only dimly comprehended, in a language he didn't speak. When World War I broke out, young Freyberg jumped into a series of swimming races in Los Angeles and won enough prize money to pay for passage to England. He enlisted and quickly made his mark by stripping naked for a suicide mission: to distract Turkish forces during the invasion at Gallipoli, he smeared his body with grease, dived off of a troop ship, and swam two miles through the bone-chilling Gulf of Saros to light diversionary flares on a beach behind enemy lines. He became England's youngest general at twenty-eight and was wounded so many times that one of Churchill's party tricks was to get Freyberg to peel off his shirt so other guests could count his twenty-seven battle scars.

But even for the Salamander, Crete was too much—or, rather, too little. Freyberg should have at least had some local troops who knew the terrain, but he'd been robbed of even that slim advantage: the Cretan division was still stranded back on the mainland.

The drug-enhanced Hunters were on the ground and moving fast, wriggling free of their harnesses and breaking open the weapon crates thumping down nearby. In minutes, the *Fallschirmjäger* were better equipped than the British. Besides motorcycles and surgical equipment, the crates also had specially designed field guns powerful enough to blow a hole through a tank. Quickly, the Germans grouped into attack formation and began advancing, cutting telephone lines to British headquarters as they moved.

But hold on a moment. Up on his hill, Kippenberger noticed one German squad was going the wrong way. Instead of advancing, they were edging backwards. Suddenly they were running, falling, shouting—and being chased by the 8th Greek Regiment.

Kippenberger couldn't believe his eyes. When he'd first spotted the 8th Greeks, he cringed; they were so dangerously exposed, he thought, "it was murder to leave such troops in such a position." But now look at them! Outgunned and outmanned, they improvised from a stand-your-ground defense to a hit-and-run guerrilla offense, flipping the element of surprise back to their favor. The Greeks had only vintage rifles and a handful of shells, but that's all they needed. As soon as their fire drove the Germans back, they raced to the dying paratroopers, stripped away their weapons, and charged on.

And the 8th wasn't outnumbered for long. A mob of villagers armed with sickles and axes ran to join them. One farmer fashioned a bayonet by lashing a knife to the end of his shotgun; another old Cretan used his cane to beat to death two paratroopers who'd gotten snarled in their harnesses in his back garden. A priest named Father Stylianos Frantzeskakis rang the church bell to summon his parishioners, then grabbed his uncle's hunting rifle and led his congregation into combat. A teenage boy followed him, dragging an old Turkish sword that was so long it scraped along the ground. "My mother sent me," the boy told Father Frantzeskakis. A monk headed into the fray with a rifle in his hand and a hand ax in his belt; later, the same hatchet-wielding holy man reappeared with a German submachine gun, presumably after killing the German who'd carried it.

A bewildered young British officer named Michael Forrester found himself at the head of "a weird counter-attack," as he called it. Forrester had gotten separated from his unit and stumbled across a leaderless band of Greek soldiers under fire from a German platoon. With their backs against the sea, the Greeks were trapped. Forrester decided to take command, even though just about the only Greek word he knew was *Aeria!*—"Charge!" Maybe he could toot commands on a tin whistle? Sure, why not. Forrester hurriedly taught his new force a signal code—one tweet to stand by, two to move—and then fixed his bayonet for a do-or-die attempt to break through the German net.

"I decided that the time had come for action and alerted my force with my whistle," Forrester would later say. "We had not gone very far before I realized that we had been substantially reinforced by a considerable number of the inhabitants of Crete—men and women—

armed with old shotguns, garden tools, sticks, broom handles, some with kitchen knives strapped on to the end of them." With Forrester shrilling away on his whistle, the mob charged. The Germans dropped their weapons and put up their hands.

Back at his command post in Athens, General Kurt Student was getting minute-by-minute updates by radio. He unsnapped his holster. "I waited with my pistol continuously by my side," he said, "ready to use it on myself if the worse came to the worst."

CHAPTER 7

FRANCE FELL IN FIVE DAYS,
WHY IS CRETE STILL RESISTING?

—ADOLF HITLER, in a message to General Kurt Student

TOO LATE, General Student was discovering that on Crete heroes aren't an accident.

For more than a thousand years, in both fact and fable, the island has been a battleground between tyrants and rebels, gods and monsters. Crete was the birthplace of Zeus, the home of the Minotaur, the launch site of Daedalus and Icarus, and the homeland of canny backwoodsmen who, for generations, refused to bow to Turkish or Venetian warlords. From those myths and struggles emerged not only the heroic ideal but the means to achieve it—a folk science of mind and body that's ancient, alive, and very teachable.

"They are good archers, every one with his bowe and arrowes, a sword and dagger, with long haire and bootes that reach up to their grine, and a shirt of male," noted a British trader in the 1500s, who was just as intimidated by the festivals as the fighting: "They would drink wine out of all measure."

Jack Smith-Hughes learned firsthand about the Cretan art of the hero during the German invasion, and it kept him breathing long after he should have been dead. Jack had pink cheeks and a bit of a belly—no surprise, since his greatest contribution for much of the war was running a field bakery and supplying bread to the front lines. Jack didn't want to lose his supply trucks to enemy ambush, so he decided to reroute by water—and it was then, while dispatching a boatload of food to troops farther up the coast, that he found himself standing next to the Allied commander.

General Freyberg had gotten word that an Australian detachment was under fire without a working radio, so he'd sent a messenger by boat with orders to retreat. Instead of pivoting to other emergencies, Freyberg began pacing the waterfront. It was as if the fighting that raged elsewhere across the island had melted away and the only thing that mattered was one small pocket of beleaguered Australians. The baker wasn't sure what to do and found himself pacing the jetty alongside his brooding commander. Was Freyberg cracking under the pressure? He was famous for keeping his cool during Gallipoli and the Somme, two of the most horrific bloodbaths of World War I, but now that he was on the verge of a stunning victory, he looked distracted and defeated.

We're about to defeat Hitler's best fighters, Jack thought. *Aren't we?*

Freyberg's underdog troops had rallied magnificently once the shock of the air attack had worn off. Many of the New Zealanders were country boys, and their confidence grew as they realized this was their kind of fight. A Hunter dropping from the sky wasn't much different from a wild boar blasting from the bush back home in Kaikoura, so Kippenberger's Petrol Company quickly adjusted their fire to the paratroopers' four-meters-per-second drop speed, aiming for their feet to make kill shots to the chest.

So sharp was their marksmanship, one *Fallschirmjäger* battalion was convinced it had dropped into a den of supersoldiers. "It was particularly noticeable that a very large proportion of our casualties had been shot in the head," a *Fallschirmjäger* sergeant-major would report. "The controlled fire and discipline of the enemy led us to believe that we were up against a specialist force of picked snipers." Two of the New Zealanders held down the entire western side of a hill on their own—*for six days.*

Springtime on Crete is hot and dry, and German uniforms were wool. So it wasn't long before the Cretan shepherds faded from the fray, settling in behind stone walls with sight lines on cool springs. "The only well where we could get water," paratrooper Sebastian Krug would recall, "was being shot at all the time." The New Zealanders caught onto the idea and set ambushes of their own, lying in wait near the paratroopers' supply boxes. From the olive groves, the same cry began to ring out over and over:

"GOT THE BASTARD!"

This isn't warfare. This is ritual suicide. Long past midnight, General Student was still at a table in his command room, stubbing cigarettes into an overflowing ashtray as he read the battle dispatches. His Luger remained ready by his hand.

Because of him, the Third Reich's finest fighters were being slaughtered by shepherds and pig hunters. More than half of Student's ten-thousand-man invasion force was dead, wounded, or captured. Many of the rest were lost or hiding for their lives. All three Blücher brothers, from the fabled fighting family whose patriarch led the Prussian army against Napoleon, were gone. Max Schmeling's photo op nearly did him in; he'd parachuted through machine-gun fire, passed out after landing hard and injuring his back, then hid till nightfall and eventually crawled back to his unit. If there was a way out of this fiasco, Student didn't see it.

Then something caught his eye. Amid the bad news, one thing should have been worse. Why hadn't the Brits blown up Maleme, the small airfield on Crete's northwest coast? That's the first thing Student would have done if he were defending Crete: he'd have packed Maleme with dynamite and blasted it into a moon crater the second he saw a parachute pop open.

Crete is basically a rectangle, with two good-sized airfields along its northern coast. Master the airfields and you master the island. The Brits could get in and out by sea, thanks to its Royal Navy, but the Germans weren't as strong in the water. With no place to land their planes, the Hunters would be stranded.

The airfield was well defended at Heraklion, in the center, but Maleme, in the west, was a different story. That's where Student had thrown his biggest punch, swarming Maleme with fifty gliders full of Storm Regiment commandos and three companies of *Fallschirmjäger*. It was a gruesome operation: both gliders and paratroopers dropped right into a hail of burning flak that tore through flesh and parachute silk. By the time the survivors hit the ground, the trees were littered with their comrades' bodies. "All over the place you could see dead and wounded *Fallschirmjäger*, some still hanging from their parachutes," a *Fallschirmjäger* survivor named Helmut Wenzel later jotted in his diary. "There had been a lot of bloodshed and you could hear the crying and shouting of the wounded and dying."

That's when the Hunters showed what they were made of. Gathering and advancing through that nightmare of moaning men, attacking only with handguns and grenades, they managed to grab their heavy weapons from the drop boxes. Wenzel, with two severe wounds and just a pistol, staggered to his feet to join them. One force headed for high ground overlooking the airfield while the other charged the antiaircraft battery. By late afternoon the Germans had knocked out the big guns and captured the hill, but at a brutal cost: their officers were dead, their ammo was low, and only fifty-seven men were still alive. Most were so hurt and weak, they could barely stand. They prepared themselves to die. They had no hope against the Allied counterattack that was about to come storming up the hill.

Except . . . it never came.

The Allied commanders on Crete were so braced for defeat, they didn't realize they'd already won. Without Maleme, the Germans had no lifeline back to the mainland. It was only a matter of days—hours, even—until the invaders ran out of food and bullets. But with phone lines down and radios failing, with Allied officers in the rear out of contact with fighters on the front, assumptions took over for action. When the colonel defending Maleme didn't see the reinforcements he requested, he assumed headquarters wanted him to pull back; when headquarters learned he was pulling back, it assumed Maleme was a lost cause and diverted the reinforcements.

You don't beat Kurt Student by giving him a second chance.

Before dawn of Day 2, German troop planes were taking to the sky, one after the other, roaring toward Maleme. Student had decided to "stake everything on one card." He committed the 5th Mountain Division and the last of his *Fallschirmjäger* reserves to a final, all-or-nothing assault on the airfield.

Only a few New Zealand troops were still within firing range of the eastern end of the runway when they heard the first Junker approach. They blazed away, riddling the plane with bullets as it skidded down just long enough to drop off forty Mountain Division soldiers and then disappeared back over the Mediterranean. The New Zealanders shifted their aim toward the Germans sprinting for cover, gunning many of them down before they got a few steps across the runway. But a few reached the trenches and returned fire, creating cover for the next Junkers screeching down. More Germans tumbled off, scrambling into the gullies as a third plane approached, then a fourth. . . .

The New Zealanders were stunned. Ten minutes ago, they were in a nice holding position against an exhausted enemy, waiting for orders to either mop up or march off. Now, suddenly, they were burning through the last of their ammunition, shooting helplessly against an enemy that was doubling, tripling, by the minute. Time was still on their side, but not for long. They had to attack immediately and put an end to the job they should have finished yesterday. They had to storm the hill before the Germans landed any more troops and fortified their hold on the airfield. This was their chance.

Bayonets were fixed. Grenades were handed around. And then the order came from the rear: *Stand down.*

Back at headquarters, Freyberg was still convinced that the *real* invasion was coming by sea. All these planes and paratroopers? Just a feint to lure Allied troops into the hills and leave the coasts undefended. *Absolutely correct*, agreed Brigadier James Hargest. Like Freyberg, the beefy old brigadier was a survivor of the Great War and thought he was still fighting it. Hargest spent the boat trip over to Crete reading *War and Peace*, and from the old Russians he took his cue. "In war," Hargest preached, "steadiness and endurance are more important than any amount of strategic flair." The key to Crete, he urged Freyberg, was caution and the coastline.

Which could explain why, days later and long after the golden opportunity was gone, Freyberg was walking the waterfront alongside a bewildered young bakery manager, watching for an enemy armada that would never appear.

"They were brave men, but no longer bold," lamented Antony Beevor, the British military historian who wrote the definitive account of the invasion. "The Battle of Crete, a revolutionary development in warfare, was to be a contest in which fast reactions, clear thinking and ruthless decisions counted most." Freyberg still had his boots sunk in the mud of the Somme, while Student—so feverishly inventive that he could use German parts to rebuild a shot-down French plane and fly it straight back into action—had no interest in refighting a war his country had already lost.

But still, there was a moment when the past might have prevailed, when trench-style tactics could have choked the Germans into submission. And that's the moment when Freyberg flinched. "A single platoon, even a single Bren gun left in place on the airfield," Beevor concludes, "could have swung the course of the whole battle."

As waves of German troops fanned out from Maleme, Jack Smith-Hughes was soon scrambling to stay one step ahead of his friends and two steps ahead of the enemy. The Royal Navy couldn't risk many ships on yet another Dunkirk, so anyone who didn't reach southern Crete quickly wasn't leaving. "Orders are every man for himself!" a sergeant shouted. Thousands of Allied soldiers scrambled frantically up and over the White Mountains, clinging to a crumbling trail that skirted "a near vertical wall of the road on one side and a drop fall of hundreds and hundreds of feet on the other," as British infantryman Edward Frederic Telling would recall. "All with no lights."

Jack Smith-Hughes was footsore and starving when he limped into the port at Sfakiá, and surprised when he was told he didn't need to line up right away. More evacuations were planned for the next day, an officer promised, before climbing into a skiff himself. The next morning, Jack Smith-Hughes was staring into the barrel of a German rifle. Along with thousands of other Allied troops abandoned on Crete, Jack was forced at gunpoint to hobble back over the mountains he'd just crossed. When the prison gate closed behind him, Jack knew he had two choices: he could escape and get shot, or stay behind the wires and waste away. Already, men all around him were dying of wounds and disease.

Well, better a quick bullet than a slow death. One night, Jack followed a Cretan prisoner through the wire, and together they escaped into the hills. Before sentries could track them, they were grabbed by villagers and pulled out of sight. Jack was hidden and fed, nursed back to health on a Cretan villager's diet of wild greens, dark bread so hard it had to be soaked in wine before biting, and *fasolakia me katsiki*—beans simmered with goat.

Jack was still too weak to hide out in the mountains, so his new friends came up with a Plan B: turn the pudgy blond Brit into a Cretan. The villagers renamed him Yanni and drilled him on the peculiarities of their dialect. Like the word for "adult": on Crete, a grown-up is known as a *dromeus*, or "runner." To be considered a full Cretan, you had to be strong and resourceful enough to run to someone's aid. Until then, young Cretans are just *apodromos*—"not quite a runner"—and the ritual passage into adulthood was celebrated with the festival of Dromaia—"the Running."

Gradually, Jack's strength returned. By his standards, at least; keeping pace with a geriatric *dromeus* was a different story. Jack was taken under the wing of a bald and blue-eyed Cretan in his fifties who was so buoyantly unkillable that the Brits would code-name him Beowulf. Beowulf was once shot between the lungs but "suffered no visible ill effects." Beowulf guided Jack to fresh hiding places, keeping him a jump ahead of German search parties and subjecting him to the ego-crushing experience of following an old Cretan into the mountains. Instead of struggling, they seemed to fall *upward*, bouncing from rock to rock for hours with an odd, effortless-looking elasticity. It wasn't just the men; Cretan women could likewise carry heftier packs, cover longer distances, navigate through snow and dark, and thrive on a diet plucked from the ground as they passed.

Strength didn't explain it—it was as if the Cretans were drawing on something else, a martial art of energy mastery. Under any kind of pressure, physical or mental, they seemed to become more pliable. Near Jack's hiding place, for instance, a teenage boy who'd blown up a German plane by sticking a burning rag into the gas tank turned himself in when the Germans threatened to murder his family. George Vernadakis was beaten and starved, then dragged naked into the village square to be executed. Dazed and weak, he had a last request: could he please wet his lips with a glass of wine and sing a farewell song? The wine was produced, and George's hands were unchained. He drank it down and took off, darting naked from lane to lane through the village. George not only got away but kept on fighting; the next time his family saw him, he was in an air force uniform.

After five months in hiding, Jack was introduced to George Psychoundakis, a young shepherd with frenzied hair and impish eyes. George thought he knew a way to get Jack off the island and to safety in Egypt. It was risky, but if Jack was willing to trust him, they could give it a try. Jack figured they'd slink invisibly through the backcountry and rendezvous with some patriotic fisherman in a hidden cove. Instead he found himself the main attraction of a bizarre parade. The two men were escorted by fifteen armed shepherds, and every time they passed through a village, more eager rebels rushed out to join them.

"Wherever we went, the villagers, seeing us carrying arms, almost exploded with joy," George would later recall. "Everyone thought something important was afoot and prepared to take up their guns and follow us. We calmed them down and told them they would be warned in time when the moment came."

Despite nearly inciting insurrection, Jack and his gang managed to dodge German patrols and make it to the Preveli monastery, a stone sanctuary on a cliff tended by monks since the Middle Ages. A few weeks earlier, the monks were in the middle of High Mass when a British submarine commander with a pirate's gold hoop in his ear burst through the door. He'd been prowling the coast for stranded soldiers, and when he spotted an SOS beacon flashing from a bluff near the monastery, he came ashore personally to check it out. Word soon spread along the Cretan whisper network: any Brit on the run who could make it to Preveli—*fast*—had a chance of escape.

A few nights later, Jack Smith-Hughes was being paddled out toward the sub in a rubber raft. Watching from the beach were George Psychoundakis and other descendants of the world's first heroes, waiting for Jack—and any other Brits who dared to join them—to return.

CHAPTER 8

We were totally amateurish, totally one hundred per cent
amateurish, and it couldn't have been otherwise.

—BASIL DAVIDSON, one of Churchill's original "dirty tricksters"

WAIT. George is still alive?

Chris White hung up the phone, stunned. It was the summer of
2004, and Chris had just gotten a call from a friend whose son was a
journalist in Greece. Her son had gone to Crete in search of World
War II survivors, Chris's friend said, and there, among the backcountry villages, he came across the old Resistance runner himself, still
roaming the high mountain ranges.

Good Lord. How was that even possible? The odds of survival in
the dirty tricks squad was appalling. Half of the recruits were captured or killed in the first year alone, and of all their assignments,
none was riskier than George Psychoundakis's. Other Resistance
fighters spent a good deal of their time in hiding, but runners lived in
the red zone, zigzagging through enemy patrols while carrying documents that guaranteed a death sentence if discovered. Runners were
an especially high-value target for the Gestapo, who knew they rarely
carried weapons and could lead them directly to nearly every guerrilla
hideout. Two other shepherds from George's valley became runners

along with him; they were soon captured, tortured, and shot. "The job of a war-time runner in the Resistance Movement was the most exhausting and one of the most consistently dangerous," observed Patrick Leigh Fermor, who relied on them during his own tour of duty on Crete as a dirty trickster.

So George somehow made it through not just one bloodbath but two, first enduring four years of relentless manhunts and then the vicious civil war that engulfed Greece immediately after the German occupation. Every decade since then, some fresh killer had swept across the island—famine, drought, epidemic disease—yet George survived them all, not to mention the constant Cretan peril of vendetta attacks. (Even Patrick Leigh Fermor, whose wartime derring-do made him one of Crete's most beloved adopted sons, was startled to discover he'd barely escaped the crosshairs of a sniper rifle after a friend's nephew swore a blood oath of vengeance against him for an accidental death.)

For Chris White, the news of George's survival couldn't have come at a better time. Because the more he learned about George's life, Chris had discovered, the better he felt about his own.

Chris lived in Oxford, and although the city, with its ancient university and cozy cottages, looked utterly tranquil, it attracted an unusual number of homeless. Chris worked with the unstable and depressed, and the despair he dealt with every day had begun to infect him. "The backdrop of any Monday or end of holiday would be hearing that someone you'd been working with was dead," Chris says. "I'd say 'Hi' to my secretary and she'd say 'Hi, Chris!' and then tell me about what we call 'incidents'—someone killed themselves or tried to kill one of your staff. Once, two staff members went to check on a guy in his home and he picked up a knife and stabbed them both in the lower back. They survived, though."

By the time he turned fifty-six, Chris had been managing mental-health services in Oxford for eight years. He lived in a charming farmhouse just outside town with his wife, Cath, and their eight-year-old twins. He had a gang of pals he joined for sailing expeditions and a great friendship with Rich, his twenty-two-year-old son from a previous relationship. He had a little log cabin he'd built out back for his books and sailing charts and music, and a delightful mother-in-law who'd bubble by to share a pint of ale and stories about living across the garden from Roald Dahl. Chris was easygoing and fun-loving, and utterly baffled when, in the middle of the night, he began to wake up in sweaty panics.

How can you close your eyes to rest when you know they'll pop open in terror? Soon, Chris wasn't sleeping at all. He lay there, heart hammering and bone weary, helpless against fears he couldn't identify, desperate for dawn but dreading the leaden day ahead. The more exhausted he became, the less he saw the point. Why keep dragging around like this? Why go on feeling so awful? So stupid. So easy to fix. Such a short walk to the cabin, where he could sling a rope over the rafter and—

Cath, Chris told his wife, *I need help.* Together they saw a physician, who made Chris understand how close he'd come to becoming an incident himself. He'd built a life he thought would protect him from depression, but instead it blinded him to the fact that he was edging deeper and deeper into danger. Chris needed to make some changes, beginning with a prescription for antidepressants and at least four months off from work.

During the time at home, Chris rested his mind by focusing on a peculiar story he'd first heard years before. An elderly friend had asked him to trim some of her overgrown trees, and as a thank-you she'd given Chris a book about the strange adventures of Patrick Leigh Fermor, known to everyone as Paddy. Paddy was Chris's kind of adventurer—gallant, literary, madcap, merry. Chris dug around for more and soon learned about Paddy's daffy scheme to kidnap a German general.

"I've always been a man who's had projects, always tunneling into something," Chris says. Paddy's saga was just the thing to get him drilling. The extreme adventure was intriguing, but what really hooked him was the surreal gentleness.

"It was the kindest, most bloodless scheme you'd ever encounter in military history," Chris marveled. In the midst of carnage and cruelty, "everyone in this operation was trying to be brave, kind, diplomatic." Chris couldn't help feeling a pang of kinship. The tilting at windmills of Paddy's plot reminded him of his own job, of the challenge of helping people he knew were headed for ruin. When you're doomed to fail, how do you avoid living in doubt and despair? By living, not doubting.

Living and not doubting had always been Chris's navigational star, at least until his recent troubles began. Back when he was a first-year student at Durham University in the seventies, Chris wrote a story about psychiatry for the school paper. It earned him a spot on the features staff and just enough credibility, Chris felt, to make a ridiculous request: he contacted Harold Evans, editor of Britain's prestigious *Sunday Times*, and asked if maybe Evans had any unused stories lying around? Something Chris could print in the Durham University *Palatinate*?

"And by return post we got an enormous article, ready to print," Chris told me. "The *Times* was investigating thalidomide"— a drug prescribed for morning sickness, later linked to horrific birth defects—"but the manufacturers had slapped Evans with another injunction. He had this massive article he couldn't publish in the *Times*, so he just gave it to our little university paper." It was a brilliant coup, and Chris's golden ticket; that article guaranteed he'd be appointed the *Palatinate*'s next editor and likely find a juicy journalism job right after graduation. Naturally, for Chris that meant it was time to quit. He couldn't imagine spending the rest of his life behind a typewriter; he'd always seen himself on the move, bopping about as some kind of roving mental-health healer. So he turned his back on writing and got his master's in psychology instead. When he was close to his Ph.D., he jumped ship again: this time, his dissertation research had taken him to Miami Beach, where he found such a bizarre buffet of mental disorders on the streets that he decided to stop studying and start helping.

For the rest of Chris's life, that was his pattern: if the easy road led toward a desk, Chris backed up and found another one. He liked being in the field, traveling from home to home each day to work with elderly and not-quite-stable outpatients. On vacation, he'd take his then girlfriend to a beach resort but persuade her to forget the sea and head inland with him, turning it into a weeklong ramble. Boating buddies could count on Chris whenever a last-minute mate was needed for *anywhere*, even a freezing sail to Scandinavia. When I first went to meet him in Oxford, I got off the train expecting lunch first, maps second, beers last; instead I found myself trotting behind him on a spontaneous, double-time, four-hour walking tour that included bell towers, underground pubs, and a muddy stretch of his neighbor's backyard. That's what happens if you tell him it's your first time in town.

Chris's natural inclination to *move*, all the time and for any reason, has made him something of a natural-movement savant. You'll never catch him working out (Repetitions? Routine? Forget it), yet he's never *not* working out. His ever-bubbling brain won't let him sit, so Chris just flows along behind it; his distractions lead the way, and his body figures out how to keep up. Like Paddy, Chris's intelligence and curiosity have made motion his natural state, his way to both push hard and rest easy. When he finally came inside as a manager, the promotion nearly killed him.

Luckily, Crete was waiting.

When Chris's friend called with the update that George was still alive, Chris's thinking abruptly changed. Until that moment he'd been dealing with history; now, suddenly, it was a *story*, alive and ongoing. How many other survivors were back in those hills? What did they know that Paddy never revealed?

Because when it came to the kidnap scheme, Paddy remained strangely quiet. He'd come close to perfectly executing one of the most daring heists of the war, but even when it was safe to talk, the show-off who could tell stories all night was reluctant to share this one. Maybe it was because of the man he killed. Maybe it was because of the other he couldn't save. Something was silencing him; even after others told their version, Paddy went to the grave with his.

But as long as Crete was alive with eyewitnesses and evidence, Chris could do more than just try to get inside Paddy's head: he could get inside his boots. By tracking Paddy's movements, he might still have a chance to track down people who'd seen everything. First he got in touch with Tim Todd, a former Oxford police detective who'd become the Mycroft Holmes of amateur Cretan espionage enthusiasts. Like Sherlock's smarter, less mobile brother, Tim's brain reached further than his legs; he knew elderly escaped POWs in New Zealand and dead soldiers' daughters in Australia. He got copies of military documents as soon as they were declassified and photos of others that weren't supposed to leave the archives. He became friendly with Stelios Jackson, the Greek book hound who can find anything in or out of print, and the husband-and-wife historians Artemis Cooper and Antony Beevor, who between them know more than anyone alive about the Cretan Resistance. Tim Todd is a hearty and resourceful investigator, but unfortunately his health isn't great. He can't really get out there in the field.

Chris can. He turned his backyard cabin into a command room, and it was there—amid the black-and-white photos, stacks of World War II memoirs, and blown-up copies of Wehrmacht maps—that we met in the winter of 2011. There is no official history of exactly what the British agents got up to on Crete, but there is Chris White. Chris had turned himself into a formidable amateur detective, and to solve the lingering mysteries of Paddy's plot, he knew exactly what we had to do next:

Go to the scene of the crime.

A few months later, Chris and his brother, Pete, were waiting for me on a notch of pebbly beach on Crete's southern coast.

"Welcome to bandit country," Chris said, as I shucked my sweat-soaked backpack and looked back at the snarl of hills I'd just hiked over. Chris and Pete had arrived a week earlier because, frankly, they weren't sure they could trust me. They hated the idea of accidentally turning the Resistance's secret hideouts into tourist attractions, so until they sized me up they'd be cautious about what they'd share. They wanted to search for some sites in private, so I gave them a week's head-start before I flew to Crete and set off to catch up.

From Heraklion I rattled over the mountains by bus to the end of the line and got a room for the night above a village taverna. At daybreak I set off on foot, the sun on my back as I headed due west along the coastline. A shepherds' trail climbed the cliffs high above the shore, occasionally wandering into stone gullies before veering again toward the water. By late afternoon, I was dead-legged and wondering if I'd find my way out before dark when I suddenly found myself a step away from empty air: far below at the bottom of a long drop was a small cove, invisible until I was right overhead. A jagged switchback led down to a solitary guest house, where Chris and Pete were bunking after hiking in the night before.

"You're seeing something Paddy never did," Chris greeted me after

I'd scrambled on down. "He could only come here by dark, guided by shepherds." It was a good place for British subs to surface without being spotted, and for British agents to disappear once they made it to shore.

Outlaws and rebels have been hiding in these parts as long as there's been anyone to hide from, bursting from the trees in hit-and-run rebellions against centuries of seagoing bullies who tried to make the Sliver their own. Thorny tangles and abrupt cliffs make pockets of the southern coast labyrinthine enough to stash a Minotaur, especially when the usual blanket of sea mist creeps in. Even George got himself into trouble around here in a fast-rolling fog, thinking he was walking down a familiar hill before discovering he was a few feet from disaster. "I wore myself out all night trying to get away from that accursed precipice," George would grumble.

Chris never got a chance to meet George; shortly before Chris' first trip to the island, the Cretan runner had died in 2006 at age eighty-five. But Chris and Pete had paid their respects by visiting George's lifelong home, the tiny and notoriously defiant village a few miles north of us called Asi Gonia. The name means "unconquerable" in Arabic and was bestowed by the Turks as an honor of sorts, during their two-century occupation of Crete. The only natural way into Asi Gonia is through a narrow gorge, and George's forefathers defended it so stubbornly that the great Ottoman Empire decided the little hornet's nest wasn't worth the trouble and mostly just left the Asi Gonians be.

"Some of the old Turkish bridges are still standing," Chris told me. "You know about the one that saved George?"

"Sure." It was one of George's most nerve-wracking adventures. A traitor had given up George's name to the Gestapo, so before dawn one morning, they came looking for him. Ordinarily George slept in a cave, never indoors, but he'd wrenched his ankle and decided just that once to rest for the night in his parents' house. The Gestapo grabbed George before he could get out the door. But because the clan had various George Psychoundakises, everyone in the village was marched to the church, where the informant—muffled in a raincoat, his face covered—was waiting to finger the elusive Cretan runner.

"I was in front," George would recall, "and I whispered to my parents and brothers and sisters, 'Fall into line, and the ones at the back, dawdle.'" The line bunched, allowing George to casually move about forty yards ahead. As soon as the path curved, he jumped into a brook and took off, counting on the brush to cover his escape and the water to mask his scent. The other Psychoundakises were interrogated and eventually released while George ran for his life, dodging up and down the mountain on his aching ankle as he tried to find a way through the German cordon. After three days without food or sleep, he nearly walked into a dead end: just as he was about to cross a stone bridge, he heard a search party approaching on the other side. Instead of bolting for cover, George slid under his end of the bridge, then silently waded in the opposite direction as German boots stomped past overhead. On the far side, he scrambled out and escaped into the woods.

"We found it," Chris said.

They found what—*George's bridge?* I felt twin stabs of envy and admiration. George had never specified where the bridge was or what it was called; to him it was just another handy hideout in a pinch. So Pete and Chris plotted the reference points in George's account, and then trekked village to village, café by café, asking around for anyone who could help them locate landmarks. Gradually, they connected the dots in George's twisting escape route until they finally found themselves on the bank of a stream, staring at a span of ancient stone. "We had a fantastic celebration," Chris said. "We jumped in."

It was a triumph of sleuthing, all the more impressive because neither of them speaks Greek. Pete is head gardener at Furzey Gardens, in the south of England, where learning-disabled adults help care for fairy houses and miniature donkeys and artisanal beehives. He is fifty-four and has the graying good looks of an aging folk singer, which is handy, since he moonlights as a ukulele strummer and ceilidh guitarist. Between them, the brothers White had mastered nearly every humanist talent except foreign languages, so they'd pretty much pinned their hopes of communication on an introductory letter that Chris drafted and got a Greek buddy in Oxford to translate:

We are historians researching the Resistance, the letter begins. *We are hoping to find caves in this area used by freedom fighters. . . .*

"Historians"? The truth was, we were totally amateurish, one hundred percent—and to follow in George and Paddy's footsteps, it couldn't have been otherwise.

. . .

The next morning, I caught Chris eyeing my feet. He looked worried, and I knew why.

We were at the spot where it all began, the beachhead where Paddy and his fellow agents of mayhem first sloshed ashore. They could smell the island before they saw it, the musky scent of wild thyme carrying far out past the breakers. Paddy hopped out of the raft before it beached, and by the time he hit land he was in trouble. The Sliver's terrain is among the harshest in Europe, and not just because of the vicious climbs; beneath a dusting of sand and soil lurk strips of razory rock that can shred leather like piranha teeth. Just walking those few yards through the surf tore Paddy's boots to tatters, so he had to spend his first week on Crete hiding in a cave until sturdier footwear could be found. He wore those out in a few weeks, and continued tearing through boots at a rate of a pair every month.

"Are you okay with those?" Chris asked, his tone making it clear I shouldn't be.

"There's this idea—" I began, but decided I'd better shut up. Chris and Pete had rugged mountaineering boots, but mine were super-lights with a thin sole designed for desert sand. Ever since I found out how often Paddy's boots were destroyed by the rocks, I'd wondered why the Cretans' held up so much better. Maybe the difference wasn't the footwear; maybe it was the feet. Instead of depending on leather, the Cretans relied on skill.

Soldiers are trained to march, but George was free to tap into an older form of movement now known as Parkour, or freerunning. Freerunners don't walk across the landscape; they bounce off it, ricocheting along in a steady, hip-hopping, acrobatic flow, treating planet Earth more like a launchpad than a landing point. Xan Fielding, one of Patrick Leigh Fermor's comrades on Crete, encountered exactly that kind of antigravity gait as he struggled to keep up with an older, heavyset Cretan who "tripped daintily along from boulder to boulder, his body bouncing with every step like an inflated rubber beach toy." Beefy old Stavros was so springy he seemed weightless and, Xan felt, a little sadistic. "I go much better uphill," explained Stavros, who then found another gear as the slope got steeper and went even faster. Xan lasted thirty minutes. "After half an hour of crazy racing, tearing through scrub and stumbling over loose earth," Xan grumbled, "I insisted on stopping for a cigarette."

Stavros was using the same technique that a doctor from Boston had observed more than a hundred years earlier when he served as a volunteer during the Greek Revolution. Samuel Gridley Howe was used to watching American troops tromp along in rhythmic formation, but the Greeks were hopping all over the place. "A Greek soldier," Howe commented, "will march, or rather skip, all day among the rocks, expecting no other food than a biscuit and a few olives, or a raw onion, and at night, lies down content upon the ground with a flat rock for a pillow."

Wait. Skipping all day on olives and an onion—mathematically, how's that even possible? The calories going in can't equal the energy going out. George Psychoundakis would sometimes shuttle between the caves for twelve hours a day on a starvation diet, yet his mind stayed sharp, his muscles strong, and his endurance unshaken. During one escapade, his only meal was hay soup, made by boiling and reboiling scrounged-up animal fodder seven times to remove the toxins. Yet even on that zero-calorie concoction, he shot off the next day to summit a peak that would stagger an adventure racer.

The only explanation, I believed, was freerunning. The Greeks were getting free fuel *and* extra leg protection by relying on an ancient, elastic gait that looked playful but was deadly effective. I'd gotten my first look at freerunning back home in Pennsylvania, when I was in line at a drugstore and suddenly saw two bodies go sailing past the window. These guys had to be six feet in the air, flying by one after the other like they'd been slung out of a catapult. Moments later they reappeared outside the glass doors, this time swinging through the railings of the handicapped ramp. By the time I got to the cash register, I'd watched them hurdle, vault, tightrope-walk, and otherwise wring a crazy amount of movement out of those green bars. I hurried outside to catch them, but they weren't leaving anytime soon.

"You start practicing Parkour," one of them told me, "and whole nights disappear."

That I could believe. From what I'd seen through the window, freerunning was anything *but* free; it looked like a ton of fun, but way too showy. All those jumps and vaults seemed too complicated to allow any kind of flow, like skateboarders who kick-flip their decks over and over and never get the thing to land on its wheels. But that's because I was making a rookie mistake, my new drugstore buddies explained. You can't judge Parkour with your eyes; you have to judge it with your body. Once you learn Parkour's basic moves, the world around you changes. You don't see *things* anymore; you see movement. Take that alley across the street, one of them said. What's in it?

Let's see. A Dumpster; some busted bottles; two cars; a cement wall with a fence on top.

For *you*. For us, there's a catpass precision, two Kongs, a running arm jump, and a step vault.

All I had to do was get some Parkour under my belt, they promised, and I'd see the world the same way. I'd look at a gnarly goat trail on a Mediterranean island, and the crashed trees and tumbled boulders would transform from stuff in the way into stuff to bounce off of. I'd handle the trail the way water handles a riverbed. I'd skip all day on olives and an onion.

That was the plan, at least. It seemed like a good one, so I threw myself into Parkour and followed it from that Pennsylvania parking lot back to a housing project in London, where an out-of-shape single mom was becoming one of the sport's finest instructors. But now that I was on Crete, it seemed smarter to keep it to myself for a while. I didn't want Chris and Pete worrying that I was about to walk into something I couldn't walk out of—even though, as we squinted up at the snow packed into the high gorges, I was wondering about it myself. Theory, meet mountain.

We shouldered our packs and set off, following Chris across the slick stones above the black sand beach. "Harsh here," Pete commented. "See the plants, all covered in thorns? That's because goats eat everything. Only the prickliest survive."

CHAPTER 9

PHILIP II, WARLORD OF MACEDON:

If I bring my army into your land, I will destroy your farms, slay your people, and raze your city.

SPARTANS TO PHILIP II: *If.*

WHEN THE BAKER Jack Smith-Hughes got off the boat in Egypt after his escape from Crete, no one gave a hoot what happened to his boots. He was met by mysterious men from London who were intensely curious about two things: tongues and talent. As in: could the Cretans keep a secret? Were they just wild men with muskets, or could they unite into a serious fighting force? In other words, could Jack trust them with his life?

Because back in London, in a small townhouse on Baker Street with no name or number on the door, a new kind of fighting force was being organized. Officially, it was the Special Operatives Executive, but it was better known by its code name: the Firm. Rumor had it the Firm was authorized to carry out sinister ops like murder, kidnapping, safecracking, booby traps, and sex-for-secrets intrigues. According to one story, the Firm had already deployed fake French prostitutes to stock a German army brothel with condoms soaked in flesh-eating chemicals.

British officers, after all, were no strangers to sneak attacks; they'd learned from the bitter experience of their own body count just how effective black ops could be. For centuries, the King's men had been ambushed by Scottish rebels, potshot by American revolutionaries, raided by Boer horsemen, castrated and beheaded by Pashtun tribesmen, sabotaged by Burmese jungle bandits, and bewildered by the IRA's urban camouflage. Britain was the greatest imperial force on earth, but even giants are vulnerable to the thousand nicks of stealthy amateurs who know the terrain and ignore the rules. It was a lesson that a young cavalry officer named Winston Churchill had barely survived forty years earlier. Britain's colonial force "can march anywhere, and do anything," young Churchill realized as he galloped for his life from Pashtun sharpshooters, "except catch the enemy."

Now—*finally*—Churchill was ready to steal a page from Britain's underground enemies and put a dirty-tricks squad into the field.

Churchill got lucky. He found two British officers who loved the idea of a dirty-tricks squad so much, they came up with it before he did. Colin Gubbins and Jo Holland had been friends for more than twenty years, ever since they'd met as young officers in Ireland, dodging rooftop gunfire from Michael Collins's IRA snipers. Nothing makes you appreciate a teacher more than the possibility that he'll shoot you, so Gubbins and Holland became rapt students of "Mick" Collins's approach to extraordinary warfare.

One thing that made the IRA so elusive was a neat trick that Michael Collins picked up from *The Man Who Was Thursday*, G. K. Chesterton's classic espionage novel about bomb-throwing anarchists who avoid suspicion by acting exactly like bomb-throwing anarchists. "If you didn't seem to be hiding," Chesterton wrote, "nobody hunted you out." So Mick taught his fighters to draw *more* attention to themselves, not less; the more visible they were, the less likely they'd be searched and questioned. Mick himself was Public Enemy No. 1, yet he cycled all over Dublin in a sharp gray suit, on an "ancient bicycle whose chain," as guerrilla-warfare expert Max Boot notes, "rattled like a medieval ghost's."

To Gubbins and Holland, the IRA chieftain was as much a mentor as an enemy. "Forget the term 'foul methods,'" Gubbins decided. "'Foul methods,' so called, help you to kill quickly." They were so on fire with the possibilities of irregular tactics, they'd already spent years reading up on Apache warriors and Russian revolutionaries before Churchill approached them at the beginning of the war with the task of creating a dirty-tricks squad.

Every guerrilla band, they discovered, relied on the same cheap and devilishly effective weapon: doubt. Create enough uncertainty in your enemy and you can paralyze him. Officers will freeze when they should charge; soldiers will flinch when they should fire. "To inflict damage and death on the enemy and to escape scot-free has an irritant and depressing effect," Gubbins realized. "The object must be to strike hard and disappear before the enemy can strike back."

Okay, that's fine if you're a Comanche slipping through your native forest and trained from birth in silent stalking. But how—and this is where Churchill's generals smelled disaster—*how* does a tweedy London gentleman pull off the same thing in some village in the Balkans?

Gubbins knew exactly where to begin. As soon as he was tapped to head Churchill's new dream force, he went hunting for misfits. Combat vets and tough guys he didn't need; anyone who looked like he could actually take care of himself was red meat for Gestapo spy hunters. When one candidate promised to "blow the head off the first German he sees," he was immediately dumped. "We don't want these sort of heroes," a dirty-tricks trainer explained. "We want them to live and do actions."

No, the type Gubbins wanted was . . . well, it wasn't something you could put into words. "I say Class X because there is no definition for it," explained Geoffrey Household, a traveling ink salesman who became one of Gubbins's early agents and drew on his adventures to write *Rogue Male*, the classic thriller about a British sportsman who eludes Nazi pursuers by using only his wits and, in a pinch, a dead cat. Class X wasn't about wealth, title, or power. "We are an oligarchy with its ranks ever open to talent," Household writes in *Rogue Male*. It was an invisible *something*, detectable only by ear. "Who belongs to Class X?" he continues. "I don't know till I talk to him and then I know at once. It is not, I think, a question of accent, but rather of the gentle voice."

The gentle voice? Yes: the tone of someone who, when asked to do and die, would quite like to know the reason why. Geoffrey Household and his generation were young enough to escape the trenches of the last war, but old enough to witness the terror and carnage that comes when countries throw millions of bodies with bayonets at one another. For this new kind of warfare—and this new kind of warrior—there would be no Light Brigade charges into the jaws of death. Class X was all for service, but not for suicide. If you wanted their bodies, their brains were part of the bargain.

Gubbins knew that trying to transform these skeptical, gentle-voiced intellectuals into icy cold operators was going to be tricky, especially since he couldn't expect much help from the military. "We've only fought decently in the British Army," one disgusted general sniffed in response to Gubbins's desire to teach "silent killing." When the Firm sent out feelers to Edward Shackleton, an air force lieutenant (and son of Ernest, the fabled Antarctic explorer), Shackleton asked his squad commander what it was all about. "Don't touch it," the commander warned him. "They're not the sort of people you want to be mixed up with."

So Gubbins bypassed the army and instead looked for help from "the Whore of the Orient"—Shanghai, where the world's dirtiest gutter fighters did battle in the world's most dangerous city. Shanghai in the 1930s was ruled by jungle law, to the extent that jungle creatures specialized in gambling, sex slaves, dope dealing, and gang warfare. As Asia's busiest port, Shanghai bustled with so many addicts, pirates, and waterfront hustlers that by 1936 it could comfortably support an estimated 100,000 criminals. Even its name meant trouble: get "shanghaied" and you'd wake up with a bad headache and a worse surprise, often a few miles out to sea as free labor on a merchant ship. One crime boss bragged that he'd fed a troublesome girlfriend to his pet tiger; another dealt with rivals by slitting their arm and leg tendons and heaving them, alive but helpless, into the middle of a busy street.

Into this madness strode Bill Sykes and William Fairbairn, the Heavenly Twins. Fairbairn was originally a Royal Marine who arrived in 1907 after answering a worldwide recruiting call by the beleaguered Shanghai police. His welcoming gift was a beating so savage he had to be hauled to the hospital in the back of a rickshaw; during foot patrol along the waterfront, a gang of hoodlums nearly pummeled and booted him to death. During his long recovery, Fairbairn ruefully reflected that none of the training he'd ever gotten—not as a boxer, not even as a frontline soldier—was of any use in the panicky, ferocious chaos of a real street brawl. So once he was back on his feet, Fairbairn began to immerse himself in the science of true gutter fighting. He began by apprenticing himself to "Professor Okada," a jiu-jitsu expert who trained the Japanese emperor's security force. Fairbairn gradually became such a skilled knifeman and sharpshooter that his innovations are still in use by Special Forces a half-century later.

Fairbairn's turnaround was so dramatic that he was picked to head the Shanghai Riot Squad. During his thirty years along the waterfront, Fairbairn survived more than six hundred fights, including the time a Chinese bandit's bullet scorched by his face and singed his eyebrows. His favorite sidekick was Bill Sykes, a slight, friendly gent who looked like he'd be happiest with a quiet pipe and a couple of grandkids. Sykes was a true oddity in Shanghai, partly because his real name was Eric A. Schwabe but mostly because he was an amateur hobbyist in a city of professional badasses. Sykes insisted he was nothing more than a sales rep who liked to hang around cops, and only went by a fake name because the real one sounded too German. Maybe. But whispers of spy service are hard to deny when you go through life with an alias and a talent for stabbing men to death with a sheet of newspaper. (*Just fold it diagonally until it tightens into a point*, Sykes would shrug, *then drive it in right under the chin. Simple, really.*)

By the time World War II began, Sykes and Fairbairn were nearly sixty years old; their hair had gone white, and their sharpshooting eyes now needed spectacles. Still, Gubbins wanted his first class of dirty-trickster recruits to see the old-school stuff in action, so he invited Sykes and Fairbairn to a training camp he'd set up at a hidden estate deep in the Scottish Highlands. "We were taken into the hall of the Big House, and suddenly at the top of the stairs appeared a couple of dear old gentlemen," recalled a recruit, R. F. "Henry" Hall. The recruits watched, aghast, as their would-be mentors stumbled and fell, "tumbling, tumbling down the stairs" . . . and then sprang to their feet in a battle crouch, each with a dagger in his left hand and a .45 in his right. The "dear old gentlemen" had gotten the drop on an entire roomful of aspiring secret agents. *Pit-pit-pit*—a few squeezes of the trigger and the room would be full of corpses.

"A shattering experience for all of us," Hall admitted.

The Heavenly Twins, so dubbed for their saintly demeanor when not demonstrating how to claw a man's testicles while dragging a bootheel down his shin, got right to work. They demonstrated thirty-six ways to knock someone cold with an open hand and nifty tricks for turning office supplies into weapons. "A clipboard for example," said Henry Hall. "You can strike somebody with it across the side of the neck, on the head, on the nose, under the nose, you can hit him in the parts, you can hit him in the solar plexus. . . ."

The Twins even introduced their own weapons: the icicle-thin Fairbairn-Sykes Commando Knife, which slides in and out of a man's heart as neatly as a hypodermic needle, and the swordlike "smatchet," a Bronze Age throwback that can crush through your rib cage and split you to the groin. "We were to be gangsters," commented new dirty trickster Robert Sheppard. "But with the behavior, if possible, of gentlemen."

CHAPTER 10

It's craftsmanship over showmanship.

—DR. THOMAS AMBERRY, a retired and overweight
seventy-one-year-old podiatrist, on why he can sink 2,750 consecutive
free throws and no NBA player can

THE TWINS HAD MADE THEIR PEACE with an ugly truth: when it comes
to raw weaponry, we're the biggest wimps in the wild. Humans don't
have fangs or claws or horns or venom. We're not strong, we're not
fast, we can't see at night or crush with our jaws. Luckily, we're really
wobbly—and that's what makes us deadly.

The best way to learn about wobble power—the same power that
helped school principal Norina Bentzel overpower a maniac with a
machete—is to strip down to your underwear in front of a bunch of
strangers. At least that's what I discovered in Tempe, Arizona, where
I became a test subject for fitness experts from across the country
who'd gathered to learn from Thomas Myers, a pioneering researcher
in human connective tissue and author of the landmark text, *Anatomy
Trains.*

"Just relax," Myers tells me as I strip down to be analyzed. "And
stand naturally," which might be the most useless advice you can give
someone whose pants are on the other side of the room. I push back
my shoulders and stiffen my back, trying to make it look as if military

attention is my everyday posture. About thirty students, including a trainer for pro baseball's Arizona Diamondbacks, gather in front of me in a semicircle and begin jotting notes on their clipboards.

"Andria," Myers says after a few minutes. "Would you?"

An athletic young woman sets aside her clipboard. She strips down to her sports bra and panties and joins me in front of the group.

"Head: anterior shift," one of Myers's students calls out. She checks her clipboard. "With a posterior tilt."

Andria juts her neck like a tortoise, and then lifts her chin.

"Shoulder girdle: anterior tilt," adds James Ready, the Diamondbacks' trainer.

Andria hunches her back as if she's been punched in the gut.

The group continues feeding instructions until someone yells, "Freeze!"

"Perfect!" one of Myers's students says. She turns to me. "That's you."

I look at Andria. "That's me?"

"You to a T," Ready agrees.

Yikes. One of Andria's shoulders is caved, her hips are off-kilter, and her head is jutting like a silverback gorilla's. That's *me*? I was ordering my body to stand Marine Corps straight, but as I look at my reflection in Andria's body and wince, one thing is obvious: something more powerful than mind and muscle is telling my body what to do. That mystery force, Tom Myers explains, is the unstoppable pull of elastic tissue.

When it comes to raw strength, muscle is only a minority partner. The real powerhouse is our *fascia profunda*, the stretchy tissue that encases our organs and muscle. Until recently, fascia was considered no more important than the gooey film around a chicken breast. But in 1999, Myers was assisting in a cadaver dissection when he became intrigued by the "rubbery gunk beneath the skin," as he describes it. The anatomists he was working with were slicing right through it because they wanted a good, unobstructed view of the muscle underneath. But fascia was *everywhere*, and getting through it wasn't always easy. In some spots, it was as tough as a car tire.

Maybe this is more than just sausage casing, Myers thought. There was one way to find out. "All I had to do was turn my scalpel sideways," Myers recalls. Instead of slicing through the gunk, he sliced *along* it, gently freeing it from skin and bone. By the time he'd finished, he was looking at a full-length body sleeve that resembled a lumpy wetsuit. Myers was intrigued to see that the flesh suit wasn't simply a slick sheet of tissue; it was more like a crisscross of fibers and cables, an endless circulatory system of strength. Under magnification, the fascia was so latticed, it seemed to have the tensile strength of storm netting.

Myers's twist-of-the-wrist technique revealed another surprise: internally, your body is shaped like your DNA. Fascia connects muscle to muscle, forming two continuous spirals from your feet to your forehead, which twirl around each other like the strands of a double helix. Meaning? Your body is rigged like a compound archery bow. Superstretchy tissue links your left foot to the right hip, the right hip to the left shoulder, and it's much tougher than any muscle.

"Think of a ladder twisted on itself," Myers explains. The spiral line of fascia crisscross your abdomen, drop over your hips and down your shins to your foot, where it loops under the arch like a stirrup. So next time you watch LeBron James blast off the paint for a dunk, observe him with Tom Myers's eyes. While everyone else is focused on the ball in LeBron's outstretched hand, Myers is zeroing in on how LeBron's trailing arm stretches wide behind his body; how the toes of his lead leg point upward; how the fingers of his idle hand splay wide. Individually, they're details. Together, they're fused elements in the same explosive act, all as crucially connected as match, fuse, and gunpowder.

Hold on. The part about the fingers. I get how they'd improve balance—maybe—but vertical leap?

Absolutely, says Steve Maxwell. And with the little device in his pocket, he can prove it. Steve is a former world champion Brazilian jiu-jitsu fighter and now a strength-and-conditioning coach who specializes in recovering lost innovations. "The old-timers knew what was up with fascia long before we even had a word for it," he explains. "You'll always be safe if you go back to the mighty men of old, the guys before the 1950s. Look at the old gyms, with their Indian clubs and medicine balls. What's that all about if not balance, range of motion, being fluid, using elastic recoil?"

Steve could have stepped out of a vintage fight poster himself. He's over fifty but still has the build of a bare-knuckle boxer, all menace in motion with no meat to spare. If an eccentric billionaire were hunting humans for sport on a desert island, you'd put money on Steve to get away. Every morning, even in subfreezing winters, he begins the day with the ancient Hindu wrestlers' tradition of stepping outside in the nude and dumping a five-gallon jerrycan of cold water over his head. Back when he was a star wrestler at West Chester University, Steve had such reverence for the sport's ancestry that he once staged a throwback Olympic Games, complete with naked events. He managed to graduate anyway and went on to found Maxercise, a Philadelphia gym that became one of the country's most respected conditioning centers for mixed martial arts fighters. Even the Gracie clan, the Brazilian dynasty that rules Ultimate Fighting, sent up-and-comers to Maxercise to be burned into shape.

One thing Steve is always searching for is elastic-recoil energy, because fighters have no margin for error. You can be the strongest He-Man ever to enter the ring, but if you run out of gas before your opponent, you're cooked. That's why even human mountains like heavyweight boxing legend Sonny Liston spent as much time skipping rope as they did hitting the heavy bag. "Jumping, bouncing, skipping—it's all free energy that comes from fascia, not muscle," Steve explains. Get that bounce right and you can pogo-stick around while barely using any muscular force. Liston weighed 220 pounds and was powerful enough to win three out of every four professional bouts by knockout, but he learned to move his feet as rhythmically as a schoolgirl, usually to James Brown's "Night Train."

"Strength is a skill," Steve says. "In the old days, every Celtic village used to have its 'manhood stone.' You didn't pass into adulthood until you could move that stone. But it wasn't about brute force; strength was knowing how to use all the tools inside your body. Here, this will blow your mind. . . ."

Steve roots around in his pocket and comes out with a rubber band. "Put this around the fingers of one hand, right up there near the fingernails. Now spread your fingers as wide as you can. Really fight it. Good. Close them and open again." It's so easy I'm getting a little embarrassed for Steve, and that's when he pulls his big reveal.

"It would be stupid to throw an arrow, right?" he says. "Better to use your muscles to pull back the string and let the string do the work." He tells me to strip off the rubber band, drop to the floor, and get ready for push-ups. But instead of lowering my chest to the floor and straining my way back up, I'm to reverse it: I'm supposed to spread my fingers as wide as they were with the rubber band, mash my palms hard into the floor, and *pull* myself down. When I do, I surprise even myself when my elbows straighten with barely any effort.

"See?" Steve says. "You tightened the spring on the way down, then it popped you right up." I try it again, and it feels like I'm being sprung from a toaster. I'm not sure how it's working—I'm not even sure if Steve knows—but those were the easiest twenty push-ups of my life.

"What if everything we thought we knew about muscles was wrong?" Tom Myers concludes. "Are there really six hundred muscles, or only one?" Bruce Lee always said his best punch came from his big toe, and now it seemed he wasn't kidding. Lee could position his fist a finger length away from a 250-pound man and with the tiniest flick, he'd send the guy flying. Left toe triggers right hip; right hip pulls back left shoulder; left shoulder catapults right fist, all that power building like a tiny ripple at sea until—*wham!*—it crashes down far from where it started. Martial artists call Lee's punch "long-distance *ging*"—strength from afar.

"For many people, fitness is still all about lifting weights to build bulk," Myers says. "But what does that make you fit for? I'd argue that this"—he taps a key on his laptop and brings up a slide—"is a much more physically fit human than a bodybuilder." On the screen is a photo of a baby rolling on its back, drinking from a bottle held between its hands and feet. Like Bruce Lee, the infant used fascia to solve a problem its muscle couldn't. "You are fit if you can adapt to the demands of your environment with ease and imagination," Myers says.

Your mind rebels against the image—a baby more fit than a bodybuilder—but by 2007 it wasn't even the most jarring statement about fascia. Imaging technology had caught up with Myers's scalpel, and Dr. Robert Schleip, head of the Fascia Research Project at Germany's Ulm University, had discovered something remarkable: your fascia isn't just taking orders—it's giving them.

·   ·   ·

Dr. Schleip is a ponytailed, hipsterish professor and about as different from Steve Maxwell as possible, except for one thing: he also keeps his best tricks in his pocket. When I meet him in the training room at a London medical clinic where he's come to present fresh fascia research, he goes into one side of his jacket for a fat bunch of keys and the other for a spring. He hooks the keyring to the end of the spring and sets it bouncing. Up and down, effortlessly and endlessly—until Schleip shifts his hand a fraction and the keyring goes wild, flying in all directions till it slows to a stop.

"Posture and rhythm," Schleip explains. "Your body operates the same way. When you're in alignment, your elastic tissue stores that energy and returns it. But when you're off-balance, it comes to a halt. For health, for strength, this has serious consequences."

Schleip is the one who first figured out how to thread ultrasound sensors into living fascia, and there he found something amazing: nerve endings. Your fascia is more than a bunch of wobbly rubber bands, he realized; it's actually an intricate network of observe-and-report outposts, all of them gathering input from across your body and relaying it back to your brain. Fascia is as rich in sensory input as your tongue and eyes—even richer, possibly, since it's getting info from *everywhere*.

"Fascia reacts and remembers," Schleip says. Every move you make is a physical experiment; if the experiment works—if, say, you swish a jump shot while sticking out your tongue—that experiment becomes a habit. All those habits get locked in as posture. Over time, posture becomes structure. "Connective tissue is the Saint Bernard dog of the body—it's slow and loyal," Schleip explains. "Once it's formed into position, it'll stick there."

That's why you can recognize a friend from a distance before seeing her face. Harvard biologist Francisco Varela liked to call fascia the "organ of form," because it creates your postural fingerprint; try to straighten your shoulders or change the way you walk and you'll soon feel not only physically off-balance but emotionally uncertain. Fascia knows where you are in the world; it's loaded with position sensors that contribute to your sense of balance and feeds those bearings directly to that fear-conditioning corner of your brain, the amygdala. Any movement grooved into the fascia feels soothing, gratifying, efficient; try to unlearn it, as any batting coach or ballet teacher will tell you, and you're in for a struggle. New movements, no matter how necessary or logical, just feel wrong.

"Isn't that a terrible evolutionary flaw?" I ask. Humans are extremely adaptable, so why isn't our fascia?

Because it would have killed us, Schleip explains. For most of human existence, consistency is what kept us alive. Before we had bows or spears, we depended on all that springy elastic tissue in our legs, plus the superior cooling of our sweat glands and furless bodies, to run other animals to death. We were able to chase antelope across the African savanna for hours at a time until they overheated and collapsed. In that kind of race for survival, there's no room for tinkering; you either hit your efficient stride and stuck with it or you died.

Until, of course, we turned our wobble power into an even deadlier weapon.

"Close your eyes," Joe Darrah says as he slaps a tomahawk into my hand. "Keep them shut. Don't think. Just throw."

Joe is a former circus performer and master knifesmith. In the basement of his home in suburban Philadelphia, he's got old sawmill blades he's shaping into competition throwing knives. On his front lawn he's got a half-dozen tree-stump slices bolted to an old table he's placed uncomfortably close to his neighbor's swing set. Joe got his start in the flinging arts in kindergarten, when his father, a U.S. Army Airborne Ranger, put a commando knife in his hand and taught him the rules of chicken. By the time Joe was a teenager he was good enough to go pro, and he got hired by a traveling circus to fling knives around showgirls. Now, at age fifty, he's a seven-time world champion with both knives and tomahawks, and he's also deadly accurate with the blowgun, bullwhip, and atlatl, an ancient spear-throwing weapon.

Luckily, Joe lives in the outskirts of Philadelphia in America's coolest suburb, judging by the fact that none of his Berwyn, Pennsylvania, neighbors seem to care that Joe likes to practice on his front lawn and often spends his afternoons hurling highly tempered pointy things past their cars. They're not even freaked when he hones his skills on human targets: next to the old door with the bolted-on log slices is a homemade body shield that Joe built by sawing a hole out of another old door and covering it with bulletproof glass. Joe gets friends to step behind the door and press their faces against the glass; it's a whole different level of nerve control when the target you're eyeing is eyeing you right back.

Joe hands me a 'hawk and then stands back and watches. I take my time and run through his pointers. Left foot forward; wide stance; easy overhand motion; tap the car keys in my right pocket on the follow-through to make sure I'm staying straight; and . . .

Clank!

The tomahawk shanks off the edge of the target, dropping into the dirt. Joe hands me another. Left foot forward . . .

Clank!

"What am I doing wrong?" I ask.

"Here comes the Zen stuff," Joe says. "You're trying to control your throw, and you can't." That's when he tells me to try throwing with my eyes closed.

All righty. I squeeze my eyes, wind up, and let fly.

Thwock!

My tomahawk is buried in the log a few inches from the playing card.

"Wow, that's—"

Before I can finish, Joe pivots. He windmills his arm and—*thwock! thwock! thwock!*—buries three 'hawks in three different targets. One splits the playing card right down the middle.

Joe grins. "You have to enter yourself and let the rhythm come. Once you do that, you can do all kinds of crazy things."

"Humans are amazing throwers. We are unique among all animals in our ability to throw projectiles at high speeds and with incredible accuracy." So says Dr. Neil Roach, of George Washington University, lead author of a 2013 study that tackles the mystery of why, out of all other primates on the planet, we're the only ones who can kill prey with a lethal throw.

It's not our muscles. Chimpanzees are extraordinary athletes and proportionately much stronger, but even though they're our closest genetic cousins, they're rotten pitchers. You can train a chimp to throw, but the most heat he'll ever muster is about twenty miles per hour. For a Little Leaguer, that's a joke; twelve-year-old boys can throw three times as fast, with much sharper precision. Softball star Jennie Finch routinely tops seventy miles per hour, and that's underhand.

So what do we have that chimps don't? A shoulder full of "rubbery gunk"—fascia and ligaments and stretchy tendons. Cocking your arm, Roach explains, is like pulling back a slingshot. "When this energy is then released, it powers the very rapid rotation of the upper arm, which is the fastest motion the human body produces—up to nine thousand degrees [of rotation] per second in professional pitchers!" A fast throw isn't just muscular effort, but a three-stage uncoiling of elastic force:

Step with the foot opposite the throwing hand.
Rotate your hips, then your shoulders.
And *whip*, by popping the joints in the arm, wrist, and hand.

We weren't always equipped with such howitzers, Roach adds. About two million years ago, our ancestors developed a few key structural changes that changed us from climbers and scavengers into living catapults: our waists got a little wider, our shoulders a little lower, our wrists more flexible, and our upper arms a bit more rotated. Once we got the hang of our wobble power and learned to put a point on a stick, we became not only the deadliest creature on the planet, but the smartest. The better we threw, the more intelligent we became.

"This ability to produce powerful throws was crucial to the intensification of hunting," Roach explains. "Success at hunting allowed our ancestors to become part-time carnivores, eating more calorie-rich meat and fat and dramatically improving the quality of their diet. This dietary change led to seismic shifts in our ancestors' biology, allowing them to grow larger bodies, larger brains, and to have more children."

Bigger brains led to a revolutionary new skill, one that would become the foundation of all human achievement: we learned to aim not only where food was, but where food *wasn't*. Kudus and rabbits dart off in mad zigzags, meaning a hunter has to mentally process the timing and distance of three different bodies moving through space—his own, his prey's, and his weapon's—to calculate the exact point where spear meets quarry. Or where Allied gunshot meets German paratrooper, on Crete.

"That kind of sequential thought requires intellect of a higher order," says William H. Calvin, Ph.D., a professor of neurobiology at the University of Washington and a specialist in the evolution of the human brain. Specifically, he's talking about imagination: the ability to project into the future, visualize possibilities, think in the abstract. That's why Calvin believes language, literature, medicine, and even love are all connected to our ancient ability to hit a hare at twenty paces. "Throwing is about finding order in chaos," he says. "The more you're able to think in sequence, the more ideas you're able to string together. You can add more words to your vocabulary, you can combine unrelated concepts, you can plan for the future, and you can keep track of social relationships."

But wait: aren't sequence thinking and idea combining the kind of tinkering there's no time for in a race for survival? Exactly; and that's why, when it came to throwing tomahawks, I was better off with a blindfold. With primal functions, education and execution don't mix. Your brain processes the movement, but your body carries it out. So once you've grooved a move into your fascia, get out of its way. It reacts—and remembers.

CHAPTER 11

Things you do,
Come back to you,
As though they knew the way.

—RODGERS AND HART, "Where or When"

TOMAHAWKS AND SPEARS weren't the weapons of choice for the Firm, but luckily, wobble power works just as well with a finger. When the Heavenly Twins began training Churchill's first class of dirty tricksters, Bill Fairbairn showed them how it's done.

Fairbairn yanked his pistol and clenched it like . . . well, like an idiot. He didn't even aim the thing. Everyone knows you have to lock out your arms and steady the pistol with both hands as you peer down the sights. But Fairbairn just stood there, his knees bent as though they were about to buckle. He clutched the pistol as if he were trying to crush it in his fist and barely raised it to his waist. He looked nothing like an expert marksman or a seasoned cop. He looked more like a confused old man who suddenly found a pistol in his pocket and had no idea how it got there.

Now this, he said, *is how you win a gunfight.* You're crazy if you think you won't be terrified when you face a man who's trying to kill you, Fairbairn explained, but that's okay; humans are terrific at turning terror into a weapon. You just need to tap into your natural ability to aim by instinct. Fairbairn believed "instinctive aim" is what made Wild West gunslingers so deadly, and one of his protégés actually went west to find out. Rex Applegate was a U.S. Army lieutenant with unusual credentials; as a boy in Yoncalla, Oregon, he'd chucked bricks in the air as targets for his uncle, a professional trick-shot artist. "These people did not use the sights for many of their acts," Applegate noted—yet when he joined the Army, he found that old-timers like his uncle were better shots than his instructors. Frontiersmen like Wild Bill Hickok had heavier weapons and no formal training, but their quick-draw skills were astonishing.

"Wild Bill was an authentic Western gunman who actually killed a lot of men in combat," Applegate learned. "I was still searching for that essential fact: how did they do it?" The Army assigned Applegate to study close-combat techniques, and one of his first stops was Wild Bill's final stomping grounds, in Deadwood, South Dakota. In the county courthouse, Applegate found a packet of Wild Bill's papers. "One was a letter from an admirer asking in effect, 'How did you kill these men? What was your method or technique?'" Applegate relates. "That was exactly what I was looking for." Luckily, Hickok had never mailed his response. In Hickok's own handwriting, Applegate read: "I raised my hand to eye level, like pointing a finger, and fired."

Like pointing a finger . . . "This was very intriguing," Applegate would recall, "but it wasn't made clear to me until I started my training in combat handgun techniques under a couple of gentlemen named William E. Fairbairn and Eric A. Sykes." The Twins, it turned out, had come up with the same technique after a lucky accident. One night, fifteen of their Shanghai policemen had raided a crime gang's headquarters. When Fairbairn inspected the building the next morning, he found it ringed with head-high booby-trap wires. His officers had passed right under without seeing them. In a flash of insight, Fairbairn understood why: whenever they tensed, they instinctively dropped into a crouch. It must be the same reason, Fairbairn realized, they also clutched their pistols in a death grip.

"You will be keyed up to the highest pitch and will be grasping your pistol with almost convulsive force. If you have to fire, your instinct will be to do it as quickly as possible, and you will probably do it with a bent arm, possibly even from the level of the hip. The whole affair may take place in a bad light or none at all," Fairbairn predicted. "It may be that a bullet whizzes past you and that you will experience momentary stupefaction, which is due to the shock of the explosion at very short range of the shot just fired by your opponent."

What Fairbairn was observing would be identified years later as the Sympathetic Nervous System response, more commonly known as the fight-or-flight reflex. Your knees bend, your heart pounds, your hands clench and jerk up in front of you, your vision tunnels toward one threat, and your body squares to face it. This is your lower brain—your animal self—coiling you like a spring to either strike or sprint for cover. Before Fairbairn arrived in Shanghai, police guidelines dictated you should ignore your animal self and get composed before shooting. But while you're composing, the other guy is firing. "If you take much longer than a third of a second to fire your first shot," Fairbairn warned, "you will not be the one to tell the newspaper about it." No wonder nine Shanghai patrolmen were killed in a single year. "There is not time," Fairbairn realized, "to put yourself into some special stance or to align the sights of the pistol, and any attempt to do so places you at the mercy of a quicker opponent."

You can't fight natural instinct, he decided. But you can make natural instinct fight for you. So the Twins came up with a new, fear-as-a-weapon approach, and brought it with them when they returned to Britain. "The man who can use his weapon quickly and accurately from any position without using the sights is the one who will stand the best chance of not going out feet first," the Twins announced. "It *can* be done and it is not so very difficult." The trick is making your pistol an extension of your fascia. And for that, you only need to point your finger.

When you sense menace, your body craves balance. That's why a scare puts you instinctively into the pose of a tightrope walker—knees bent, hands up—but there's another effect: your arm can locate a threat like a compass needle finding true north. The biomechanics make sense: to avoid getting knocked over by an attacker, your body weight has to be ready to instantly shift from two points of support—your feet on the ground—to three: your feet plus the attacker you're about to hold at arm's length. Your hand can't wait for a command; it needs its own defensive directional system, a fascia-based response.

Fairbairn called it "the impulse of the master-eye." Pick a spot on the far wall, he'd instruct his recruits. Cock your thumb and finger like an imaginary pistol. Now *pull*—yank up your hand and quick-draw toward your target. Don't think, don't aim; just move. "Observe carefully now what has taken place," Fairbairn would say. "Your forefinger, as intended, will be pointing to the mark you are facing squarely." To convert that impulse into deadly force, Fairbairn concluded, you just need to point your gun the same way.

"We were not taught to hold the gun out at arm's length or with two hands but to draw the gun and hold it tucked into your navel with the gun pointing straight ahead," one of the Twins' students, Robert Sheppard, would explain. "Wherever you looked, your gun moved round towards the target you were looking at." SOE recruits who'd handled a gun before bristled at the point-and-shoot system. It was ugly and humiliating. They didn't look like brave lawmen, aiming carefully with locked-out arms and two firm hands. They looked like scared punks trying to sneak off a shot without getting spotted.

But Fairbairn's partner, Bill Sykes, knew how to deal with doubters. "I've seen that chap turn round with his back facing the target and hit the bull's eye from between his legs," Sheppard would recall. "I've seen him do that."

CHAPTER 12

Now, Ah Hing, I'm going to teach you
how to fight like a woman.

—GRANDMASTER IP MAN, Bruce Lee's teacher

REX APPLEGATE got off to a bumpy start with the Twins. He was a massive guy—six foot three inches hardened into 230 pounds of muscle from a boyhood in Oregon logging towns—and so skilled with his fists and trigger finger that even as a young second lieutenant, he was handpicked by Colonel "Wild Bill" Donovan to teach stealth fighting to the espionage-and-sabotage unit that would become the Central Intelligence Agency.

Word had it that two old Brits were the best gutter fighters in the world, so Wild Bill sent Applegate to find out what the Twins were up to. "We soon sized each other up," Applegate recalled, and he was unimpressed. Maybe Fairbairn knew a little judo and was flashy with a pistol, but in a real scrap, Applegate would smother the shrimp. Fairbairn must have sensed what he was thinking, because during a demonstration he invited Applegate to come forward. "I want you to attack me," Fairbairn offered. "Just like you were going to kill me."

Applegate was thirty years younger and nearly a hundred pounds heavier, but, more important, he knew how to dismantle these so-called martial artists: you psych them out with some noise, then run 'em over before they have time to set up any of their little flippy moves. "The first thing to do when on the offensive is to weaken the opponent's balance mentally and physically," Applegate explained. "I let out a roar and went for him." The soldiers in the front row had to scramble out of the way as Applegate came sailing back at them. "I had been in some bar room brawls and held my own," a stunned Applegate would recall. "It got my attention."

Whatever the Twins were teaching, it was different from anything Applegate had seen before. "We are reverting to the type of individual warfare of earlier times," Fairbairn explained. Your strength won't help, he told Applegate. Neither will boxing, wrestling, or most anything you might have learned in a karate dojo. Those are just games, with made-up rules and show-offy skills. You can break a board with your foot? Big deal; try it on the Twins and you'll go home with that foot in a cast. You're a Greco-Roman wrestling champion? Super; Fairbairn could cripple a wrestler as easily as he'd manhandled Applegate.

"Stay on your feet," Applegate learned. "A cardinal rule of this kind of combat is *never* go to the ground."

But wait—wouldn't mixed martial artists later claim that 90 percent of all fights end up on the ground and win bouts all the time by bringing the action to the mat? Very true, Fairbairn would reply— and if you find yourself inside an octagon with a cushioned floor and a Brazilian in surf shorts, then go ahead and grapple. But in a *real* fight—with no rules, no ref, no tap-outs, no guarantee the other guy doesn't have a weapon—the ground is where you go to die. If an attacker gets you down, you'd better grab his testicles, jam a thumb in his eyeball, tear his ear off with your teeth, whatever it takes to kick free and scramble back up so you can use the "Bronco Kick," one of Fairbairn's pet moves: jumping on the guy's chest until his ribs are jelly. Real violence isn't about sportsmanship, Fairbairn stressed; it's about survival. You're not shaking his hand and wishing him well. You're hoping he's still lying there when you leave.

Boxing and wrestling aren't natural forms of combat, the Twins explained. They're natural forms of peacocking, created by and for men to showboat two unique male attributes: bulk and upper-body strength. Otherwise they're useless. No human in the wild would ever throw a punch if he could avoid it, not even against another human. Why risk breaking all those fragile bones and knuckle joints, or jabbing out an arm that can be trapped, twisted, and snapped?

But that's not even the big red flag. There's a more glaring giveaway that boxing and wrestling are just recreation: girls and old guys aren't good at them. As a rule of thumb, performance aberration in a basic skill is a good way to evaluate whether it's natural to a species. When you spot a giant ability gap between ages and genders, you know you're looking at nurture, not nature. Male and female geese differ in size but not in speed; otherwise, migration would be mayhem. Same with trout: if males rocketed past the females, they'd always be first to eat, last to be eaten, and on their way to a disastrous shortage of spawning partners. Gender and age differences don't disappear, of course, but they're tremendously diminished.

Especially among humans. Compared with other animals, men and women are remarkably alike. We're roughly the same size and shape, and share the same biological weaponry. Men aren't specially equipped with horns, fangs, or giant racks of antlers, like the males of other species, and they don't dwarf women; men are only about 15 percent bigger, not 50 percent, like male gorillas. We need to be similar because for most of our existence we shared similar jobs. Humans survived for millions of years as hunter-gatherers, ranging across the terrain together in search of edible plants, digable roots, and catchable game. We worked together, and as couples we stayed together: humans choose one mate at a time, and we do it peacefully.

That's why our courtships are a dance, not a death match. Apes and elks battle for the right to reproduce and take multiple mates by force, but humans have a more runway-model approach: rather than fight, we flaunt. Men primp themselves up to look like hearty specimens and sturdy providers, then wait for the women to make their choices. That's one of the necessities of monogamy: apes can afford to tear one another apart, since the alpha male ends up with a harem. But in a system of one-to-one mating, courtship can't conclude with half the males on life support.

We're creatures of restraint—of endurance and elasticity—and that's where men and women, old and young, are most alike. When it comes to tests of endurance, like distance running and swimming, the performance difference between ages and genders is even smaller than the difference in our size: it's only about 10 percent. A twenty-five-year-old man wasn't the one who battled through fifty-three hours of jellyfish stings and bruising currents to become the first to swim from Cuba to Florida without a shark cage; it was a senior citizen, sixty-four-year-old Diana Nyad. The fastest female ever to swim the twenty-three-plus-mile English Channel was just thirty minutes behind the fastest man, and a thirty-year-old bankruptcy lawyer named Amelia Boone nearly won the World's Toughest Mudder obstacle race in 2012, covering ninety miles and more than three hundred obstacles to finish second overall and ten miles ahead of the guy in third. Middle-aged women are likewise no strangers to the lead pack in ultramarathons. Pam Reed was forty-one when she outran all the men to win the 135-mile Badwater ultra across Death Valley in 2002; the following year, she returned and did it again. Diana Finkel was just shy of forty when she led for the first ninety miles of the brutally hard Hardrock 100, finishing second overall.

With a little more practice, the same *could* be true for throwing. Anatomically, there's no reason women can't fire a ball as hard as men. Strength and physique aren't the issue: when researchers tested Aboriginal Australian girls who grow up hunting alongside boys, they found the difference in top-end throwing velocity was only about 20 percent. Mo'Ne Davis, the thirteen-year-old South Philadelphia schoolgirl who pitched shut-outs against all-boy teams to lead her squad to the Little League World Series, routinely fires 70 mile-per-hour fastballs even though she's only five feet four inches tall and weighs 111 pounds. Hip rotation is the key: whipping a rock is simple but sequential, so if you don't practice the link between opening the hips and releasing the arm, you'll lose the knack or never learn it in the first place. The reason women don't throw as well as men, it seems, is because they don't throw as *much*. But the raw weaponry is still there, and it's the best weaponry we've got.

That was the Twins' special talent. For men and women alike, they found a way to turn throwing into fighting.

What's the worst fix you can find yourself in? Fairbairn asked Applegate.

Jumped from behind, Applegate replied. Someone gets the drop on you. Now you've got a gun in your back and your hands in the air.

Fine. Show me.

Fairbairn offered himself up as a prisoner, turning around and clasping his hands behind his head. Applegate approached warily. He pulled his sidearm, jammed it hard into Fairbairn's spine, and—

Fairbairn helped Applegate up off the floor and handed him back his gun. Care to see it again?

For the second time, Fairbairn turned and put his hands in the air. He spun around more slowly this time, sweeping the gun away with his left hand and grabbing Applegate's chin with his right, finishing him off with a knee to the groin and a shove to the ground. Even though Fairbairn was moving at demonstration speed, Applegate couldn't stop him. "Strange as it may seem," Applegate learned, "the gunman cannot think fast enough to pull the trigger and make a hit before your body is out of the line of fire."

Now look right at me, Fairbairn ordered. Applegate stuck the empty pistol in Fairbairn's belly and curled his finger around the trigger, watching Fairbairn's eyes for a flicker of intent. Fairbairn twisted and slapped, knocking the gun away before Applegate could click the trigger. He bent back Applegate's wrist, driving the big man to his knees and yanking away the gun. Fairbairn's feet never moved. All he did was dip his knees, pivot his hips, and bend his elbow.

"The body twist is the basis of all disarming," Applegate realized, but that was just the beginning: for the Twins, the body twist was the basis of *everything*. In the jungle, body twist is so potent that baboons use it as a white flag of surrender; to avoid a fight, they let their trunk and abdominal muscles sag, indicating their most powerful weapon has been deactivated.

Humans, Fairbairn demonstrated, come pre-equipped with the same primate power. Fairbairn ran Applegate through a series of gutter-fighting moves—breaking free from a stranglehold; recovering from a knockdown; bringing a bigger man to the ground; and, of course, the "Match-Box Attack." All Fairbairn's tactics had three things in common: they were quick, easy, and appalling. "Any individual in combat in which his life is at stake very quickly reverts to the animal," it dawned on Applegate. "After a few seconds, and especially after he has been hit or jarred by his opponent, the blood lust is so aroused that from then on his combat is instinctive."

Take the Match-Box. Once you know it, you can walk down a

dodgy street at night or escape from gunpoint in the back of a car with nothing more lethal in your pocket than a cell phone—or, in Fairbairn's day, a small cardboard box of matches. If you find yourself in an apprehensive situation, stick close to the walls on the right side of the street and casually slip your right hand into your jacket pocket. Wrap your fist around the phone, with the top just below your thumb and index finger. *Damn!* You were right to be nervous, because here comes trouble. Someone's moving in fast with—what? a gun? a knife?—in his hand.

The phone will now save your life, but only because of body twist.

"Parry the gun away from your body with your left forearm," Fairbairn instructs. Now bring out the phone; by clenching it in your fist, the bones in your hand compress into a hard block. "Turning your body from the hip, strike your opponent hard on the left side of his face, as near to the jawbone as possible." You barely need to move your arm; keep your shoulder pinned to your side and come up hard with the forearm, letting your hips do the work. "The odds of knocking your opponent unconscious by this method are at least two to one," Fairbairn adds. "The fact that this can be accomplished with a match-box is not well-known, and for this reason is not likely to raise your opponent's suspicion of your movements."

Applegate quickly grasped the power of Fairbairn's discovery. Body twist, like instinctive aim, works for anyone and can be mastered fast: you can pick up the basics in an afternoon and perfect them with just ten minutes or so of daily practice. You don't need years of training in a dojo and a drawerful of colored belts. What you need most, Applegate realized, is to remember what it's like to fight for real. In our quest to become more humane, we've forgotten that self-defense is a survival skill, not a spectator sport. Fighting has been turned into entertainment and toned down so much, it's more about what you *can't* do than what you can:

You can only fight guys your size, with padded gloves, under a referee's supervision and a physician's care, for three minutes at a time before taking a one-minute break and sitting on your own stool in your own corner of a roped-off ring. You've got to keep your feet on the judo tatami and tie back your hair, and you can't lock your fingers together or kick your way out of a grip. Even in the Wild West of Ultimate Fighting, it's forbidden to bite, spit, curse, claw, pinch, throat-strike, head-butt, flesh-twist, eye-gouge, hair-pull, fishhook, groin-grab, heel-kick a kidney, head-kick a grounded opponent, or fake an injury. You must wear officially sanctioned shorts and "be clean and present a tidy appearance."

Clean and tidy? We've become so civilized over the past hundred years, we're denying what it was like for the previous two million. Worst of all, we've mothballed our deadliest weapon and taken our fascia out of the fight.

Except, as Fairbairn discovered long ago, when the sun went down on a certain Chinese waterfront.

Fairbairn first heard about Wing Chun while recovering from the beating he suffered when he first arrived in Shanghai as a new policeman in 1907. The name means "humming a song in the springtime," and it nicely captures Wing Chun's ease and apparent languor. Your stance is barely recognizable as a stance. You don't put up your dukes to protect your head or clench your hands into tiger claws. Your hands are so loose and open, you could be playing patty-cake. But beneath that effortless appearance is a shrewd insight into the science of elastic energy.

If you've heard of Wing Chun, it's probably thanks to Hollywood star Robert Downey Jr., who credits it with saving his life. Downey was one of the most promising young actors of the 1980s, but by 1996 he'd become a toxic menace. He was arrested for cocaine; for heroin; for crack; for carrying a concealed Magnum pistol; for breaking out of court-ordered rehab. One day he was arraigned on drug charges, then arrested again hours later for stumbling into a neighbor's home in an apparent heroin stupor and passing out in his underwear in one of the children's bedrooms. "It's like I have a loaded gun in my mouth and my finger's on the trigger, and I like the taste of the gunmetal," Downey said shortly before he was sentenced to a year in prison and led off with his hands shackled to his waist. After he was released, Downey discovered Wing Chun and began training for hours at a time, often five days a week. Something about Wing Chun made him feel balanced and *alive*. It wasn't the discipline; it was the sense that his body was finally doing what it was supposed to.

"Wing Chun teaches you what to concentrate on, whether you're here or out in the world dealing with problems," the actor explained once when a reporter joined him for a workout. "It's second nature for me now. I don't even get to the point where there's a problem."

"You don't want to fight the truck," Downey's instructor added. "You want to step out of the way."

Legend has it that Wing Chun is the only martial art invented by a woman. Ng Mui, it's said, was studying at the Shaolin Temple when it was attacked by Qing dynasty soldiers. The temple was destroyed and monks were slaughtered, but the Five Elders—including Ng Mui—managed to escape. While Ng Mui was hiding in the forest, she saw a crane being ambushed by a wildcat at the side of a stream. There was no way the crane, with its two awkward legs, could survive the cat's fangs, razor claws, and four-legged athleticism—yet it did, pivoting and twisting its wings until the cat was defeated by its own ferocity. The parallels to Ng Mui's own situation were unmistakable, and she began transforming the lesson into a fighting style that would make her as formidable as any man. That meant solving the toughest puzzle of any martial art: surviving inside the "trapping zone."

Whenever your opponent is close enough to grab you, you've entered his trapping zone. Boxers depend on the length of their jab and the quickness of their feet to escape the trapping zone, while karate and tae kwon do teach long, snapping kicks; the goal is to pop your opponent from a distance and keep as far from his hands as possible. The trapping zone rewards bulk and brute force; it neutralizes speed and skill. It's the big man's friend and the little guy's nightmare—yet oddly, it's where the feminine style of Wing Chun works best.

Wing Chun tells you to step right into the trap and make yourself at home. Don't bob and weave or even turn sideways to offer a smaller target: just face your attacker, square up your feet, and wait for him to do his worst. But first, make sure to "mark your centerline." The essence of Wing Chun is the belief that human power is strongest when it spirals up from your feet through the center of your body. You can access that centerline energy by following these four steps:

1. Slide your feet out to shoulder width.
2. Sink your thighs into the slightest of squats.
3. Cross your open hands in front of your crotch.
4. Then raise them chest high in that most instinctive of defensive positions—an X.

Now you're ready for Sticky Hands to turn your opponent's trapping zone into your own.

Sticky Hands is next-level wobble power. It takes your attacker's force, merges it with your own, and slams the doubled-up energy right back at him. The key is body connection; as soon as he starts throwing punches, you lightly "stick" your hands to his, deflecting the blows rather than blocking them. When he cracks a hard right at your eye, you divert it with your left wrist and use his force to pivot you like a wheel around an axle. Now it's your turn to hit, using the momentum of his push to power your right arm. He's belting himself in the face with your fist.

"The hands are swinging doors, built on the fortress of legs," the great Wing Chun grandmaster Ip Man liked to tell his students. "Ip Man did not move a great deal," one of his followers observed. "When someone punched at him, he moved just enough to avoid it, but when he attacked he went straight for his opponent's center, either striking him or making him lose his balance." Ip Man was just as stingy with his feet. The higher your foot, the more compromised your balance, so Ip Man only kicked low; never those big, crowd-pleasing head shots you see in tournaments, only short bug-stompers aimed at your knee, crotch, shin, or ankle. Wing Chun isn't a spectator sport; it's a science of crippling force, designed to end fights fast by hitting quickest where it hurts the most.

William Fairbairn was exactly the kind of guy who wasn't supposed to be learning Wing Chun. China was suspicious of outsiders even when times were good, and the early 1900s were anything but. Chinese fighting secrets were for Chinese only, not to be shared with foreigners who could use the arts against them. But even though he was a blue-eyed Brit who'd been in Shanghai only a few months, Fairbairn had a chip to play. One of the duties of the empress's security-and-intelligence force was to recover royal antiquities pillaged during the Boxer Rebellion, that disastrous uprising by Chinese militants against foreign influence in 1899. Fairbairn was a great resource for finding lost booty; between his raids on underworld dens, his contacts in the British military, and his relationship with the European nationals he helped protect, he could get leads on lost treasures the empress's men had no hope of finding. In return, Fairbairn was allowed to train with Cui Jindong, the Wing Chun master who taught the empress dowager's bodyguards.

Under Cui Jindong's tutelage, Fairbairn learned something surprising: violence has a pretty thin encyclopedia. Every way you can think of to punch a windpipe or knee a groin, someone else figured it out ten thousand years ago. For self-defense, that was great news: if Fairbairn could master Sticky Hands, he could download every conceivable attack into his fascia memory and turn his body into an Automatic Response System. Like instinctive aim, Sticky Hands takes your higher brain out of the fight and activates your animal self. When an attacker grabs your wrist, up comes your elbow; if he tries to tackle you around the waist, your foot takes out his knee before he gets there. You don't need to think or even see—just react.

For the Shanghai police, often facing long odds in dark basements, fascia-powered fighting was a lifesaver. And when Fairbairn and Sykes brought it back with them to Britain, they found it was just as effective for the women and poets and professors about to be dropped behind German lines on sabotage missions. "Sykes was the instructor who taught me silent killing," recalled Nancy Wake, the Australian party girl who became one of the SOE's best agents. Nancy's specialties were strolling past Gestapo offices in France to chuck grenades through the door and rescuing downed Allied fighter pilots by using her sex appeal and ice-cold nerve to distract checkpoint guards.

"I'd slink right up and purr, 'Do you want to search me?'" Nancy would recall. "God, what a flirtatious little bastard I was." The Gestapo nicknamed the mystery woman the White Mouse and put her at the top of its Most Wanted list, but Nancy was uncatchable. Seventeen times, she successfully led British fighters all the way across the Pyrenees to freedom. "If a German came at me I'd kick him in the 'three-piece service' and chop him in the side of the neck." Once, when her Resistance band was surrounded, Nancy shot her way out and stole a bike, pedaling more than 125 miles through the night to safety. When a German sentry blocked her escape during an arms plant raid, the Mouse's hands came up just the way Sykes had taught her. "*Whack*," recalled Nancy. "It killed him, all right."

Miraculously, Nancy Wake survived the war and lived to a fiery age ninety-eight. During a postwar dinner in France, she heard the waiter mutter under his breath that he preferred Germans to "the rotten English." Nancy followed him to the kitchen, hit him Sykes style, and knocked him cold. When the manager rushed over, Nancy's dinner companion advised him to walk away or she'd drop him next. "There had been nothing violent about my nature before the war," Nancy shrugged. "The enemy made me tough."

A Mouse who thrives inside the trapping zone: what a perfect bookend for Ng Mui, the battling abbess who three hundred years earlier proved that women could fight as well as men. Except the origins of Wing Chun, it turns out, are a little more complicated. And a lot more Greek.

Deep within the Labyrinth on the island of Crete, Theseus felt his way through the dark stone maze, nudging his feet past the gnawed corpses of men and women who'd come before. He was just a teenager, with no help or weapons. Turning a corner, he came face-to-face with the Minotaur: half man, half bull, and hungry for human blood. A new art was about to be born.

"Much weaker in strength than the Minotaur, Theseus fought with him and won using *pankration,* as he had no knife," goes the legend from Pindar's Fifth Nemean Ode. *Pankration* basically means "total power and knowledge," but the word resonates deeper than the definition: it's associated with gods and heroes, with those who conquer by tapping every talent. Pankration is a fighting style that not only combines boxing and wrestling, but exceeds them, with a savvy of its own. Some pankration techniques, like the *gastrizein* heel kick, have never been surpassed. "It's one of the most powerful offensive moves we've ever seen," a modern martial-arts expert marveled after watching a demonstration. "The attacker's knee and foot are chambered like a piston and then stomped into the opponent's stomach, genitals, or thighs. It channels some 2000 pounds of force into the opponent, more than enough to break a baseball bat."

The scariest thing about pankration is when it's not scary at all. The ready position is so nonchalant and relaxed, you could be a blink away from taking a *gastrizein* to the knee and never suspect the person across from you is poised to attack. If you're set to play catch with a toddler, you're set to fight pankration: just face forward, dip your knees, and raise your open hands. It looks less like art and more like an accident, which speaks to pankration's ancestral authority: it feels so natural because it is. Pankration refines raw impulse, chucking out everything that doesn't help and focusing on the three things that do: ease, surprise, and stopping power. You activate without thinking. Attack without signaling. And strike, like any other animal in a fight for its life, without mercy.

Pankration is so frighteningly true to real violence that for years it wasn't included in the original Olympics. "To get his opponent down and by throttling, pummeling, biting, kicking reduce him to submission is the natural instinct of the savage or the child," explained E. Norman Gardiner, D. Litt., the Oxfordian ancient sport specialist. "But this rough and tumble is not suitable for athletic competition; it is too dangerous and undisciplined." Pankration finally made it into the 33rd Olympic Games, in 648 B.C., with two rules: no biting, no eye gouging. Otherwise, it was anything goes; the entire range of human cruelty and creativity were at your disposal. The Spartans still grumbled and refused to participate: if you can't blind your opponent and chomp his nose, then what's the point?

But for everyone else, pankration became "the most exciting and worthiest of all sports in ancient Olympia," as the Greek chronicler Philostratus put it, even though some bouts didn't last much longer than a sneeze. There were no points or pins; you won as soon as you put the other guy into unbearable agony. One champion won three Olympic titles by getting really good at snatching his opponent's fingers and bending them back. Matches could end only in death, submission, or—as in one epic contest—both: the great champion Arrhachion was in a choke hold when he managed to grab his opponent's foot. Ankle breaking is a classic pankration move, and so effective that thousands of years later it would be the reason the Twins protected their feet by never risking anything higher than a crotch kick. But Arrhachion locked on too late. His opponent begged for mercy, forfeiting the match, but not before Arrhachion suffocated. Victory went to the dead man.

Pankration's creation myth is peculiar, and not just because it has two. Storytellers couldn't agree on the original event: was it Theseus against the Minotaur, or Hercules versus the Nemean Lion? But they were unanimous on one key quirk: while boxing and wrestling were fruits of the gods passed down from Apollo and Hermes, pankration was born from human weakness. Theseus was just a boy out to prove himself when he went to Crete, and Hercules wasn't exactly the hulking He-Man we've come to assume. Hercules was never the strongest guy in the fight; in fact, Pindar even went hard the other way and chalked Hercules's achievements up to little-man syndrome: Hercules was "of short stature with an unbending will." The heroes were still plenty powerful, but muscle alone would never get them out of a jam. Their real strength was their ears: Theseus and Hercules were lifelong learners and equal-opportunity students, always seeking advice and just as happy to get it from women. That was the mark of a hero and the signature of pankration: total power *and* knowledge.

And that knowledge has been around a *long* time. History actually has a dog in the fight in the Battle of the Pankration Myths. When archeologists cracked open sealed caves on Crete—the site of Theseus's showdown with the Minotaur—they discovered pottery and wall paintings from 1700 B.C. with the earliest depictions of pankration. King Minos really did rule Crete, and his ships often returned from Egypt with hot new discoveries—like the peculiar Hittite religious rituals of bull leaping, boxing, and grappling. On Crete, these rites were honed into martial arts, then exported to mainland Greece. Naturally, anything involving total power and knowledge was irresistible to a combat scientist like Alexander the Great, who still slept with the *Iliad* under his head. Alexander became a true believer as soon as he saw his best Macedonian warrior defeated by Dioxippus, a pankration fighter from Athens. Alexander's armies learned pankration, and as they marched east into Persia and India, it's believed pankration spread toward Asia and became the inspiration for all modern martial arts.

So—no Ng Mui? No Five Elders, no cat-whomping crane?

Nope.

There's no evidence that the origin myth of Wing Chun is any more real than the Minotaur. But just because it's make-believe doesn't mean it's not true. Wing Chun took the crucial elements of pankration and improved the backstory: if you're really out to prove that natural movement and elasticity can make anyone a fearsome fighter, don't use a couple of monster-killing heroes to make your case; use a fightin' nun on the run from an evil dynasty. Ng Mui wasn't dreamed up just to repackage Greek fashion for a Chinese audience; rather, it took pankration off the battlefield and away from the oiled-and-naked manly Games and steered it back to its original message: that when it comes to real strength and self-defense, muscle power isn't the path.

Despite the revamp, the art that could help everyone was taught to almost no one. Dynasty warfare and clan secrecy kept it underground in China, while for everyone else it was ruined by the Romans. Under the Caesars, pankration was degraded into a gladiatorial spectacle and became so savage it was eventually banned by the Christian emperors. No one really had the stomach after that to revive something so closely associated with the blood-crazed Colosseum. "It may be suggested that the Pancratium is too terrible to serve any useful purpose in these modern times," conceded a British sportsman who failed to bring pankration back to life in 1898.

And so the greatest Olympic sport faded away and vanished. . . .

Except on the island where it was born. In the mountains of Crete, pankration was passed down between generations of rebels who never forgot what it could do and why it was created. After the German invasion, an odd photo made its way back to British Intelligence: it showed three German soldiers being ambushed by a trio of Cretan freedom fighters, one of whom has his legs scissored around a German's back. It's classic pankration, and exactly the message the Twins were trying to get across to their students back in the dirty-trickster training camps:

All the strength, speed, and suppleness you need, you already have. You just need to release it.

CHAPTER 13

The name of Crete is for me—the man who
conquered it—a bitter memory.

—LUFTWAFFE GENERAL KURT STUDENT

CRETE was the perfect test. The mountains were honeycombed with
caves, and with all those German supply planes transiting through on
their way to Russia, the targets were ripe. But the Firm couldn't go in
blind; someone first had to find out whether George Psychoundakis
and the rest of the Cretans really wanted to take a bunch of amateurs
under their wings. If not, the Brits wouldn't last a week.

So within days of his escape from Crete, Jack Smith-Hughes was
asked to head back. Returning a man to the same island he'd spent
seven months trying to get off was harsh, but what choice was there?
The Battle of Crete had lasted ten days, but the battle *for* Crete was
just getting started. Hitler needed to lock the Cretans down, but he
couldn't . . . quite . . . stop them. The Russian attack was already
months behind schedule, but instead of speeding every available man
to the Eastern Front, five entire divisions were still chasing shepherds
around that *gottverdammten* island.

Brilliant. This was exactly what Churchill had been hoping for:
that somewhere, a band of irregulars would catch the giant off guard

and make it stumble. Before the British even had a chance to get the Firm off the ground and spread its own Resistance operation, one had suddenly burst into existence by itself. "The Cretan Resistance, unlike those underground movements in the rest of Europe which did not start to develop until a year or so after the German occupation, began literally in the first hour of the invasion," noted Antony Beevor, who would write the definitive history of the Battle of Crete. As if they'd been rehearsing it for years, the Cretans quickly assembled armed militias, mountain-running messengers, and a folk-song emergency alert system: anytime a German patrol was spotted, a warbling tune would pass from villager to villager across the valley and up to where their men were hiding in the hills.

But realistically, how long could the Cretans withstand the fury of General Kurt Student, who for once was even more enraged than Hitler? The Führer had ordered his troops to terrorize the upstarts, but Student wanted more than just fear; he wanted blood. The Germans had lost more troops in the Battle of Crete than in France, Yugoslavia, and Poland combined. Student himself had almost committed suicide and all because of those savages. The Cretans were "beasts and assassins," Student decreed, who should be treated like all dangerous animals. Anywhere a hint of rebellion was detected, Student ordered "extermination of the male population of the territory in question" and "total destruction of villages by burning." There wouldn't even be the pretense of a trial. "All these measures," Student commanded, "must be taken rapidly and omitting formalities."

Freed from any restraint, the Germans on Crete erupted in a rampage of revenge. In the town of Kastelli Kissamou, two hundred men were selected at random and slaughtered. In tiny Fournés, 140 more. Entire villages were surrounded by tanks and put to the torch, with women and children running for their lives into the mountains. Not that every woman escaped; many had their dresses torn down, and if a shoulder bruise was spotted that could have come from a rifle recoil, they joined their brothers and husbands in the death pit. The manhunt was pitiless and relentless; German foot soldiers ransacked farms and towns while recon planes growled low over the mountains, machine-gunning anyone who looked suspicious and snapping aerial photos of every visible cave and goat trail.

So one night in October, Jack boarded a camouflaged trawler and returned to Crete with a promise. He slipped into a black blouse and pantaloons to disguise himself as a shepherd—well, sort of. "Anyone could pick him out as an Englishman from a mile away, especially when he was dressed in those clothes!" grimaced George Psychoundakis, who once again stepped in to sneak Jack past German patrols. Together they trekked up the cliff to see Abbot Lagouvardos, the three-hundred-pound, fire-breathing, Friar Tuck–like head of the Preveli monastery. From there, they visited the hideouts of local Resistance fighters Beowulf and old Uncle Petrakas and "Satan" Grigorakis, so nicknamed because only the devil could have survived all the bullets in him.

If the Cretan fighters could hang on a little longer, Jack told them, they wouldn't be alone. Britain's new masters of mayhem were just about ready for action.

Jack had just returned from this recon mission to Crete when a penniless young painter named Alexander Fielding was brought to meet him. Call me Xan, the fellow said, pronouncing it "Chan." Xan's father was a major in the 50th Sikh Regiment, so as the son of a career soldier, Xan had known exactly what to do when the war broke out:

Run and hide.

"My first reaction," Xan would admit, "was flight." He'd done a pretty good job of it, too. Before the war, he'd tried making a living by sketching diners in fancy London cafés, then he pushed east to study German classics and take up painting. When Hitler invaded Poland and most of Xan's university friends stepped forward to enlist, Xan stayed put in Cyprus, where he'd landed a nice gig as a bar manager. "I was not afraid of fighting," Xan recalled, "but I was appalled by the prospect of the army." Did anyone seriously expect him to shove into an officers' mess three times a day and make small talk with a guest list not of his choosing? "I could not bear the idea of an enforced and artificial relationship with a set of strangers chosen to be my comrades not by myself but by chance," he complained. Call me a coward; just don't call me "Sir."

German subs were about to close the sea-lanes, so Xan hopped a boat to a tiny island off the coast of Greece owned by his old friend Francis Turville-Petre—the world-famous archeologist, sexual adventurer, and, of late, wild-haired recluse. Francis made history when he was fresh out of Oxford by uncovering "Galilee Man," one of the first Neanderthal skulls to be discovered outside of Europe. But Francis was soon spending more time partying than digging (one fellow archeologist wrote home in disgust about "the empty whiskey bottles that were tossed out of Francis's tent and the Arab boys who crawled into it"), and when a bout of syphilis sent him to Germany for treatment, he decided to abandon the deserts of Palestine and switch his specialty to "sexual ethnology." "Der Fronny," as he was known, became such a legend in the Berlin boy bars that he inspired both the musical *Cabaret* (by way of Christopher Isherwood's *Berlin Stories*) and W. H. Auden's play *The Fronny*. Then, abruptly, Francis vanished. Word got around that he was in seclusion on a Greek island, sleeping till dark, wandering by night, and surviving on a diet of brandy and bread fortified by a weekly cup of Bovril.

By the time Xan arrived, in 1939, the once bright star of British archeology looked like a shipwreck survivor. "Long straight Red-Indian hair framed a sad sallow face so lined that it was impossible to guess its owner's age," Xan would recall. "Below it an emaciated body, always clothed in bright colors, stretched six feet down to an almost freakishly small pair of sandaled feet." But Fronny's mind was as keen as ever, and during their long moonlit hikes together, he shared the secret of how he beat the world to the Galilee skull.

Early in his career, Francis realized that when it came to archeological knowledge and geological mastery, it would take him decades before he could compete with senior scientists. He needed a short cut, so he began hanging around the villages, sipping tea and trading chit-chat, soaking up scandals and dialects and ghost stories. Legends have long tendrils, Francis believed, that eventually twine back to solid earth. If kids believe a patch of woods is haunted, they may really have seen spooky shadows . . . which, with a little investigating, could turn out to be goatherds taking shelter for the night in a cliffside crevice with an invisible entrance and terrific campfire ventilation. A warm snug today could have been just as cozy in the Stone Age, which means that in a vast desert with thousands of caves, an afternoon spent listening to old wives' tales could help you eliminate false leads and point you straight to the find of a lifetime. Francis's nose for gossip eventually led him to some chatty Bedouin traders who tipped him off to the cave where the Skull would be found.

"The companionship and conversation of a man like Francis did much to dispel my increasing sense of guilt, so that the report of the evacuation from Dunkirk and the account of the Battle of Britain caused me no more than a passing twinge of conscience," recalled Xan, who wasn't gay but regarded Francis as "one of the most stimulating and rewarding companions" he had ever known.

Xan spent his days painting landscapes and practicing Greek with Fronny's six servants, waiting for his night-stalker host to awake at dusk. Together they'd huddle around the radio and listen to evening war news from the BBC.

Shouldn't we be ashamed? Xan wondered. *Maybe it's time to do our duty.*

Francis snorted. "What good do you think *you* could possibly be?"

Hitler took the choice out of their hands. Xan and Fronny got off the island ahead of the German invasion and reluctantly went their separate ways. Fronny opted for Egypt; he had a taste for erotic adventure, and wartime Cairo was sizzling with sexual intrigue. Fronny soon reclaimed his throne as master of back-alley revels, but collapsed within a few months. By age forty—"bored with love, with sex, with travel, with friendship, even with food," as one friend recalled—the man who'd inspired Xan with his genius for learning secrets from the past was dead.

Xan returned to Cyprus, where he found an even better way to hide from the war: he joined the army. Xan got a commission as a junior officer in the 1st Cyprus Battalion, the biggest joke in the Mediterranean Theater. "The Cypriots had never had a military tradition, and it soon became clear that they were not going to break a habit formed before the first century by taking kindly to soldiering in the twentieth," he observed. Many of Xan's fellow officers were disciplinary problems who'd been chucked out of other details, or pacifists and shirkers desperate to avoid action. "Our unit, then, was understandably free from any sense of regimental pride."

Since neither officers nor enlisted men had any interest in engaging one another, let alone the enemy, they agreed to stay out of one another's way: the troops spent their time in Nicosia's brothels, while the officers lingered in the casinos. Within a few weeks, new recruits were less combat ready than the day they arrived. "The incidence of venereal disease among the men rose to a height that was only surpassed by the officers' drunkenness," Xan admitted.

Xan's official assignment was to visit fake platoons. The Cypriots figured their best defense was trickery, so they built a bunch of phony barracks to make it appear as if the island were jammed with troops. "All those phantom units," Xan would recall, "were represented only by myself." He roared around all day on a motorcycle delivering messages to these invisible brigades in the hope that, somehow, Hitler would believe Cyprus was too heavily fortified to attack. What a delightful surprise war turned out to be! Military service on Cyprus, Xan would later acknowledge, was "one of the most carefree periods of my life."

Until refugees from Crete began to arrive. "The island was expected to surrender in a day," Xan noted, but when it didn't—when reports came through of shepherds and farmwives and village priests defending their island with barn tools and rabbit guns and, in one case, an old man's walking stick, when these peasants and a battered rank of British troops somehow held off Germany's fiercest fighters until the sun had set on Hitler's deadline and rose again on another day—Xan began feeling a strange sensation: envy.

"I felt that if I had to fight, the least ignoble purpose and the most personally satisfying method would be the purpose and method of the Cretans," he'd recall. The Cretans weren't taking orders and wearing uniforms; they were thinking and fighting for themselves, using their own skill and ingenuity and natural weapons to defend their homes and families. No one had to train them or tell them what to do; their own traditions had prepared them all their lives for this moment. "My own position as a member of an organized army," Xan recalled, "became increasingly galling."

Xan began haunting the Cyprus waterfront, greeting refugees from Crete as soon as they arrived so he could get firsthand news about the Resistance. Word of his interest must have spread, because one morning a stranger came looking for him. He gave Xan directions to a building in Cairo and said if he was serious about Crete, he should go to Egypt at once. Xan would find out more—maybe—once he got there. Soon, Xan was touching down in Cairo and hailing a taxi.

"Ah," the driver responded when Xan gave him the address. "You mean 'the secret house.'" The Firm might be invisible to the rest of the world, but not to Cairo cabbies; whatever the organization was up to, it was attracting so many mysterious visitors that the cab ranks had marked the address as an eerie but profitable fare. Xan found the building, and was shown into a back room. There he met Jack Smith-Hughes, who was already in charge of finding recruits for the Firm to send to Crete.

"Have you any personal objection to murder?" Jack began.

Xan had to admit the only time he had come close to acting like a hero—the only time he'd come close to a fight—was when he tried to stop a gang of drunk Australians from bullying a Jewish family. One of the Aussies grabbed him by the jacket and yanked him off his feet, snarling, "Whose side are you on, Galahad?" That did it for Xan's chivalry.

To be honest, Jack was okay with that. The army didn't make him a hero; the army made him a baker. It was only when Jack was abandoned, when he was on the run and in the hands of the Cretans, that he turned into a force to be reckoned with. And that gave Jack an idea. . . .

In Scotland, Fairbairn and Sykes were trying to reconstruct the art of the hero and pass it along to their students. But on Crete, Xan could skip the middlemen and learn the same ancient skills directly from the source. If Xan put himself in the hands of Beowulf and that canny young shepherd George Psychoundakis, maybe he would learn more in action than he would at any school. He'd get pankration from the source. He'd discover how shepherds climbed mountains all night on a starvation diet, and learn instinctive shooting from shepherds and bandits who could split a man's skull from a quarter-mile away without any sights on the rifle.

Jack knew it could be done, because one man had already done it. John Pendlebury was a British archeologist who'd come to Crete well before the war. Pendlebury was missing an eye, had never served in the military, and was nearly twice Xan's age, so of course he had to get off the island as soon as Hitler pivoted toward the Mediterranean. Except Pendlebury stayed put. "It required more resolution in an Englishman to stay behind voluntarily and be submerged by the German tide than to return later," reflected Nicholas Hammond, a Cambridge archeologist and one of Pendlebury's friends. "But for John the choice did not exist." Before long, the Oxford academic had been transformed into a legend whose name would send Hitler into a rage.

That's because strange things can happen on that island, Jack discovered—fierce, audacious, brilliant things that no one should be expected to pull off, least of all a baker and a one-eyed archeologist. That tiny rock in the sea had made Hitler bleed, and it changed the Third Reich's military strategy forever: never again would the Hunters from the Sky lead an invasion. "Crete has always been a theatre for strange and splendid events," Paddy would later agree, marveling at Crete's "indestructible old men" and their "extremely handsome" sons, the way "their eyes kindle and their grins widen at the suggestion of any rash scheme."

"Especially," he added, "if the scheme involves danger."

Two weeks later, Xan poked his head out of a submarine hatch and into a howling gale. He tried to speak, but nothing came out. "The shriek of the wind," he realized, "drowned every other sound." Waves smashed against the side of the sub, shattering and sinking a collapsible canoe—the canoe Xan was supposed to be in.

Instead of four months of round-the-clock training at SOE school, Xan had spent three days blowing up abandoned trains. "The knowledge that no railway existed in Crete did not dampen my immediate ardour for demolition work," he'd comment. "Those daily explosions in the sand represented all the training I received before being recalled to Cairo a few days after Christmas."

As soon as Xan got back from his bomb-blasting holiday, he was told to pack a duffel and get to the waterfront. First they set off toward Crete in a camouflaged navy trawler, but twice fierce seas forced them to turn around and return to Egypt. Finally, sub commander Anthony "Crap" Miers offered to bring them in beneath the waves. They got within sight of the island, but just as they launched the first man in his canoe, a storm blew in and swirled him off into the darkness.

After that . . . nothing. For half an hour they scanned the churn, hoping for a sign he was still alive and afloat.

Crap couldn't linger any longer. *Bad business*, he finally said. *Your man is either dead, adrift, or surrounded by Ger—*

A pinprick of light flashed. *Good old Guy!* He and his canoe had made it. Guy Delaney was an Australian staff sergeant in his fifties with bushy eyebrows and bristling whiskers, a survivor of the *Fallschirmjäger* invasion who, like Jack Smith-Hughes, had managed to hide for months in the mountains and escape by way of the Preveli monastery. If a battered piece of army surplus like Guy Delaney could survive that surf, Xan figured, so could he. The sailors quickly readied another canoe, but the waves crushed it, then the next one. Xan and his partner had one last chance of making it to shore, Crap told them: a rubber raft would swamp if they sat inside, but they might be able to straddle it like a rodeo bronco, clutching it between their thighs as they thrashed like hell with their paddles.

Three sailors fought to hold the raft as it lunged alongside the sub like "a grey monster-fish cavorting in and out of the surf," as Xan put it. "Not courage, I think, but fear prompted the decision," Xan continued; he dreaded the thought of cramming himself back inside the stifling sub. He threw himself onto the raft, followed by a man he'd recently met and already hated. Captain Guy Turrall was even older than Delaney; he was a World War I vet who'd spent the years since then pip-pipping around the British tropics in a pith helmet. Turrall was driving Xan nuts, trying to speak to Greek crewmen in his colonial *français* and constantly repeating, "You see, I've lived so long in the bush . . ." and "offering advice that was more applicable to a peace-time safari than a clandestine naval operation." True to form, Turrall had shown up for the undercover mission with a pack stuffed with pajamas and an enamel washbasin. He was also in full military uniform and his pith helmet, which Xan chucked overboard as soon as Turrall wasn't looking.

The sailors released the rope, and the current sucked the raft away and began spinning it in circles. And at that moment, as the raft twirled "like a buoyant saucer trapped in a whirlpool," Xan and Turrall achieved a kind of perfection: the two novice secret agents were the perfect expression of everything that Churchill's generals told him was foolish about his plan. *This* was going to stop Hitler—Capt. Right-Ho splashing around the Mediterranean with some smart-ass slacker, an obnoxious little "artist" whose first order of business as a member of an ultrasecret force behind enemy lines was to prank the only man who could cover his back? Face it; Turrall might be handy with explosives and had a drawerful of dusty medals, but how was he going to infiltrate hostile territory when he kept forgetting that in Greece they don't speak French?

Xan and Turrall chopped at the water with their paddles and finally managed to stop spinning. Crap's sub submerged behind them and disappeared, leaving them adrift on a squishy raft in a sea as dark as the sky. Guy Delaney, bless his bristly Aussie mug, was still flicking his flashlight on the beach. Xan and Turrall spotted him through the waves and began digging toward shore. For half an hour they paddled through the surf, slowly getting closer to Delaney's light—until suddenly it went black.

Was that a pistol shot they heard? A shout? Impossible to tell. Xan and Turrall waited, floating . . . but the light never reappeared. With no other choice, they pushed on toward the beach.

CHAPTER 14

Θά πάρωμεν Τ' άρματα νά Φύγωμεν στά Μαδάρα.
TRANSLATION: "We will take our arms
and flee to the White Mountains."

—JOHN PENDLEBURY,
in a last letter to his wife before the German invasion

XAN'S BOOTS scraped pebbly sand, then a wave cracked and sent him tumbling. He stumbled to his feet, and together with Turrall he struggled through the surf and up onto the beach. There was no sign of Guy Delaney.

"Something must have gone wrong," Turrall said.

"But he signaled OK."

"That doesn't mean a thing. The Germans may have intentionally let him make his signal before nabbing him, in the hope of nabbing us as well."

Xan knew Turrall was right. Their original plan was to come ashore a few miles away and rendezvous with another British agent in a hidden cove, but rough seas had forced them farther down the coast. More than likely, they'd landed near a German lookout, which meant Guy was a goner. Delaney would be lucky if the Germans didn't open fire the instant they spotted his light, thanks to that whole Operation

Flipper fiasco: a few weeks earlier, a British commando assault team using the same rubber rafts as Xan and Turrall and launching from the same sub came ashore on another Mediterranean beachfront, this one in Libya. They were hunting Erwin Rommel, "the Desert Fox," whose unstoppable Afrika Korps panzers were threatening to over-run Cairo. The Brits burst through Rommel's bedroom door with grenades flying and guns blazing . . . except Rommel, famous for his *Fingerspitzengefühl*—"fingertip feel," or sixth sense—had already moved base. But the fact that Allied raiders got within pistol range of a top general's bed, even an empty one, left a lasting impression of what to expect from strangers in the night in rubber rafts.

The storm; that's what must have saved Xan and Turrall. They must have blown past the sentries, who couldn't spot their gray raft in the dark chop. They had to get to cover—fast—but where do you run when you don't know where anyone is? Xan saw a faint strip of light in the distance. *Let's crawl in for a look,* Turrall urged. It was risky, but shrewd: they could at least figure out where *not* to go, and hopefully confirm Guy's whereabouts.

Xan pulled his pistol and slipped off the safety. "I started creep-ing up the beach towards the light, which as I approached revealed itself as a gap in a shuttered window." Xan inched closer and picked up a snatch of conversation. He listened intently, then got to his feet. "Be ready to give me covering fire," he whispered to Turrall. "I'm going in." Before Turrall could grab him, Xan charged. "I kicked open the door, at the same time flourishing my pistol and flashing on my torch." And there, "sitting by a twig fire in steaming long-legged underwear," was Guy Delaney, drying his clothes and chatting with the fisherman who owned the hut.

"You've been bloody slow getting here," Delaney grumbled.

Xan had recognized Delaney's voice and understood the fisherman's Greek, so he'd only mock-attacked, to get Turrall's goat. Delaney was just as relieved; he'd been chilled to the bone on the beach and finally had to get warm or risk hypothermia. Even the fisherman was delighted; he wanted to call the whole village to arms, and was just a bit crestfallen when Xan explained that the three midnight guests were alone and not the advance team of a full Allied invasion. Only

Turrall was in a foul mood—he'd been through too much in his life, not to mention that night alone, to tolerate any more of Xan's shit.

But the fisherman had a little gift to cheer him up: a prisoner!

"There's a German here in Tsoutsouros!" A deserter had turned up a few days ago and kept hanging around, hoping to find someone he could surrender to. He couldn't have wandered into better luck: that little cove was too barren and inaccessible for the Germans to bother with, so Xan and his team were the only outsiders anyone had seen for weeks. Crap was supposed to surface again the following night to offload rifles for the Cretans and supplies for the British agents, so Turrall could paddle the forlorn German out to the sub and notch himself a capture.

By the time Xan dried and warmed himself, dawn was breaking. He'd only seen Crete through the sub's periscope, so as the sun rose, he went outside for his first good look. You'd expect to be dazzled by sea views on a skinny sausage of an island like that—161 miles long and 37 wide at its thickest, 12 at its thinnest—but even those turquoise shimmers are overshadowed by the startling explosion of mountains. From the beach it all looks so easy, so summery, Alpine and inviting. It's only when you push into the hills and find yourself twisting through gorges and smacking into sheer rock faces hidden by trees that you discover why there was no coast-to-coast road and why a two-mile trek could take four hours and leave you where you started.

No wonder Crap's sub was able to come within a mile of the beach without being spotted: all that elevation meant Xan was nicely hidden by a giant stone fence. Most of Crete's mountains run right through the middle of the island, creating a jagged belt separating the Germans in the north from the rebels in the south. Just east of Xan, ablaze in the early-morning sun, was the skyscraping prenatal unit of the world's first guerrilla fighter: Zeus, greatest of the Greek gods.

Zeus wasn't born to the throne; he scrapped his way there, Cretan style. Zeus's father was Kronos, the Titan who ruled the earth and swallowed his children so they wouldn't overthrow him. When Kronos's wife was pregnant with Zeus, she snuck away to Psychro Cave, in Crete's easternmost Dikti Mountains. After giving birth, she returned home and fooled Kronos into swallowing a stone wrapped in a baby's blanket, while the infant—"safe in Crete, strong of limb and crafty"—was raised by Diktynna, the cunning and elusive goat-nymph. A tribe of mountain warriors, the Kouretes, guarded the baby and performed a shield-clanging war dance so Kronos wouldn't hear him crying. When Zeus was big enough, he cut his brothers and sisters free from Dad's belly and led them in bringing down the tyrant.

Some insist Zeus's birth cave was farther west of Xan on Mount Ida, Crete's highest peak, which made a lot of sense. Ida is snow-crowned and glorious, home to golden eagles and the kri-kri, the rare and magnificent Cretan ibex. Sure enough, searchers located a palatial cave on Ida overlooking the Amari, Crete's lushest valley. Buried inside this natural throne room were ancient offerings: bracelets, Egyptian pottery, bronze knives. Pythagoras was even said to have made a pilgrimage to the Idaean Cave, and Euripides mentioned "Idaean Zeus" in his play *The Cretans*. The Idaean Cave is majestic enough for a king—but the infant Zeus was a fugitive with a death sentence. That's one reason why, in 1901, the British archeologist D. G. Hobarth decided to take another look at Psychro.

The Dikti range is dark and rough, exactly the kind of place where a wild child could disappear from the world and be raised by a band of loyal mountain men and a mystical she-goat. Hobarth pushed deep into the rocked-off recesses of Psychro. Blasting his way with dynamite into an "abysmal chasm," he discovered a treasury of other devotional gifts, including Cretan double axes, believed to be a sacred emblem of Zeus—far more than the trinkets discovered in the Idaean Cave, but more important, far *older*. "The Cave of Ida, however rich it proved in offerings when explored some years ago, has no sanctuary approaching the mystery of this," Hobarth wrote. Visitors assumed regal Mount Ida was the place for a god, but true Cretans knew the Dikti is where a hunted man would hide.

The killers were coming for Xan, too. German troops may have spotted the sub and could already be closing in, so the longer he lingered in Tsoutsouros, the more he risked himself and everyone in the village. He now had to search for Monty Woodhouse, the other British agent stationed on the island. Luckily, the solution soon appeared, high on a ridge behind him.

Trotting down the rock slope came two Cretan highlanders, both dressed in black shirts and old-time shepherd's breeches, with the knee-length crotch for easy running. The highlanders hurried into Tsoutsouros with news: they could lead Xan to Monty, but they had to leave at once. Xan had been on the move for nearly two full days by that point and eaten little more than bread crusts, but rested or exhausted, fed or famished, go-time for a guerrilla is non-negotiable. Xan set off behind one of the highlanders and got his first taste of the Cretan Bounce.

"As soon as we reached the foothills and started climbing he was in his element at once," Xan noted, "bounding from stone to stone with a speed and precision which defied our breathless attempts to emulate him." Monty's man was patient but relentless, slowing his uphill rock hopping long enough to keep Xan in sight but pushing steadily through the afternoon and into the evening. Finally, at nightfall, Xan trudged out of the mountains and into a bizarre dream world.

"Through the open door of the village coffee shop I saw a horde of frenzied giants in tattered khaki and slouch hats," he observed. "The chorus of *Waltzing Matilda* filled the dusk." More than a dozen drunk Australian soldiers were sloshing about, guzzling Cretan moonshine. After months on the run, the fugitive Aussies had heard that Crap was on the way and came out of hiding to slip down to the beach. When they discovered Crap had come and gone without them, their determination to remain invisible gave way to desperate drinking. For one night at least.

Xan slunk past, head down. "The sight of them reminded me of the last time I had to deal with drunken Australians," he'd remark, recalling his quick surrender when he tried to defend a Jewish family from some Aussie bullies. Xan was led to a small house and entered to find his boss: a twenty-four-year-old Oxford classics scholar who not only looked like a college boy on spring break, but not long ago was. Montgomery Woodhouse was tall and gawky, so blond and pink-cheeked in that roomful of ferocious stubble that he almost looked albino.

Still, Monty had style. Xan had to admire the "superb shepherd's cloak" Monty had chosen for his disguise. "Clandestine life came easily enough to me," Monty would explain. "My Greek was good enough to deceive the enemy, though my appearance was against me. Of course no Greek was ever deceived either by my accent or my disguise, but that was an asset, because as soon as I was recognized a spontaneous conspiracy sprang up to protect me."

Seven weeks behind enemy lines had also hard-sharpened him, so Monty got straight down to business. Hitler suspects Crete is his Achilles' heel, Monty explained; Xan's job was to convince him. Only four or five thousand troops should be necessary to secure an island of Crete's size, but the Resistance had done such a superb job of making Hitler nervous that more than *eighty thousand* Germans were still stationed there. Hitler desperately needed that manpower in North Africa and the Russian front, but he couldn't risk shifting them if it meant that an underground army would overthrow his Mediterranean base.

Which makes you, Monty told Xan, *the master of mayhem in the middle.* Clans and villages across the island had turned themselves into small guerrilla forces, each under the leadership of its own chieftain. And every Cretan who wasn't carrying a gun was still armed with eyes and ears: no German plane could leave the island without being spotted, and no German soldiers could board a troop ship without being counted. Xan would be the spider in the center of the web. He'd have to race back and forth across the island, bringing in weapons by parachute for Cretan bandits and radioing German plane coordinates for British fighter pilots.

Every day that Xan could stay alive, Monty told him, was another day that Field Marshal Rommel's panzers might have to wait for fuel, Russian fighters could hold out in Leningrad, and entire German regiments would be lost in the Cretan mountains in pursuit of a few dozen invisible men. But for now, Xan would have to do it alone. Monty was heading back to the mainland, so Xan would basically be on his own until a new man could be recruited.

And his first challenge, Monty warned, could be his last. Xan's only contact with the outside world would be his radio operator, who was in a hideout on Mount Ida. Between them lay some of the most treacherous terrain on the island: the Messara Valley, which led right to the Germans' main airbase. To establish radio contact with Cairo, Xan would have to trek across a hundred some miles of mountain and slip through crisscrossing German patrols.

If he could do that, then it was on to even trickier territory: the White Mountains, a favorite lair for bandits, rebels, and John Devitt Stringfellow Pendlebury, the one-eyed archeologist who'd become one of the great enigmas of the war. No one on Crete was more hated by the Germans or more hunted. Stories had spread beyond the island of "Pendlebury's Thugs," a band of Allied evaders led by a tall, pale man with a patch over one eye and a silver dagger in the sash around his waist.

"The small force of British, New Zealand, and Australian troops who evaded capture in Crete and are conducting vigorous guerrilla warfare against the Germans," Reuters news agency reported, "are commanded by a British officer well known to the islanders." In broadcasts from Berlin, the German military fumed, "It is undoubtedly to be attributed to Pendlebury's activities that large numbers of the population turned guerrilla."

The Thugs were said to fight like desperadoes—sniping from the dark with deadly aim, taking no prisoners. If Pendlebury's exploits were real, Churchill and those two old Shanghai hands, Fairbairn and Sykes, would be delighted; it meant at least one swashbuckling Brit had come up with a way to give Hitler a taste of total war. The Führer was reportedly so intent on seeing Pendlebury killed that he demanded the glass eye be plucked from Pendlebury's skull and sent to him as a war prize. Greek prisoners were forced to search through piles of corpses, poking their fingers into eye sockets. But as of Xan's arrival on Crete in December, Pendlebury's whereabouts were still unknown.

Monty finished his briefing. Xan was desperately tired and needed a solid meal and a good rest before making his attempt on Mount Ida. On the other hand, there were those Australians. . . .

"Since I felt no particular urge to remain in Akendria," he judged, "I decided to set off at once."

CHAPTER 15

The friend of wisdom is also a friend of the myth.

—ARISTOTLE

HORRIBLE IDEA.

"Had we known what was to come," Xan complained, brushing by the fact that he'd been warned *exactly* what was to come, "we would never have started out immediately after two consecutive days with little rest or food." Still, maybe Monty could have been more specific about the weather. Xan and Delaney hadn't gotten far from Akendria when it started to rain, building to a downpour that continued all night. Finally, after hours of stumbling in the dark on wet stones and pulling his boots out of gluey mud, Xan gave up. If he was caught, so be it.

"Even the threat of capture and its inevitable outcome, the firing squad, were not sufficient to induce us to keep walking," he'd recall. "I found myself longing for the sudden appearance of a German patrol to put an end to our increasingly unbearable muscular fatigue and sleeplessness."

That did it for Costa, too. As Xan's guide, he'd done his best to live up to *xenía*, the Cretan code of hospitality. *Xenía* speaks to the heart of Greek identity, because every Greek at some point has been a stranger; in ancient Greek, "stranger" and "guest" are even the same word. In a nation of seafarers and shepherds and traveling scholars, of earthquakes and warfare and overseas trade, relying on an occasional unexpected handout is necessary and inevitable. "All is performed with simplicity and lack of fuss and prompted by kindness so unfeigned," one British traveler still marveled after many trips to Greece, "that it invests even the most ramshackle hut with magnificence and style."

Xenía isn't even a virtue, really; it's a law enforced by thunder-god Zeus himself. Much the way Christianity adopted a pay-it-forward policy as its "Greatest Commandment" and reveres a homeless savior who got by on handouts, the Olympian myths are all about the immortals quality-controlling *xenía* by wandering about in human form and seeing how they're treated when they show up in disguise. The *Iliad* and the *Odyssey*, the two Greek pillars of Western literature, are *xenía* written in blood—a pair of epic thrillers that explore what happens when you (a) abuse hospitality by monkeying with your host's wife and (b) depend on it during a twenty-year road trip to hell and back. A Cretan is measured by her *xenía*, and the three rules are very clear:

You offer food.
You offer a bath.
You ask no questions.

Not, at least, until the traveler has been refreshed. That way, he'll at least get a bite and a breather in case you discover you can't stand him. You can think of *xenía* as compassion, but only if you get rid of the notion that compassion is based on sweetness, or charity, or even trading favors. Compassion is a battle instinct, a jungle-law alert system that lets you know when someone, or something, is closing in on you for the kill. We like to pretty it up with a halo and call it angelic, but compassion really springs from our raw animal need to figure out what is going on around us and the smartest way to respond. It's your social spiderweb, a protective netting of highly sensitive strands that connects you to your kinfolk and alerts you the instant one of them runs into the kind of trouble that can find its way back to you. Compassion requires you to be a wonderful listener, much like psychiatrists and FBI profilers and for essentially the same reason. The goal is to get inside someone else's head, and in that regard Rule #3 of *xenía* was way ahead of both crime detection and psychoanalysis; peppering someone with questions, as any police interrogator will tell you, isn't nearly as effective as letting him relax until the words flow on their own. And when they do—when you get access to someone else's feelings— you can put aside your own and see the world through a new set of eyes. That kind of insight is crucial to what combat soldiers call "situational awareness"—a constant mental scan of your environment so you're always up to the second on the best and worst way out of any situation. That's really the unvarnished essence of *xenía*, and it's the reason Darwin and Andrew Carnegie could never quite grasp what heroes are all about. They thought it was crazy to risk yourself for a stranger. But to someone truly tuned into situational awareness—into *xenía*— treating a stranger like a brother can be the only sane response.

Many years after the war, Americans rushed to their televisions to watch *xenía* in action when Air Florida Flight 90 crashed into the icy Potomac River on January 13, 1982. To horrified viewers, it seemed impossible that anyone could be alive inside the mangled steel carcass slowly vanishing into the water. But one by one, six survivors gasped to the surface and grabbed at the tail of the plane. Freezing rain and winds were so brutal, it took twenty minutes before a rescue chopper finally arrived. It dropped a life ring into the hands of one survivor and plucked him from the water. Then something peculiar happened.

The next person to receive the ring handed it over to someone else. The chopper lofted her to safety, then wheeled back.

The man gave away the ring again.

And again.

He even gave it away when he knew it was his last chance to live. He must have known, because when the chopper thundered back seconds later, he was gone. The man in the water had vanished beneath the ice. He was later identified as Arland "Chub" Williams Jr., a forty- six-year-old federal bank examiner who hated water and spent his life, until the day he lost it, playing it safe.

"Arland never called a lot of attention to himself," says Peggy Fuesting, his high school sweetheart from Illinois, whom he'd begun dating again shortly before the crash. "He'd had that fear of water his whole life." Arland was trusted by bankers and borrowers alike, his boss would say, because he was careful and discreet and never took risks. But there was another side of Arland, one that was formed nearly a quarter-century earlier when he was a cadet at one of the country's most demanding military colleges: the Citadel. "They make a man out of you," I was told by Benjamin Franklin Webster, Arland's Citadel roommate. "The job of the upperclassmen is to remake you from a boy to a man in one year. They push you, physically and mentally. We lost thirty cadets before we even started classes."

When Webster heard about the crash, he was perhaps the only person who wasn't surprised that a risk-averse accountant would suddenly emerge as the Hero of Flight 90. The Citadel has one iron law: "Always take care of your people first," Webster says. "That's an unbreakable code. You go last. Your people go first." Some of the survivors said Arland seemed to be trapped by the wreckage and unable to free himself. But instead of clinging desperately to the life ring or clawing out for help, he assessed the situation and realized there was only one best decision. To Arland, the survivors around him in the water weren't competitors in a battle for survival. They were family.

Of course they were, agrees Lee Dugatkin, Ph.D., a professor of biology at the University of Louisville who specializes in altruistic behavior. After all, *xenía* is the military's specialty. For most of our evolutionary history, our ancestors moved in such tight family circles that the only people they'd ever see were members of their own hunter-gatherer clan. "If you saved someone's life under those conditions, you were very likely saving a blood relative," he says. But now our relatives are scattered all over the place, so the military has made a science out of reviving that lost feeling of fellowship.

"The armed forces always use the language of kinship to condition soldiers to think of one another as family," Dugatkin points out. "They're not 'strangers'; they're a 'band of brothers.'" Consider what happens when a bus full of strangers of all races and backgrounds pulls into Fort Benning for boot camp. As soon as you arrive, your head is shaved, your clothes are replaced with a uniform, you're taught to walk and talk and eat and make your bed *exactly* the same way as everyone around you. Because the more alike you look, the Army understands, the more likely you'll look out for one another.

Lawrence of Arabia underwent the same transformation during his first trip abroad as a young archeologist. He arrived in Egypt as a fussy Brit and made one crucial decision that would change his life: instead of spending his nights in the English compound, he began camping at the dig site with the Arab workers. He shared their meals of sour goat's milk and warm hearth bread. He traded his khakis for a tunic and a Kurdish belt and joined the singing and storytelling around the fire. Mostly he listened, absorbing "the intricacies of their tribal and family jealousies, rivalries and taboos, their loves and hates, and their strengths and weaknesses," as one biographer would put it. When the Arab Revolt began, Lawrence's *xenía* knew exactly where he had to be. He saw himself in them, and them in him.

So when Xan and Delaney began lagging, Costa remained true to the *xenía* code. For as long as he could. He slowed his pace and carried their supplies, and he even bit his tongue when Xan weirdly insisted on bolting out of Akendria the same day they got there. But take a bullet for them? Forget it. *Xenía* says you have to be hospitable; it doesn't say you have to be an idiot. When the young Brit and the aging Aussie sergeant sank down and refused to get up, Costa tore into them.

"Delaney and I would have willingly succumbed but for Costa's example and exhortation," Xan would admit. The relentless Costa dragged his two charges to their feet and got them moving again. By dawn he'd harried them as far as the southern foothills of Mount Ida. There, at last, they could hole up in a little village and get some rest before pushing on that night.

Except . . . something didn't feel right. Something about the valley was making Costa uneasy. It just seemed . . . wrong. He hunted up a local and discovered his suspicions were correct: Germans were ransacking the villages in search of a local guerrilla. Costa had to get Xan and Delaney out of sight before the sun came up, so he led them into the cliffs and found a snug spot between some brush-covered rocks. They burrowed in while Costa slipped off for provisions, soon returning with goatskins of wine, a pot of cold beans, and some friends in the Resistance. By the time he got back, Xan was already out cold. While the other men ate and whispered, Xan slept through the day on the cold, wet stone, too exhausted to eat.

Turning himself into John Pendlebury was turning out to be a lot tougher than Xan had expected. Of course, Pendlebury had an advantage: he'd been practicing the art of becoming John Pendlebury his entire life.

When Pendlebury was two years old, his parents left him one evening in the care of friends. When they returned, one of his eyeballs was punctured. Maybe the boy poked himself with a pen, maybe he was scratched by a thorn—no one saw it happen or could ever figure it out, not even his father, a surgical professor and house surgeon at St. George's Hospital. Pendlebury didn't seem to mind at all; he liked to dress up the glass replacement with a monocle, or pluck it out when going on a hike and leave it behind on his desk as a way of saying he'd be gone awhile.

His taste for masquerade followed him to Cambridge, where he became an excellent high jumper, despite poncing around between jumps in a white cloak. Although he was the university's preeminent archeology student, Pendlebury liked to "play the buffoon," according to a friend's recollection. He'd scrawl endless doodles of knights in armor in his notebooks, and he founded a drinking club he called Ye Joyouse Companie of Seynt Pol, a sort of boozing fantasy league for make-believe Merry Men. He and Lawrence of Arabia loved the same favorite book, which is an even odder coincidence because it's so awful. *The Life and Death of Richard Yea-and-Nay* is the story of Richard the Lionheart, except told with more stabbings, straining bosoms, and wild-eyed killers than a Mexican telenovela. Lawrence read it nine times before he graduated Oxford, while Pendlebury was always raving about it to his friends. When a classmate dropped by before returning to Australia, Pendlebury "pounced on his *Richard Yea and Nay*, by Maurice Hewlett, which he gave me with instructions to think of him when I read it. This was a much bigger gesture than it appeared, for this grubby little book was, to John, a symbol of heroism and romance."

Wrong! That's what his friends didn't get. To Pendlebury, those mace-and-maiden tales weren't symbols; they were real voices from the past with important lessons to teach. Chivalry and the art of the hero were the fading lights of a train he'd just missed, and Pendlebury was obsessed with finding a way to catch up. *Yea-and-Nay* was his inspiration, and soon after he graduated Cambridge, he found his path.

Pendlebury spent his twenty-fourth birthday as a visiting student at the British School in Athens, and it was there that a strange book with a blue-and-gold cover came into his hands: *The Palace of Minos*. Inside, he found a thrilling proposition: was he willing to believe that all those myths he'd loved as a boy—King Minos and the Minotaur, Theseus and Ariadne, the *Iliad* and the *Odyssey*—were based on real people, real places, real events? Could he accept that they weren't just make-believe, but a snarled thread of history that, once untangled, led back to a time when heroes roamed the earth? Because if he could, fantastic new discoveries awaited him.

And they began on the island of Crete.

Pendlebury was so electrified, he left Athens within days of reading *The Palace of Minos* and went in search of its author, Arthur Evans, the eccentric adventurer and antiquities collector. Evans claimed he'd found hard proof that the legend of King Minos—son of Zeus, stepfather of the monstrous half man, half bull who ate fourteen of Athens's best-looking teenagers every year—was based on a true story. Evans said he'd located not only Minos's lost kingdom and the Minotaur's fabled Labyrinth but also the remains of a fabulous Minoan culture that dominated the Mediterranean two thousand years *before* the pyramids were built.

Was it a hoax? If so, Evans was going all out. To believe his story, you had to believe he'd found the birthplace of, well, *everything*. This lost world he described was so old, it was already *dying* by the time the Egyptians began making words out of dog and bird drawings. Science, literature, politics, advanced math, philosophy, sports, theater—according to Evans, it all sprang from Crete, that craggy little cinder in the sea. It also meant that this nearsighted amateur, a fiery, squinting little man who strode about London smacking carriages with a hiking staff he called "Prodger" and set entire teams of diggers to work because he'd caught a whiff of fennel, had stumbled across a new chapter of human history nearly as long as the span from the birth of Julius Caesar to the death of Steve Jobs.

Pendlebury's excitement grew as he got off the boat in Crete. Just walking along the waterfront was like seeing Evans's book come to life. In the frescoes Evans described, Minoan women were curiously graceful and attractive, "gaily dressed in the height of fashion, with elegantly coiffured hair, engaged apparently in gay chit-chat," as Evans put it, while Minoan men had the sinewy physiques of aerial acrobats. "They were quite unlike the classical Greeks, unlike the

Egyptians, unlike the Babylonians, unlike any ancient people whose painted or sculpted representations had survived from the ancient past," archeological researcher Leonard Cottrell would note. There's something very right, Evans reflected, about a culture that portrays itself with such sass and strength.

And here they were, alive and well and strolling the streets. "I know of no sight finer than a well-dressed Cretan peasant, and with the dress goes a swing and a lightness of foot which always sets me thinking of the slim athletes of Minoan days," Pendlebury would write. From the port of Heraklion, Pendlebury made his way three miles south to Knossos, Evans's spectacular six-acre restoration of an ancient Minoan city. Inside the great palace, Evans had found marvels of sophisticated design: a plumbing system, chess games, four-story architecture, locking doors, a trademark registry, a system of weights and measures, and an astronomical calendar. But deep belowground were hints of darker arts: sinister catacombs with mysterious piles of children's bones.

Pendlebury got lucky; he found Evans on the porch of the Villa Ariadne, the stone compound that served as his home and a kind of youth hostel and teaching hospital for wandering archeologists. Students from all over the world were constantly bustling through, enjoying Evans's excellent food and wine before setting off into the mountains or creeping through the thousand interlocking crypts and throne rooms of Knossos. Unlike most scientists, Evans was rich; between his family's paper mill and his late wife's estate, he had the cash to entertain scholars and bankroll an army of architects, artists, builders, and diggers in pursuit of his hunches.

And his wildest notion was this: maybe Homer's and Virgil's tales about Trojan Horses and man-eating Cyclopes weren't fairy tales, but historical fiction: fiction, sure, but still historical. Evans knew he was risking a firestorm of ridicule, but at least he was following in a cock-sure set of footsteps. Back when he was getting his start in archeology, Evans had been spellbound by Heinrich Schliemann, another rich rebel who sought more than proof that heroes existed; he wanted to visit their homes. Schliemann had been fixated by the idea that the *Iliad* and the *Odyssey*, despite their magic and monsters, were far too realistic to be just make-believe stories about superhuman warriors and bewitched boat rides. His critics smirked, but that's because, unlike Schliemann, they'd never amassed a fortune after being broke, homeless, and shipwrecked in a foreign country; they weren't living proof, in other words, that average people are capable of epic feats.

As a teenager in Germany in the 1830s, Schliemann had hoped to improve his weak lungs by working as a shiphand on a voyage to South America. The boat went down off the Dutch coast, and Schliemann barely made it to shore. Sick and penniless, he slept in an unheated warehouse while running messages by day for a Dutch merchant. By night, he studied so feverishly that by age twenty-two he'd mastered bookkeeping and seven languages. By thirty-three he was boss of his own company and spoke *fifteen* languages. He became such a financial dynamo that during a short trip to San Francisco to recover the body of his dead brother, Schliemann learned about gold prospecting; quickly set up a frontier savings and loan; and pocketed another pile of cash before heading home.

But Schliemann's true love was antiquity, and there was something about the Greek classics that always nagged at him. Was Homer really such a creative wizard, or had his stories lasted so long because they gave off a whiff of the real? Take Agamemnon, King of Men. He sounds too operatic to be true, the way he butts heads with Achilles, blood-sacrifices his own daughter, leads an army of warriors in battle for Helen of Troy, and then comes home victorious, only to be murdered by his wife. But if it's all fantasy, why did Homer crowd his narrative with so many directional details that it reads like a pirate's map to a treasure chest?

So Schliemann treated it like a map, and treasure is what he found. After decades of puzzling over Homer's description of, for instance, a stone wall just past a windswept fig tree and not far from an icy-cold spring next to a steaming thermal pool, Schliemann finally sleuthed his way not only to the lost city of Troy but to the ruined palace and hidden jewels of Priam, its king. Triumphantly, he crowned his wife with "Helen of Troy's tiara," a stunning headdress of cascading gold he'd uncovered that was certainly worthy of the fabled beauty, if not owned by her.

And Schliemann wasn't finished; he followed his success at Troy by hunting down palaces that matched to an uncanny extent Homer's descriptions of the homes of Agamemnon and Odysseus. "Here begins an entirely new science," one converted scientist admitted. All this time, a written road map had been *right there*, right in two of literature's best-read texts. No longer would archeologists have to search for the stones and then figure out what happened; they could now read what happened and go in search of the stones.

Schliemann was sixty-four and wearying of a lifetime of underdog battles when he met young Arthur Evans, so he was inclined to pass along a tip: no one had ever solved the mysteries of Crete. Homer told of "a great city called Knossos, and there, for nine years, King Minos ruled and enjoyed the friendship of almighty Zeus." Thucydides backed up the story, describing Minos as a world shaker whose fleets dominated the mainland and controlled the seas. So Evans followed Schliemann's lead; relying on myths as his guide and his detective's eye for landscape clues (Evans knew, for instance, that fennel has long roots and often sprouts where the ground had been deeply disturbed), it wasn't long before he zeroed in on a pair of dirt mounds not far from the coastal city of Heraklion.

Evans was soon burrowing into a kingdom older and wilder than anything he'd imagined. The Minoans were so remarkable, Evans began wondering if all those awful legends about King Minos weren't just sour grapes and gossip. "The fabulous accounts of the Minotaur and his victims are themselves expressive of a childish wonder at the mighty creations of a civilization beyond the ken of the new-comers," Evans would write. "The ogre's den turns out to be a peaceful abode of priest-kings, in some respects more modern in its equipments than anything produced by classical Greece." Of course, King Minos didn't help his public image any by conducting a weird basement ritual that had teenagers somersaulting over the horns of charging bulls. "It may even be that captive children of both sexes were trained to take part in the dangerous circus sports portrayed on the Palace walls," Evans had to admit.

By the time Pendlebury arrived at the Villa Ariadne, it was Evans's turn to withdraw from the hunt. He was seventy-seven years old and secretly in some serious hot water. He'd been arrested in London's Hyde Park for public indecency with a seventeen-year-old boy, and only eased his way out of the scandal by turning over ownership of Knossos and the Villa Ariadne to the British School on the day he appeared in court. John Pendlebury's timing couldn't have been better. He arrived at the Villa Ariadne in 1928 as an unknown student and a year later was hired to run the entire operation.

Pendlebury knew right where he wanted to start: with the Minotaur, which he suspected was a lot more sinister than Evans realized.

CHAPTER 16

1,058 POUNDS: weight of boulder discovered on the Greek island of Thera, inscribed in the sixth century B.C. with *Eumastas, son of Kritobolos, lifted me from the ground*

1,015 POUNDS: heaviest weight any human has raw-deadlifted in the subsequent 2,600 years

TWO THINGS bugged Pendlebury about Evans's Everybody-Was-Just-Jealous-of-the-Minoans theory.

First, you've got to stick to your guns. If you're going to claim that myths have their roots in reality, then you can't back away once they get bloody.

Second, King Minos *had* to be evil, or Theseus couldn't have been great. Crete was where Theseus came alive as a hero, where his legend was formed and defining characteristics were revealed. *Something* must have happened, some kind of epic challenge that would test a man who'd become known as both a genius of self-defense and a true champion of the hurt and hopeless.

"He showed himself the perfect knight," the master mythologist Edith Hamilton would declare. Except where girlfriends were concerned, of course; no matter your excuse, you just don't strand the princess who saved you from the Labyrinth on a rock at sea, or try to win the love of both an Amazon queen *and* the future Helen of Troy by dragging them off by force. Theseus's heart was his weakness—and his strength. He was always pulling his bonehead buddy Pirithous out of some desperate scrape, and when the world turned its back on disgraced and blinded Oedipus, Theseus took Oedipus in and cared for his daughters. After Hercules recovered from a spell of madness to discover he'd murdered his own family, Theseus alone stood by him, talking Hercules down from suicide and bringing him home to heal from his horror. At war, Theseus refused to pillage his defeated enemies. In peace, he granted power to the people and made Athens a true democracy.

So couldn't there be more to the Minotaur story? Isn't it possible that some kind of dark deeds really were afoot on Crete, something nefarious involving Athenian teenagers who were saved by a "perfect knight"?

As new curator of Knossos, Pendlebury began his own investigation into what really went on down in King Minos's basement. According to legend, Minos's son, Androgeos, was a superb athlete who was murdered after winning all the events at the Athenian Games. To avenge his death, Minos forced Athens to send fourteen of its finest young men and women every year to be sacrificed to the Minotaur, the monster born after Minos's wife had a fling with a magical sea bull. The Athenian teens would be shoved into a labyrinth, where they'd wander in darkness as the Minotaur sniffed them out and devoured them. Until Theseus, prince of Athens, volunteered to go.

Theseus was clever enough to increase his manpower by persuading two young men to masquerade as girls, but his big break came when he caught the eye of Minos's daughter Ariadne. Her heart fluttered at the sight of Theseus, so she snuck him a ball of string and whispered some advice: if he tied one end of the string to the entrance, he could follow it back out of the maze if he defeated the Minotaur. How exactly he'd handle the monster's horns and bone-crushing strength, Theseus had no idea—until they were face-to-face. The instinct of any creature with horns is to thrash its head, so Theseus got behind the Minotaur and onto its back, locking on to the Minotaur's neck as it raged and flailed and finally choked itself out.

"He presses out the life, the brute's savage life, and now it lies dead," Edith Hamilton writes of that epic battle. "Only the head sways slowly, but the horns are useless now." Theseus followed the string back to the exit and set sail. The trip home was a disaster; Theseus somehow lost Ariadne along the way and caused his father to commit suicide by raising the wrong signal-sail, so his father, waiting on shore, believed Theseus had died. But he brought the Athenian teenagers home, along with a new way they could defend themselves from future monsters: when the Minotaur died, pankration was born.

Could "circus sports," as old Arthur Evans insisted, really be the basis for such a dramatic and enduring legend? Pendlebury didn't buy it. Spectacles come and go, but cruelty lasts forever. Only something horrible would linger so long in the collective memory, and Pendlebury believed the hint was right there in the language.

"Names have a habit of being remembered when the deeds with which they are associated are forgotten or garbled," Pendlebury mused in his masterpiece, *The Archeology of Crete*. Theseus means "the one who sets things straight," while Minotaur is "Minos's bull." *Labyrinth* comes from *labrys*, or "double-edged ax." Add the children's bones discovered in the Labyrinth—"chamber of the double-edged ax"—and a scenario like this takes shape: A priest-king who's been stampeding across Greece like a bull believes his power comes from a magic ceremony, so he uses captured children to represent weaker nations and kills them with his *labrys*, shaped like a bull's horns.

"Do we dare believe he wore the mask of a bull?" Pendlebury wonders. Why not? Executioners hood their heads not only to hide their identities, but to split them; to separate who they are from what they have to do. King Minos becomes a monster only when he pulls on the Minotaur mask, and once the slaughter is over, he's back to being the benevolent ruler again. Until, that is, a crusading hero storms his way into Knossos at the head of a rebel band. Guards and soldiers can't stop them, but maybe a supernatural ritual can.

"The final scene takes place in the most dramatic room ever excavated—the Throne Room," Pendlebury writes. "It looks as if the king had been hurried here to undergo too late some last ceremony in the hopes of saving the people. Theseus and the Minotaur!"

Pendlebury got his own taste of the *labrys* when he published his theory. "His imagination drove his passion for archeology," biographer Imogen Grundon would explain, but senior archeologists worried that all that passion and imagination were launching Pendlebury right past science and into science fiction. His article became "notorious," and he was urged, for his own sake, to "tone down his conclusions." Realistically, the kind of people Pendlebury was relying on to make his case—murderous bull-wizards and swashbuckling kid saviors—simply didn't exist.

Didn't—or *don't?* "My theory is not fantastic," Pendlebury fumed. Just because men and women of our era don't live up to the myths doesn't mean no one ever has, or ever will again. Pendlebury was digging into a world that few people alive have ever seen, and it was opening his eyes to electrifying possibilities. We're hardwired by nature to find common social ground, to believe that whatever we're doing today is normal and not much different from the way people have always behaved. We assume human achievement is on an *upward* slope, that learning from the past has made us stronger and smarter than anyone *of* the past.

But if that's true, then explain Eumastas.

In the sixth century b.c., Eumastas hoisted a stone so huge that no one has lifted its equal in 2,600 years. How did he get air under those 1,058 pounds without the aid of steroids, padded gloves, or gym equipment? Or is the question its own answer: was it *because* he had to rely on his own body genius and struggle with bumpy boulders, instead of smooth modern steel, that Eumastas learned more than we'll ever know about leverage, balance, and explosive power?

And if that's the case, then Pheidippides also makes sense.

In 490 b.c., Pheidippides is believed to have run more than *ten consecutive marathons*, nonstop, racing up and over mountains for three straight days. He wasn't one of a kind, either; he was one of a corps. Pheidippides was an *hemerodromos,* or "all-day runner," a foot messenger who was faster over rough hills than a horse and tougher in the heat. When Athens was under attack by Persia at the Battle of Marathon, Pheidippides ran 280 miles round-trip to ask Sparta for reinforcements. At the finish, he wasn't wrapped in a silvery space blanket and handed an orange slice; he still had enough juice to yank his sword and plunge right into the fight. As amazing as that sounds, Pheidippides wasn't even best of class. "A young boy but nine years old," Roman historian Plinius Secundus reminds us, "between noon and evening ran 650 stadia"—that's seventy-five miles—while two other couriers, Lanisis and Philonides, whipped through 144 miles in twenty-four hours: four miles more than Pheidippides's first leg in twelve fewer hours.

And John Pendlebury was supposed to "tone down his conclusions"? Please. His imagination could barely keep up with the realities he was unearthing from the buried world. Take Homer: he turned out to be right about the places he described, so why not the people? Were his heroes truer to life than we believed? Homer was no fan of perfect golden boys, after all; he was more intrigued by the guy who's off his game, past his prime, always one step closer to losing than winning.

Like Odysseus. In Homer's tales, Odysseus's best days are behind him, and the young warriors won't let him forget it. "You know, stranger, I've seen a lot of sportsmen and you don't look like one to me at all," a strapping fighter named Euryalus taunts Odysseus during an afternoon of athletic contests in Phaeacia. "You look more like the captain of a merchant ship, plying the seas with a crew of hired hands and keeping a sharp eye on his cargo, greedy for profit. No, you're no athlete."

Odysseus gets to his feet, and school is in session. "Now I'm slowed down by my aches and pains and the suffering I've had in war and at sea," he concedes, but that's all he'll concede. Swirling back his cloak, Odysseus reaches for a discus and grabs not the lightest, for more control, but the heaviest, for maximum momentum. He uncoils from his windup and lets fly, hissing the discus on a flight path so low and perfectly angled it nearly takes the Phaeacians' heads off. It lands so far ahead of the field it doesn't even need to be measured.

"And if anyone has the urge to try me, step right up," Odysseus snarls. "I don't care if it's boxing, wrestling, or even running. Come one, come all."

His young man's body is gone, but he's an expert at using what's left. Earlier in the *Iliad*, Odysseus races two younger men. He's the underdog once again, but his tactics are terrific as he slipstreams right behind the leader. "His feet stepped in Ajax's footprints before the dust settled into them, and his warm breath from inches behind streamed down onto Ajax's head." Just before the finish, Odysseus surges so suddenly that Ajax is startled and falls. Ajax leaps to his feet, flinging horse dung off his face and complaining that the goddess Athena tripped him. But the runner who came in last saw it all and tells it straight.

"Odysseus is of an earlier generation," Antilochus explains. "He is a tough old bird, as they say; it is hard for any of us to beat him, except for Achilles."

John Pendlebury was running into the same tough old birds all over Crete.

The more he wandered the island after he took over as curator of Knossos, the more of these ageless, bounding, Odyssean mountain men he ran into. He couldn't swear any were as strong as Eumastas; on the other hand, he kept coming across cheese huts high in the hills stacked from head-scratchingly huge stones. The great messenger Pheidippides was said to be Cretan; so were many of the other all-day runners, including Alexander the Great's special courier, Philonides. And Pheidippides was certainly no youngster; he held the rank of "master *hemerodromos*," so his heroic effort during the Battle of Marathon would have come during the twilight of his career.

So why should it be any different for Pendlebury? Now that he was living in an open-air performance lab, he had another way to test his theory that myths were based on real men and women: he could experiment on himself. Like Lawrence, Pendlebury loved role playing, so total immersion came naturally. He also shared Lawrence's trick for getting inside someone else's skin: first, get inside their clothes.

"Have just got a Cretan costume—perfectly gorgeous, a great show," Pendlebury was soon writing his father. For a Cambridge academic, it was quite the makeover, even outdoing Pendlebury's previous phase of wearing a white cape to high-jump competitions. Cretan shepherds dress more like buccaneers than farmhands, so Pendlebury kitted himself out almost Halloweenishly, in an embroidered black waistcoat, black breeches with a knee-length crotch, knee-high boots, a black headkerchief, a wide sash wrapped around his waist, and a black cloak with red-silk lining.

Every morning before breakfast, he did a fifteen-minute skipping drill that mimicked the light, skittering shepherd's stride. "I find it quickens the muscles which walking is apt to increase but slow down," he commented. To uncramp his body after long hours hunched over potsherds, he had masks and foils shipped to Crete and began fencing so he could stretch into full-length lunges and sharpen his balance, enlisting his plucky wife as a sparring partner. He even began high-jumping again, and gradually found he could sail higher than ever. As a university athlete, he'd barely cleared six feet, but that now looked easy. "Very fit and all the spring in the world," he wrote to his father. "I think I shall have a good chance at the Greek record, it is only 6 ft or just under."

Every afternoon, he stopped work and pushed into the hills for a ten- or twelve-mile hike. His range and curiosity were impressive—until they became astonishing. During one season alone, Pendlebury hiked more than a thousand miles across the island. One afternoon, he scrambled all the way over Mount Ida and still made it back to Knossos before sundown: "26 miles over filthy country in 6 hrs 25 m," he jotted, always exact about his journeys. Cretan highlanders who at first didn't know what to make of this eager, one-eyed stranger got used to having him ramble into their villages at night—famished, exhausted, and half-lost, yet ready to lift a wineglass and learn some new songs.

"He was making friends everywhere," recalled Dilys Powell, who met the Pendleburys and became their occasional expedition companion when her husband took over as head of the British School in Athens. "By now he had travelled on foot from one end of the island to the other. It was only natural that its people should feel affection and respect for this tireless young Englishman, his fair skin burned dark, his hair the color of stubble, who turned up everywhere, slept anywhere, drank with them, talked with them, spoke their own kind of language."

Pendlebury felt the same way about the Cretans, and he was ready to prove it. By the time Hitler had driven English forces out of Europe and was threatening London, Pendlebury had spent ten years on Crete and decided to make his stand where he was. He was pushing forty, but a decade of learning from tough old birds had left him lean and fit as a teenager. "Record time to the summit," he noted with satisfaction after speed-climbing Mount Ida. "And a resultant waist measurement, pulled in a bit, of 22½ inches."

But the War Office wasn't in the market for middle-aged, half-blind academics, regardless of trouser size. Pendlebury was convinced his Mediterranean expertise could be invaluable to naval intelligence, but they brushed him off. He tried the military attaché in Athens, then army intelligence, before finally volunteering for the job of last resort: stretcher bearer. Before he was to start duty, however, word spread along the Cambridge-Oxford old boys' network that certain, um . . . *characters* were needed for a new "special services" operation. No fighting know-how required.

"Seems tough and generally desirable" was the shrugging appraisal after Pendlebury finally got his interview, and he was soon heading back to Crete. His cover story: he was vice-consul, a midlevel, do-little diplomat. But to get a whiff of what he was really up to, Pendlebury's friends learned to check his bedside table. "On his more nefarious expeditions," Dilys Powell was told by one Pendlebury confidant, "he used to take out his glass eye and wear a black eye-patch. He would leave the eye on the table by his bed—if you found it there you knew he was away on some excursion or other."

Pendlebury regularly slipped away from the Villa Ariadne and climbed into the mountains to scout hideouts and organize rebel bands. As a student of ancient warfare, he knew Crete was critical, and his own eye for the island's defenses told him two things: the attack would have to come by air, and the real battle would be high in the hills. The Germans had crushed every ground force they'd faced, but they had yet to run into anything as elusive and unrelenting as a Cretan bandit. If Pendlebury could get ten thousand rifles into the hands of the highlanders, he was sure the Germans would have a fight on their hands.

So Pendlebury strolled about, pretending to be a diplomat while carrying an innocent-looking walking stick with a sword inside, which he judged perfect for skewering paratroopers. No matter what happened, he decided, he wasn't leaving. "He felt himself a Cretan and in Crete he would stay until victory was won," recalled Nicholas Hammond, a Cambridge don who'd been one of Pendlebury's archeology students and came to Crete to join his special operations force. For extra secrecy, but mostly to show off, Pendlebury and Hammond encoded their conversations by speaking to each other in their specialty dialects, Cretan versus Epirotic.

Hammond and Pendlebury teamed up with a swashbuckling boat captain, the gold-earringed Mike Cumberlege, who growled into Crete at the wheel of a combat-ready fishing boat called the *Dolphin*. Together, the three men hatched a scheme to glide by night out to the Italian-held island of Kasos and kidnap some Italian soldiers they could haul back to Crete and sweat for information about the looming German invasion. Just to be safe, Cumberlege decided to take Hammond with him on a last recon trip across the channel to Kasos. They tucked in beside an offshore island to hide until dark . . . and then the engine refused to start. While Cumberlege struggled to fix it, German warplanes suddenly began thundering overhead. Bomb bursts flashed across the water from Crete, followed by mushroom puffs of parachutes.

While his gang was marooned offshore during the invasion, Pendlebury threw off his diplomat's disguise and joined the street fighting alongside Satan, the Cretan guerrilla leader. When it became clear that Allied forces had given up and were ready to abandon the island, he and Satan strode into the British command cave and volunteered to cover the retreat. "I was enormously impressed by that splendid figure," recalled Paddy Leigh Fermor, who'd been deployed to Crete just before the invasion. "He had a Cretan fighter with him, festooned with bandoliers, and John Pendlebury himself made a wonderfully buccaneer and rakish impression."

Paddy was in awe, not least because, as every other Allied soldier was scrambling toward the evacuation beach, "the one-eyed giant," as Paddy called him, refused to follow. "His single sparkling eye, his slung guerrilla's rifle and bandolier and his famous swordstick brought a stimulating flash of romance and fun into the khaki gloom." Paddy managed to escape Crete, and he was still hearing about Pendlebury's adventures long after he made it back to Cairo. "The German SS got to know of Pendlebury," Paddy would say. "They called him *'der kretische Lawrence'*—the Cretan Lawrence—and rumours spread amongst Pendlebury's hillmen that Hitler could not rest until he had Pendlebury's glass eye on his desk in Berlin."

Two days into the invasion, the *Dolphin* fired back to life, and Cumberlege steered stealthily into a hidden cove near Heraklion. Hammond and Cumberlege's cousin, Cle, each grabbed a Mauser rifle and crept ashore. Dead and dying soldiers were tumbled together in the streets of Heraklion, while bullets whizzed from house-to-house firefights. Hammond and Cle realized they had no chance of finding Pendlebury, so they slunk back to the boat and pushed off toward safety in North Africa.

The *Dolphin* never made it. Cle was killed by fighter-plane fire, and

Mike Cumberlege was wounded, surviving only because another captain came to his rescue. Three weeks later, Cumberlege was recovering in Egypt when he tuned in to a radio broadcast from Berlin. "The bandit Pendlebury," Cumberlege heard, "will be caught and he can expect short shrift when he is found."

Thank goodness! That still left Cumberlege a chance to find him first. As soon he could get to his feet, he secured another boat and was off, threading his way through German patrol ships to search for his friend. The trouble was, Pendlebury could be anywhere. During his thousands of miles of archeological hikes, he'd learned the mountains "stone by stone," as he liked to say. He'd been a whirlwind of preparation before the invasion, setting up weapons stashes and hideouts in places only he and the canniest old shepherds could ever find. He'd even made a mountain more mountainous, persuading a small army of Cretan volunteers to trek to Mount Ida and, "with Herculean efforts," as Antony Beevor reports, "they shifted boulders down to its smooth areas to prevent aircraft landings."

So where was he now?

"There were persistent tales of an Englishman who had been seen at Hagia Galini, a village on the south coast near Tymbaki," Dilys Powell would learn. "What was more, it was an officer who had lost an eye." Three months after the evacuation of Crete, Britain's chief of military intelligence in Cairo personally told Churchill, "We also tried to drop a wireless set by parachute to Pendlebury, who at the moment is largely controlling guerrilla activities in the Cretan hills."

But if anyone knew how to actually find Pendlebury and his Thugs, they weren't talking. No matter where Cumberlege looked, Pendlebury always seemed tantalizingly close, yet nowhere to be found. The champion of heroic myths was turning into one himself.

CHAPTER 17

David, let's not forget, was a shepherd. He came at Goliath
with a slingshot and staff because those were the tools of
his trade. He didn't know that duels with Philistines were
supposed to proceed formally, with the crossing of swords.
"When the lion or the bear would come and carry off a sheep
from the herd, I would go out after him and strike him down
and rescue it from his clutches," David explained to Saul. He
brought a shepherd's rules to the battlefield.

—MALCOLM GLADWELL, "How David Beats Goliath"

THE LAST, BEST SIGHTING had Pendlebury heading toward Mount
Ida—bandit country. Hard to get in, easy to get lost. Same place
where, after sleeping under wet bushes all day after his long night
hike through the rain with Costa, Xan Fielding was waking up to a
double dose of good news.

The German search parties had moved on, so he and Delaney
could crawl out of hiding for a while and stretch their aching bodies.
And instead of having to scrabble another eighty miles to the radio
operator's mountain hideout, word arrived that the radio operator
was coming down to them. Xan was thrilled, since he could finally
kick back for a night after three hectic days on the move since splash-

ing ashore from the sub, but then he grew apprehensive. Why was the radioman suddenly out of his hole and on the move after he'd been safely hidden for months?

Soon enough, Ralph Hedley Stockbridge hiked into camp in the worst Cretan costume Xan had ever seen. The only thing more British than his overcoat—*seriously, an overcoat?*—were his horn-rimmed glasses. Unlike every Cretan male past puberty, he had no mustache, and instead of shepherd's boots, he was still in shoes. "In no way did he look like a peasant," Xan thought. And that, it gradually dawned on him, was Ralph's sly genius: Ralph looked exactly like a Greek trying not to look Greek. It was a stunt right out of *The Man Who Was Thursday*, and it worked brilliantly. Once, Ralph strolled right through a German checkpoint while the real Cretan beside him was grabbed and questioned. "They must have been blind not to see me trembling," Ralph would recall. During another close encounter, he blurted, "Gosh, sorry!"—in English—after bumping into a German soldier, and he still didn't attract a second look.

But the audacity of Ralph's no-disguise disguise was brutal on his nerves. Like Xan, Ralph wasn't much of a soldier. He was notorious in the War Office for making a fuss about having to wear puttees—wool wraps that twine up from the ankle and tuck in at the knee—and then quitting the Officers' Training Corps because he felt his superior officers were acting too superior. Despite or maybe due to this obsessive contrariness, Ralph was recruited by "Mike"—MI6, the Secret Intelligence Service. Mike was James Bond's outfit, but unlike 007, real MI6 agents kept their flies zipped and gadgets holstered. Their job was to live in the shadows, eavesdropping in cafés and building webs of civilian spies. That often put them at odds with the dirty tricksters of Xan's unit, the Firm, because the last thing any Mike agent wanted was a bar of soap blowing up in a brothel they had under surveillance.

But on Crete, where the tiny band of Brits depended on one another for survival, the rival spies split the work and got along like brothers. Which, biology aside, they basically were. Like Xan and Monty, Ralph was another of Geoffrey Household's Class X "rogue males"; he'd fight for his country, think for himself, and try not to hurt anyone in the process. Ralph was brainy and bookwormish, and more than a little bewildered that he'd ended up fiddling with a wireless radio set up in a Mediterranean cave. He'd studied classics at Cambridge, which meant his ability to chat with Cretans was hampered by his two-thousand-year-old vocabulary. And if you can't have a good natter, he warned Xan, undercover life was torture.

To be honest, that's why he was rambling the mountains instead of staying put at his station. He could handle hiding in the dark for days at a time, getting his drinking water from stalactite drips and eating nothing but tough seedling potatoes washed down with gulps of boiled orange-peel tea. But the conversation—that's what finally broke him. Ralph was holed up with Colonel Andreas Papadakis, the old ex-army officer who'd helped Jack Smith-Hughes during his escape and put Jack in the expert hands of George Psychoundakis, the young shepherd turned super-messenger. Since then, Colonel Papadakis had gone mad with imaginary power; with Ralph as his captive audience, he spent his days yammering about how he and his "Supreme Committee of Cretan Struggle" would clean house once he figured out how to get rid of the Germans. Finally, Ralph couldn't take it anymore. He threw his radio set onto a mule and took to the hills.

After a few days, Ralph discovered he hadn't calculated one thing: Papadakis's wind-battered hilltop turned out to be the only place he could get decent transmission strength. When Ralph heard Xan had arrived and needed a safe house, he figured he'd save his pride by using Xan as an excuse to return.

"Ah, so you're back again," Papadakis sneered when Xan and Ralph approached the door. Xan knew the old colonel had risked his life and shared his own meager food to aid the Resistance, but he couldn't help being repelled by a voice that "oscillated between arrogance and plaintiveness" or noticing the way "his hard black eyes glittered with peasant cunning and his general expression could best be described by the American term of 'sour puss.'" Between the three of them, the atmosphere in Papadakis's little hut was primed for an explosion— and it only got worse when Guy Turrall arrived.

Turrall's talent for making himself swiftly and universally disliked as he worked his way across the island was as remarkable as Guy Delaney's knack for spontaneous adoration. On the long trek up to Papadakis's home, the Cretan guide who offered to carry Turrall's pack couldn't figure out why it kept getting heavier—until he discovered that Turrall, an amateur geologist, was loading it with rock samples.

Another Cretan guide got so fed up with Turrall that he violated his *xenía* duties by storming off and abandoning Turrall when they were still a half-mile outside a village. Turrall marched in alone and got lucky: the villagers only ignored him, instead of beating the tar out of him and turning him over to the Germans. Many islanders had been executed after being tricked by Germans masquerading as Allied fugitives, so in retaliation, they'd come up with a wickedly clever response whenever they smelled a rat: they'd play dumb and attack the "Brit," getting their boots into him good before innocently dragging him off to the nearest German outpost. To a wary Cretan, nothing would look more German than a bossy stranger wearing a British captain's uniform and speaking French. Turrall never knew how close he came to a beating and a bullet.

Once in Papadakis's hut, Turrall immediately set everyone's teeth on edge. He kept up the French and bustled about every hour heating water for another pot of boiled orange-peel tea. He argued bitterly with Papadakis about how and when they should set off to plant bombs on German ships in the harbor, even though neither he nor Papadakis had any clue what the other was saying.

"This madman wants to destroy us all!" Papadakis complained. Ralph and Xan were trapped between them; with snow threatening and bitter winds blowing, it was too risky to attempt further recon in the mountains, so they were stuck inside playing endless games of gin rummy.

So this is what it's like being a rebel fighter? Xan had to wonder. *Huddling over a twig fire while two old lunatics squabble all day?*

Luckily, bad news came along to save him. Word came up from the lowland villages that German search teams were on the way. The old colonel and the Brits would have to separate and scramble— immediately. As radioman, Ralph drew the short straw and would head into the wild with Colonel Papadakis to establish a new base in a cave. For Turrall and Delaney, the time was right to pack it in. The only way to survive on Crete was to learn from the Cretans, and that was as impossible for these two regular army soldiers as it was for the British commanders who'd lost the invasion. Turrall was still grumbling about "the natives" even as one of them guided him out of the hills a few nights later and into a secret cove where an escape boat was waiting.

Xan was now on his own, and after months of being cooped up, he was aching for action. The real hot spots were down at the German bases along the waterfront, and Xan felt he was ready for a closer look. One of Papadakis's friends led him out of the mountains and down to a safe house near Rethymno, a northern port thick with Germans. Xan didn't dare venture out by day, but by night, he'd put on his disguise and slip off for tentative walks though the village.

During his weeks in Papadakis's hut, Xan had worked at mastering his new identity. He'd trained himself to answer to "Aleko" and to knot his black headkerchief so it tilted over his eye just so. His mustache was finally as credible as his cloak and high black boots, and his elfin face presented all kinds of interesting possibilities: powder the hair, crinkle the brow, and the young shepherd turned into his own grandfather. Super-close shave, sling on a head scarf and skirt, and voilà: the teenage girls had some competition.

But from the chin down, Xan still had work to do. "My wastefully energetic manner of moving over uneven ground," Xan admitted, "would give me away at a distance of a mile." Until he figured out how the Cretans got those springs in their legs, he came up with a temporary fix: dementia. Whenever they ran into someone on the trail, Xan's guide would sigh and explain that, yes, his friend was kind of a klutz, but what do you expect from a poor fellow who's deaf and deranged? Xan was so convincing, he hurt his own feelings. "Without wishing to flatter myself," Xan felt compelled to clarify, "posing as a deaf-mute imbecile did not come naturally to me. It was the hardest performance I have ever undertaken and I had to keep it up for over a fortnight."

After two weeks of fooling even native Cretans into believing he was a brain-damaged brother, Xan had all the encouragement he needed to get himself into trouble. He was intrigued by a rumor that the burly old mayor of Chania, Crete's then-capital, might be willing to go undercover for the guerrillas. The mayor's prestige and daily contact with German officers would make him a tremendous recruiter and a valuable spy; with intel and contacts like that, Xan could get down to some serious dirty trickery. So instead of waiting for the mayor to come to him, Xan decided to try sneaking into Chania. German sentries surrounded the city, but Xan's guide noticed that solitary travelers were scrutinized a little more closely than groups.

If Xan rode in the back of a crowded bus and kept his mouth shut, he might get past with just a quick glance at his fake papers.

A few days later, Mayor Nicolas Skoulas was in his office when three German officers paid a call. By midmorning the Germans had wrapped up their business and were heading out the door when they ran into a little traffic jam: two shepherds were trying to get in without an appointment. Charitably, the mayor agreed to see them, although one of the shepherds was clearly a little slow. The Germans noticed nothing, but the mayor quickly saw through Xan's disguise and "looked aghast," Xan would say. "He hardly expected to see a British agent in his own office in the Town Hall in the middle of the morning."

As soon as they were alone, the mayor heard Xan out and agreed to become his eyes and ears in Chania. Xan slipped out of the city that afternoon, eventually arriving safely at his stifling little hideout. *Unbelievable*, Xan thought. He'd just walked into the heart of German operations—he'd brushed chests with three German officers!—and enlisted a top asset right under their noses. Churchill was right: Xan really did have a fighting chance of turning Hitler's greatest weapon—fear—against him.

All Xan needed was some help. Not help exactly. What he needed was . . .

CHAPTER 18

Don't worry, Paddy's not a typical army officer
or guerrilla leader. He's not a typical anything, he's himself . . .
a sort of Gypsy Scholar.

—DAPHNE FIELDING, friend of Patrick Leigh Fermor

Leigh-Fermor does not submit willingly to discipline,
and I think, requires firm handling.

—BRITISH WAR OFFICE MEMO

"YASOU, KOUMBARO!" And then . . . *whap!*

Paddy Leigh Fermor made an entrance that could out-Greek any Greek. "His *Yasou*—'Hail' or 'To your health!'—was much louder than any Cretan's, his slap so much harder, and his embrace a danger to one's ribs," one war memoirist recalled. Paddy also liked to call total strangers "godfather"—*koumbaro*—because to his thinking, that made them instant co-conspirators in a private joke. "It strikes a note of friendly collusion," Paddy explained, and friendly collusion was the story and guiding light of his life.

Paddy snuck ashore from a camouflaged fishing boat in June, after Xan had been working with the Cretan Resistance for six months.

Paddy was immediately led to "Lotus Land"—Gerakari, a lost village in a remote mountain valley. Gerakari was a favorite place for the Resistance to stash Brits on the run, because finding it, even with a map, meant getting very wet and very lost, very often. Rivers tumbling from mountains on all sides twist together, often washing over the single dirt road and forcing foot travelers to curlicue their way through a dizzying maze of torrents and gullies. You can be close enough to see Gerakari and *still* not know how to get there. But arrive and you'll look back on the hellish hike as the gateway to paradise. The pastures are thick with wildflowers and edible greens, the orchards heavy with grapes, cherries, and *vyssina*, a luscious stone fruit that makes an even more delectable liqueur. Fugitive soldiers would stumble into Gerakari and stare, stunned, as they were handed frothy pitchers of wine and gigantic bowls of creamy yogurt smothered with syrupy cherry *glyko*.

Xan set off on the thirty-five-kilometer trek to Gerakari as soon as he heard the new SOE agent had arrived. When he got there, he was greeted by a beaming grin, a full bottle of raki, and a nagging sense he'd seen this guy before. They yanked the cork as they got acquainted. . . .

. . . And Paddy was still talking when the sun came up the next morning.

"When Paddy opens his mouth, shut yours," Lady Diana Cooper, the socialite and celebrated beauty, later advised her granddaughter, the writer Artemis Cooper. Paddy's stories crackled like fireworks; he could pop off tales about his teenage romance with a sultry married Serb in a red dress or a summer swim in Transylvania that turned into a hay-bale sexcapade with two saucy farm girls, or his ill-considered attempt to sell silk stockings door-to-door by likening them to condoms, and he seemed as alarmingly intimate with German dueling scars as he was with "unconventional young shepherds" who "may have cast a thoughtful eye among their ewes for the quenching of early flames."

Between snorts of laughter, Xan suddenly realized why Paddy looked so familiar. They'd run into each other before, back in a London café when Xan was hustling work as a wandering sketch artist and Paddy was in the midst of the best punishment any student ever served for getting thrown out of school. *Schools*, actually—by seventeen Paddy had seen two psychiatrists and been expelled three times. The only place that hadn't tossed him was Walsham Hall, an experimental program for disciplinary cases that specialized in nude dancing and free association storytelling. Walsham was run by bohemians in homespun dresses and tattered tweeds, and their approach to education suited ten-year-old Paddy perfectly: he got to run around in the woods, perform naked barn dances with his teachers and fellow students, and lie back on the floor and spin yarns instead of conjugating verbs. But after his mother heard rumors that the headmaster was personally bathing the older girls and hand-toweling them dry, Paddy was pulled out for another try at a conventional boarding school.

He was bright, no doubt about it, with a hunger for literature and a flair for languages. By his early teens, he was devouring Rabelais and François Villon in French and crafting his own translation from Latin of Horace's ode "To Thaliarchus," which, not surprisingly, spoke directly to his heart: "Spurn not, young friend, sweet love-making, nor yet the dances round. . . ." Romance and dances round weren't on the curriculum at most of the schools his mother forced him into, however, so Paddy had to skulk them up on his own.

"Patrick had an energy and individuality which the oldest public school in England could not tolerate, the real trouble being that he liked women and did something about it," recalled Alan Watts, a classmate who'd go on to write *The Way of Zen* and become an international authority on Buddhist thought. "Patrick, as an adventurer of extreme courage, was constantly being flogged for his pranks and exploits—in other words, for having a creative imagination." The floggings even became a kind of methadone when Paddy couldn't score any other kind of adventure. "I didn't mind the beatings," he'd shrug. "There was a bravado about that kind of thing."

His final offense was sneaking into town and getting caught in a back room with the greengrocer's daughter. When he was thrown out this time, Paddy didn't complain. "Far better to get the sack for something slightly romantic than for just being a total nuisance," he'd say. Paddy's fed-up parents wanted him in Sandhurst military academy, but he failed the entrance exam. So Paddy came up with a plan of his own.

On December 9, 1933, after waking up with a terrific hangover from a farewell party with his London friends, Paddy pulled on an outfit he'd assembled from army surplus: hobnailed boots, leather vest, a soldier's greatcoat, and riding breeches with vintage puttees. He shoved Horace's *Odes* and *The Oxford Book of English Verse* into a rucksack, along with a sleeping bag, which he almost immediately lost. Then he set off in a freezing rainstorm to catch the ferry to Holland.

"Paddy" was staying behind; the young man in the wandering-poet costume would be known as "Michael." And when Michael came ashore, he planned to walk all the way across Europe and keep going until he reached the "Gateway to the East," Constantinople. He was facing a journey of some two thousand miles, hoboing his way deeper and deeper into the growing Nazi storm as he followed the Rhine and Danube Rivers through Germany, Austria, Czechoslovakia, and Hungary.

"We don't get many in December," the ferry's steward told him as the boat slid from shore and rain turned to snow. Paddy was the only passenger. Winter was a terrible time to set off, and because Paddy's small monthly allowance was being mailed to post offices along the way, he'd eat only if he kept moving. Where he'd sleep, how he'd get by without speaking the languages, how he'd even get home, Paddy had no clue. Like Lawrence, he was just desperate to peel off the outer shell that had caused so many problems and start over with a new name, a new look, in a new place. Among strangers, maybe he wouldn't seem so strange.

He got off the boat near Rotterdam, then trudged through the snow all day before falling asleep watching a card game in a water-front bar. Instead of being robbed or tossed in the street, he woke up "under an eiderdown like a giant meringue." When he pulled on his boots and found his way downstairs, the bar owner wouldn't let Paddy pay for the room. "This was the first marvelous instance of a kindness and hospitality that was to occur again and again on these travels," Paddy would tell Xan—but that didn't even begin to describe the bizarre talent he'd demonstrate for hopscotching between castles and baronial estates for the next four years.

"I had meant to live like a tramp or a pilgrim or a wandering scholar," Paddy would tell Xan. Instead he found himself "strolling from castle to castle, sipping Tokay out of cut-glass goblets and smoking pipes a yard long with archdukes."

In Bratislava, a banker he met by chance hosted him for three weeks of hot meals, fireside brandies, and endless browsing in the rich family library. In Stuttgart, Paddy was watching sleet batter the café windows and wondering where he'd sleep when two lovely young women in fur boots stomped in to buy snacks for a house party. Their parents were away for the holidays, so Paddy spent the long weekend drinking "the last of a fabulously rare and wonderful vintage that Annie's father had been particularly looking forward to" and sleeping in Papa's scarlet silk pajamas. In Greece, he galloped along on a borrowed horse in the middle of a cavalry charge when his host was suddenly called to help quell a military revolt against the king.

Listening to Paddy's tales, Xan was stupefied. "Like him, I had tramped across Europe to reach Greece; like him, I had been almost penniless during that long arduous holiday—but there the similarity between our travels ended, for whereas I was often forced to sleep out of doors, in ditches, haystacks or on public benches, Paddy's charm and resourcefulness had made him a welcome guest wherever he went and his itinerary was dotted with the châteaux, palazzi and Schlösser in which he had been put up before moving on to his next chance host."

Paddy was a fine-looking young man—any Pre-Raphaelite would have loved painting those wavy brown curls and earnest eyes, always hunched in thought over a journal or the tattered Horace he'd dug from his rucksack—but smooth talk and a pretty face weren't the secret of his appeal.

"One has also to imagine the impact of Paddy on an old count from eastern Europe, barely able to live off his much-diminished lands and keep the roof on a house stocked with paintings and furniture that harked back to better days," the writer Artemis Cooper, Paddy's long-time friend, would later explain. "A scruffy young Englishman with a rucksack turns up on the doorstep, recommended by a friend. He is polite, cheerful, and he cannot hear enough about the family history. He pores over the books and albums in the library, and asks a thousand questions about the princely rulers, dynastic marriages, wars and revolts and waves of migration that shaped that part of the world. He wants to hear about the family portraits, too, and begs the Count to remember the songs the peasants used to sing when he was a child. Instead of feeling like a useless fragment of a broken empire, the Count is transformed. This young Englishman has made him realize that he is part of a living history, a link in an unbroken chain going back to Charlemagne and beyond."

The Paddy problem wasn't so hard to solve after all: once fidgety, show-offy, daydreamy Paddy was allowed to get up and walk around a little, he began soaking in languages and literature at a tremendous rate, far faster and with more command than he would have in any classroom. The same impulsive curiosity and raw animal energy that got him serially ejected from the British educational system was turning him into Europe's Favorite Guest. From then on and for the rest of his life, Paddy's motto was *Solvitur ambulando:* "When in doubt, walk."

Paddy was having such a good time that even after he reached Constantinople, he kept on rambling, only coming to a dead halt on a rooftop terrace in Athens, when he first caught sight of Princess Balasha Cantacuzene of Romania.

Balasha was breathtaking, a dark-eyed beauty who'd descended from one of the great dynastic families of Eastern Europe and looked it. When she met Paddy in May of 1935, she was thirty-six years old and had been abandoned in Greece by her cheating Spanish-diplomat of a husband. Charming as Paddy was, it was hard to imagine a worse choice for a romantic rebound. He was restless, jobless, homeless, nearly penniless, and barely out of his teens, having just turned twenty. But Balasha found him "so fresh and enthusiastic, so full of colour and so clean" that she took him back with her to Baleni, the Cantacuzene ancestral manor deep in the Romanian countryside.

There, cut off from the world as snow piled up to the windowsills, they settled into a life of artsy aristocracy. Balasha spent the mornings painting, often portraits of Paddy, while Paddy worked at translating a friend's French novel into English. By the same instinct that prompted Paddy to adopt his alias of "Michael" at the beginning of his journey, he now dropped it: his life on the road was over. Content with the woman and life of his dreams, he showed no sign of straying.

Until, four years later, a new adventure called.

CHAPTER 19

SITUATION HERE UGLY

—PADDY'S FIRST MESSAGE TO HQ AFTER ARRIVING ON CRETE

"UGLY" barely cut it.

Paddy had been surprised to find guerrillas wading past him to escape the island while he was wading in. Satan and his family were eager to get aboard the British boat, while grumpy old Colonel Papadakis was stewing on the beach because he'd just been told there was no more room for him and his followers. A lot had changed since Xan's moment of derring-do in the mayor's office, Paddy would soon learn, none of it good and much of it due to the Russians and a murderous thug known as "the Turk."

Xan filled Paddy in during their long night of drinking and storytelling in the cave outside Gerakari. The Germans had gotten off to a late start on Operation Barbarossa, exactly as Hitler feared, so instead of blitzing into Moscow they'd been socked by snow and were now stuck in a muddy, bloody, frozen-toed death slog. Hitler was facing a campaign that could last years, rather than months, so to rest some of his troops he'd begun rotating them with tours of duty on Crete. Frostbitten and battle-scarred, these frontline survivors showed up with a score to settle and zero patience for any shepherd shenanigans.

Crete was now the biggest transit depot in the Mediterranean, and the Germans intended to lock it down once and for all.

"Better to shoot once too often than once too seldom" was their standing order, and their approach to bandits was even more vicious: If you can't grab a ghost, grab his family. That's why Satan and Colonel Papadakis had to get off the island until the heat died down; their children, parents, and neighbors were in danger of being seized. "Since it was the German practice to seize the relatives of a 'wanted' man as hostages," Xan explained, "the Colonel's family had taken the precaution of leaving their home in Kallikitri to join him in the mountains, and were now living as he was, like hunted refugees out in the open."

Along Crete's northern coast, the mysterious Gestapo sergeant Fritz Schubert was operating his own reign of terror. Born in Turkey, raised in Germany, fluent in English and Greek, a Nazi true believer, the Turk was a specter who haunted cafés and village squares. With so many refugees from burnt-down villages turning up in the cities, it was hard to tell the difference between a survivor and a spy, and the Turk's walnut skin and Mediterranean savvy gave him natural camouflage. "The name Fritz Schubert became anathema to the people of Rethimnon, as he would be to all of Crete," one war chronicler reported. " 'The Turk' was now equated with barbarity."

Terrible as he was, the Turk was still no rival to "the Butcher of Crete," General Friedrich-Wilhelm Müller.

The Butcher and Paddy arrived within weeks of each other in the summer of '42, and that is where any similarity ended. Paddy's assignment was to match wits with the Butcher and undermine his command of Crete, but frankly, they couldn't be more mismatched. Müller was afraid of nothing, least of all war crimes: he starved civilians by burning their winter food, he torched their homes, he turned any village suspected of sheltering rebel fighters into a death camp, murdering *everyone*—infants, elderly, the disabled. Any survivors who returned to bury the dead were shot on sight.

Paddy, on the other hand, had quickly established himself from the start as a cheerfully useless soldier. The dirty-tricks squad wasn't his first choice; like Xan, he'd washed up in the unit only because he was so inept everywhere else. He'd originally volunteered for the Irish Guards, because he liked the snazzy cap and tunic—"I thought I might as well die in a nice uniform," he explained—but army life, according to Artemis Cooper, "came as a severe shock to his system." Paddy managed only one month of training before spending the next three in the hospital. His official assessment ranked him as "below average."

Once again, some combination of failure, death, and disgrace loomed in Paddy's future, so he decided to try a fresh path before it was too late. The regular army wasn't for him, but the irregular might be a different story. Thanks to his flair for foreign languages, he managed to follow in the footsteps of other misfits and get a transfer to the Firm. Now, *finally*, he was in a situation perfectly suited for his natural gifts, a place where imagination and resourcefulness mattered more than blind obedience. All he had to do was focus a little and learn exciting stuff like forgery, demolition, and knife fighting.

Except not even that could hold Paddy's attention. On the day France fell, Paddy's fellow trainees were in turmoil, wondering how their country would survive without its staunchest ally. Paddy, meanwhile, was working on a poem about a fishpond he'd seen in the Carpathians. He only heard the news later that night.

Xan liked Paddy immediately. Sure, Paddy was a show-off and a chatterbox, but that's because he was addicted to drama; if there wasn't any at hand, Paddy would whip some together himself. Paddy lived for romance, which meant he was up for *anything*.

"This charm of his was still apparent beneath his shabby disguise," Xan explained. "Though we all wore patched breeches, tattered coats, and down-at-heel boots, on him these looked as frivolous as fancy dress. His fair hair, eyebrows and moustache were dyed black, which only added to his carnivalesque appearance, and his conversation was appropriately as gay and as witty as though we had just met each other, not in a sordid little Cretan shack, but at some splendid ball in Paris or London."

During that boozy, all-night debriefing, Xan told Paddy how they'd take on the Butcher. They'd split the island between them, with Xan in the west and Paddy in the east. Whenever the Butcher was hot on

Paddy's trail, Xan and his men would erupt from hiding and draw them off in the other direction. They'd keep the Butcher's forces zig-zagging back and forth through the mountains, which meant German fortifications along the coast would be underprotected and ripe for spying eyes and Cretan hit-and-run attacks. Any German troops in transit to Africa or any convoys refueling for the East would be detected by Xan's operatives and become sitting ducks for Allied attack planes.

Xan and Paddy hoisted their cigarette-tin cups in a toast. "By the time the raki was finished," Xan would recall, "and as I fell asleep on my narrow ledge of twigs I could not be sure whether it was the strong spirit, Paddy's company or the prospect of Egyptian fleshpots that was responsible for the happiest night I had so far spent on Crete."

A few nights later, Paddy was burrowed into a tiny cave for the night when he heard a faint crackling in the brush. He yanked his pistol and took aim at the entrance, but before he could shoot, something scuttled in beneath his line of fire. In the dim light, Paddy glimpsed a sweat-streaked face and black eyes glinting with, as he put it, "embers of mischief." He drew down.

George Psychoundakis had just trotted fifty-some miles over the mountains in old boots held together with baling wire. His clothes were as ragged as his shoes and stuffed with secret messages he'd brought for Paddy from other Resistance fighters. As George began to dig out the tiny slips of paper, Paddy burst out laughing; George kept putting a finger to his lips and glancing mock-fearfully over his shoulder, living up to his code name—Bertódolous, or "the Clown," from an Italian comedy—because he was brave enough to make fun of how scared he was. George had survived plenty of close shaves, including being stopped by a German sentry for questioning while his boots were stuffed with secret maps. That's why, besides "the Clown," George was also called "the Changebug": he'd shown a magical ability to spirit himself out of impossible jams. So far.

Cramped by the low, dripping ceiling, Paddy and George and two local partisans stretched out to have a drink of raki and munch some almonds while George waited for the sun to set for his return trip. Paddy marveled at George's stamina and ingenuity, his ability to run for hours at eagle's height and consistently outthink, outmaneuver, and out-endure German manhunts. George didn't shrug it off—he knew the value of what he knew.

"I felt as if I were flying," he liked to say. "Running all the way from the top of the White Mountains to Mount Ida. So light and easy— just like drinking a cup of coffee."

George kept Paddy amused, sharing the only complete sentence he knew in English: "I steal grapes every day." As it got dark, George rolled Paddy's replies into tight little twists and hid them in his clothes. By day, Crete belonged to the Butcher; by night, George and the shepherds ran free again. "When the moon rose he got up and threw a last swig of raki down his throat with the words 'Another drop of petrol for the engine,'" Paddy recalled. Then he raised a finger, whispered "The Intelligence Service!" and was gone.

"A few minutes later," Paddy continued, "we could see his small figure a mile away moving across the next moonlit fold of the foothills of the White Mountains, bound for another fifty-mile journey."

CHAPTER 20

"YOU REALLY GROW to love George, don't you?" Chris White said, as we inched along a thin goat track on the cliffs above Sfakiá. Sun glare and sweat were scorching my eyes, but Chris seemed unbothered. "Such warmth and humor. He's a true Greek hero. Honest but a trickster. Brave, but goofy."

Awful climbs on crumbling footing, I'd begun to see, put Chris in a meditative mood. Several times along this same cliff face I'd been frozen in place, convinced there was no way forward that wouldn't end in freefall, while far ahead, I could hear Chris's voice fading around a bend as he motored along obliviously, chatting about his old job working with the homeless in Miami Beach or his recent fascination with clinical research into root causes of good luck. (Visual receptiveness is key, apparently, along with extensive kinship bonds.)

Personally, I was fixated on how George could handle a trail like this with a girl on his back. George couldn't have weighed more than 130 pounds, but he'd once saved a friend's daughter by piggybacking her up these mountains with the Turk and his Gestapo band hard on his heels. George had been standing sentry early one morning when he heard a patter of gunshots. The Turk had tortured a Cretan prisoner into leading them to a guerrilla hideout, but made the mistake of shooting at a villager they spotted on the trail, giving George a chance to sprint back and sound the alarm.

"In a moment all our men were gathered along the height, opening fire on a party of Germans and Italians," George recalled. One guerrilla hollered to George to alert the nearby village. George arrived to find a friend's wife fleeing with her two little girls, so George and another man hoisted the girls on their backs and ran for it.

They made the woods just in time. "The Germans, having cut off the upper villages, were streaming south from every direction," George recalled. George headed toward a hamlet he thought would be safe, but veered away when he heard distant screams and the roar of flames. The Germans had already arrived and were burning villagers to death in their own homes. Slipping and dodging, George snaked his little escape party through the dragnet and reached the remote home of one of his aunts. There, the young girl slid down from George's back to safety.

Purely on a strength and skill level, I didn't have to guess what that rescue was like; I could feel it. My boots were struggling for grip along the same cliffs—possibly the same trail—and I was carrying a pack roughly the weight of a small girl. I hadn't stood guard duty the night before or begun my day with a high-speed mountain traverse to save my friends from German stormtroopers, but already my legs were burning, my balance was shaky, and every step, no matter how slow, seemed too quick to be safe. That was the simple genius of the Chris White immersion method: it got to the bottom of the historical questions—the whos and wheres and whens of the traitor Alexiou, the guerrilla chieftain Bandouvas, the frightened young Katsias girls, the villages of Kali Sikia and Nisi—so we could then zero in on the far trickier mystery:

How? How did they actually pull it off?

David Belle had a clue. David grew up in the outskirts of Paris, in a rough neighborhood that was even rougher for half-Vietnamese kids like him. When he got tired of being roughed up by bullies, David decided to do something about it: he teamed up with a band of other mixed-race kids to create what he called a "training method for warriors." His inspiration was a mysterious stranger, someone David had heard amazing stories about and, a few times, even seen in the flesh: his father, Raymond.

Raymond Belle was born in Vietnam to a French military doctor and a Vietnamese mother. During the First Indochina War, the Belles had to flee for the border. Somehow, Raymond was separated from the family and ended up, at age seven, as a boy soldier in the French colonial army. Training was savage and effective: "It was 'Walk or Die,'" David Belle would say. "Survival of the fittest." In the mayhem of a jungle fight against Viet Minh guerrillas, the boys were told, it would be every man for himself. "He started training like a maniac," David recalled his father saying. "At night, when other kids were asleep, he would get out of bed to go run in the woods, climb on trees, do jumps, push-ups, balance. He would never stop, repeat his moves twenty, thirty, fifty times."

It worked; Raymond survived the war, and when the French were chased out of Vietnam, he escaped on a refugee boat and made his way to Lyon. There, his jungle-honed natural-movement skills qualified him to become a member of the *sapeurs-pompiers*—Paris's elite paramilitary rescue squad. Fearless and nimble, Raymond became the squad's go-to man whenever a mission looked impossible. Once, he cat-footed far out on a bridge and managed to pull a suicidal woman to safety. What perplexed David wasn't his father's heroics but his mechanics. How on earth do you balance with one arm on a spider-web of steel when a woman is trying to hurl both of you into the river?

"When I was young, I was doing *parcours*," Raymond explained.

"What is *parcours*?" David asked.

"*Parcours*, it's like in life, you have obstacles and you train to overcome them. You search for the best technique. You keep the best, you repeat it, and then you get better."

David had to figure out the rest on his own, because his superstar dad was rarely around. David teamed up with other outcast boys, and together they began re-creating Raymond's survival challenges in the streets around their homes. They called themselves the Yamakasi—a Lingala word from the French Congo meaning "Strong man, strong spirit"—and their homemade training method for warriors would go on to become the open-air, underground fight club known as Parkour.

Somehow, this back-alley art with no rules, no training manual, and—God forbid!—no competitions traveled from the mean streets of France to a drugstore in Pennsylvania farm country. Like the original Yamakasi, the two guys I met in the parking lot were using their own bodies to discover the most animal-efficient way to fly over, around, and under the hard edges of the city landscape the way monkeys tumble through the trees. "I got into it because I was so fat," Neal Schaeffer told me outside the Rite Aid. He'd begun partying after high school and by age twenty had bloated up from 175 pounds to 240. One afternoon, he was in the park watching some strangers "Kong-vault" picnic tables—they'd charge a table, plant their hands, and shoot both feet through their arms like gorillas and fly off the other side—and Neal was talked into giving it a try. Neal was shocked to discover that, even out of shape, once he got over his fear he could master skills that at first looked impossible.

Well, maybe not *master*. "You're on this endless trajectory where you're always getting better, but it's never good enough," Neal explained. "That's what's so exciting. As soon as you land one jump, you can't wait to try it again. You're always looking for ways to make it cleaner, stronger, flow into your next move." Neal became a member of a local Parkour tribe that likes to train after midnight, when the city is all theirs. Whenever a police car prowls by, they drop to the ground and bang out push-ups. "No matter what time it is, no one bothers you when you're exercising." Within a year, Neal was so fit and trim he was able to scramble to the roof of a three-story building and hang off the flagpole like Spider-Man. "You're back," he told himself.

But if I really wanted to learn, Neal pointed out, I was in the wrong parking lot. I took his advice and found myself a few weeks later struggling to the top of a twenty-foot retaining wall in a London housing project while a woman half my size and twice my strength stretched out a hand to help me over the top. Ordinarily the climb wouldn't have been that tough, but after two hours of Shirley Darlington's wild urban obstacle course, my legs and arms were jelly. Every Thursday, Shirley blasts an e-mail to the hundred or so members of her all-female crew, revealing the secret location for that night's challenge. She keeps the venue a surprise so her crew never knows what to expect, and she keeps guys away because the biggest threat to Parkour—as even the Yamakasi would agree—is testosterone.

"Young guys turn up, and lots of times all they want is the flash and not the fundamentals," says Dan Edwardes, the master instructor who gave Shirley her start. "They want to backflip off a wall and leap around on rooftops. With a group of lads, you'll get the show-off, the questioner, the giddy one. But in a women's group, there's none of that. It's very quiet. They get to it."

Back in 2005, Dan stepped in to solve a problem the Yamakasi weren't equipped to handle. No one outside the Yamakasi inner circle really knew what Parkour was supposed to be, and the Yamakasi weren't interested in explaining. David Belle is an artist, not a teacher; he wants to create new moves, not break down old ones. "The only way you could get into it was if you were determined and crazy enough to find some guys practicing and try to keep up," Dan explains. "There was no teaching, no guidance." Dan was in the same fix, but he got lucky: he met François "Forrest" Mahop, a Yamakasi acolyte living in the tough London borough of Westminster. Forrest agreed to let Dan shadow him, and at that moment a crime-fighting duo was formed.

"There's a lot of gun crime in the area, a lot of knife crime," Forrest would explain. "A lot goes on after dark that most people don't see." A Westminster rec director saw Dan and Forrest leaping around the city one day and realized they were doing exactly what kids are always told not to. In his mind, wheels started whirring. The more they tried to keep youngsters off the streets at night, the more they rebelled. Since they were going to run wild anyway, why not run wild under adult supervision? He asked if Forrest and Dan would teach a few sample classes on Friday nights, just to see whether it could keep some bodies off the streets.

"As a government body, that was visionary," Dan marveled. "In France, Parkour was vilified."

But when the rest of the Westminster City Council found out, they were appalled. "They thought we were going to train kids to escape the police," Forrest would recall. Most UK schools believed Parkour was so dangerous and rebellious, they wouldn't even allow it on the playgrounds. In the United States, a university graduate student made headlines when campus police tasered and handcuffed him after mistaking his Parkour training for a drug episode. (On a personal note, I was disinvited from a speaking event at a public library when I mentioned I'd be talking about Parkour.) Anything that wild and daring has to be a magnet for juvenile delinquents—and it was. More than a hundred kids turned up for the debut session, and it was bedlam.

Then Forrest and Dan got to work. They began hammering home the Parkour ethic—"Respect your environment. Respect other people"—and taking the young thugs out in the streets to train. "They reappropriate their city space," Dan says. "They're less likely to vandalize or litter or cause trouble if they have ownership of it." Soon, something changed.

"We saw young people that a couple of weeks ago were swearing at them in the classroom, now they're nodding and saying, 'Yes, Dan. Yes, Forrest,'" says Cory Wharton-Malcolm, the Westminster sports development officer. "To be able to watch that change over a period of weeks is amazing." The police were even more dumbfounded. "Metropolitan Police came back and said crime among that age group had dropped 69 percent, which was a mind-blowing stat," Dan says. *Sixty-nine percent!* "That was a huge validation that this actually works."

Dan felt a change coming over himself as well. "Until then, I was about improving myself. Now I thought, *Right. Let's see how many people we can reach and how far we can take it.*"

Dan's next frontier arrived in the form of a single mom playing wingman for her nervous cousin. Shirley Darlington was sixteen when she dropped out of high school to help support her family after her father died, and nineteen when she had a baby of her own. Shirley knew she'd boxed herself into a bleak future, so she began scrambling for a way out. She sold sneakers by day while getting her high school degree at night, then began university studies while creating a job for herself with the health council as a mentor for other teen moms. "I had to grow up fast," she explains. "I was working full-time and caring for an infant. I didn't have time to play." She had two other reasons for begging off when her cousin was too shy to go to Parkour alone: "Never heard of it" and "God, I haven't exercised since PE class in school five years ago."

Shirley eventually caved—and regretted it. She and her cousin arrived for the Westminster class and found themselves alone in a sea of lads pulling themselves over brick walls twice as high as their heads. But the heckling and the babying they expected never came. When Shirley and her cousin struggled with a drill, two of the lads who'd already finished silently circled back and completed it by their side. "There's no written code for Parkour, but pretty much everywhere you find the same principles," Dan says. "At some point, even the strongest person freezes on a jump. It teaches you humility and reminds you where you came from." That's why no one ever finishes a challenge alone. "Even from the beginning, with the Yamakasi," Dan points out, "Parkour was always about community."

Dan began having his own visionary breakthrough. Night after night, he watched Shirley show up for class even though she was weak and clumsy and usually exhausted from work and class and pre-dawn baby feedings. For two years, Shirley struggled to do her first pull-up. "She used to just hang from the bar," Dan says. "She'd pull and pull and she wouldn't move one centimeter." But she continued showing up and grabbing for the bar until a year later, Shirley nailed her first "muscle-up"—a challenging and essential Parkour maneuver in which you continue the pull-up until you're waist high on the bar and can vault yourself on top. By her fifth year, Shirley was not only outperforming the men, like a modern-day Atalanta—she'd become the one circling back to help struggling lads. The real obstacle wasn't strength, she discovered; it was trust. "I never knew what my body could do, so it took a long time to build the confidence to throw my full weight into a movement," Shirley says. "Once I did, it changed everything."

It's great we're winning over young guys and thinning out the predators, Dan thought as he watched Shirley's transformation. *But what if we also empowered everyone else?* In 2005, only five women in the world practiced Parkour, which Dan found insane. "The time has come for all of us, men and women alike, to adapt to the world we now live in," Dan believes. By the year 2050, after all, six of every seven people on the planet will live in a city. "We have to shape our training to fit our lifestyle," Dan says. "We're no longer surrounded by trees, so we have to learn to climb walls."

Dan began playing with an idea: What if women discovered they could be just as strong in the city as they were in the wild? What if they knew they could climb, run, jump, and adapt as powerfully as any man? Dan couldn't really make the case himself, being a man. But he knew someone who could.

On the Thursday morning I arrived in London, my phone pinged with a message from Shirley:

Kilburn tube station, 7 pm.

I got there ten minutes early, but about twenty women were already warming up, including the British movie actress Christina Chong and her sister Lizzi, a professional dancer. We set off at a jog, arriving about a half-mile later at a cement courtyard in the middle of a high-rise housing project. Shirley had us line up at the top of a long, zigzagging access ramp and drop to all fours. We monkey-walked on hands and feet about forty yards to the bottom, then bunny-hopped up the stairs and did it again backwards; then crab style; then squat-hopping, each time with a new twist and a push-up between circuits.

By the thirteenth loop, my hands were cement-scuffed and my head was spinning from being at knee height for so long, but the parade of hopping, bear-crawling, push-upping women showed no sign of slowing. I looked around for Shirley, but she'd disappeared into our midst. "The best Parkour coaches are invisible," Dan told me. "They get you started, then get out of the way." I spotted her again when three men took a seat on the wall and began sharing a smoke and loud comments on the women's bodies. Shirley quietly peeled off from the circuit and trotted over to a swingset. She leaped for the crossbar, and in a blur somehow ended up squatting on top. It's become her signature move, and it's a showstopper.

Not long ago, she'd teamed up with Felicity "Fizz" Hood and Anne-Therese "Annty" Marais for an extraordinary YouTube clip called "Movement of 3." In little more than two minutes, the three cat-leap up and over a seven-foot wall, land precision jumps on two-inch guardrails, execute a hand-to-hand traverse along a rooftop railing, and then Annty and Fizz catapult themselves through a swingset while the single mom who couldn't do a pull-up when she began Parkour squats on the bar above their heads, perfectly balanced while blowing soap bubbles.

This time, Shirley lowers herself from the bar with such slow grace and power that the three mopes on the wall shove their cigarettes in their mouths so their hands are free to applaud.

Moving on! Shirley's tribe is heading out, so I have to sling my bag on my back in a hurry and sprint to catch up. For the next two hours, North West London is our playground. Shirley leads us to metal benches, where we practice diving into shoulder rolls and popping back up on a dead run. She finds a beaut of a wall where we work on running arm jumps: running straight up the bricks, basically, and grabbing for the top of the wall, and hoisting ourselves up when momentum dies and gravity takes over. Well after dark, we're all clinging to a railing as we traverse a cement wall in a hanging squat. My feet are slipping and I'm in danger of dropping off when Lizzi Chong tucks in beside me. "Get your knees higher," she says. "You're relying on your arms, but this is about legs."

Step by step, we work our way to the end, then drop to all fours and bear-crawl on hands and feet back to the beginning; press out our fortieth or so push-up of the night; and get ready for another loop. I try to thank Lizzi for the help, but she waves me off. "I needed a hand to hold when I started because I thought it was too dangerous," she said. "If I break an ankle, that's my career." But after her first class, she was hooked. "I could see the dance in it. The flow, the rhythms, the strength and danger. You're always on the edge of fear, because your body senses it can do more than your mind will let it."

By the time Shirley cuts us loose for the night, I never want to do Parkour again and can't wait to come back. I didn't just run and climb all over North West London; I still had its cement grit deep under my fingernails. *This must be what George Psychoundakis meant when he said a true Cretan citizen is a* dromeus, *a runner,* I thought. *Someone who can handle any obstacle and circle his hometown like a guardian spirit.*

CHAPTER 21

﹄﹂
┓┏

"WE'RE HEADING into 'Evaders Country,'" Chris called back, leading
us off the crags and across some jagged stone flats toward the Samaría
Gorge: baddest of the badlands. "It's where a lot of Allied soldiers hid
after they were left behind by the evacuation."

Samaría is a thunderbolt in stone, a thin gash that splits two rock
towers and zigzags eleven miles upward from the beach until it crests
on a grassy mountain plateau. It's a terrific place to hide, because the
walls are honeycombed with caverns; tuck inside one and dislodging
you could be lethal. No one can get down to you from above, and
coming up from below means crossing your kill zone. During the
war, the Gorge became a free-for-all zone for Evaders, who could see
pursuers coming from miles away and scamper down to the beach
whenever they heard rumors of a rescue boat, and the "wind boys"—
Cretan desperadoes whose only allegiance was to their own cutthroat
gang.

George had his own run-in with the wind boys while he and another
guerrilla were crossing the Gorge with a message for the Resistance.
George played it cool, bantering with them cautiously from halfway
behind a boulder while covering them with the pistol in his pocket,
but his partner ran for it. The wind boys caught him with a rifle shot,
and in the turmoil George vanished among the rocks and slipped
off. Miraculously, George found his partner the next day, passed out
miles away from a bullet wound through his arm. George got him to
a guerrillas' den, then pushed on with his mission.

The White brothers and I slept at the base of the Gorge, but not for long. By 3 A.M. we were up and setting off for the trailhead. Climbing the Gorge is daunting on a good day, especially when you tilt your head way back and realize you'll be walking through those clouds overhead and still be a good way from the top. We took another look at the clouds, glowing in a milky moon. If they opened up, we were in trouble; we'd be pinned in a water chute where going back down would be as risky as pushing on up.

"It had to be terrifying for the Germans," Pete mused. "Jumping out of a plane over an island full of born-murderers who all hate you. Survive that, and they send you into this place"—he jerked his head toward the rain-forest foliage around the dark trail—"to hunt men who are better at hunting *you.*"

Lovely. I wasn't surprised by the scope of Pete's empathy—his chosen career, after all, is nurturing plants and teaching learning-disabled adults to create with their hands—but it was eerie to suddenly be reminded how horrifying this wilderness used to be. It's hard not to feel tiny and trapped at the bottom of a canyon, especially when you begin to sense all the invisible eyes once hidden by its caves and gnarled trees. The Gorge still has that feeling of menace and evil opportunity, at least until the sun comes up. By midmorning we were bumping into a few downhill hikers, and then a merry stream. Samaría has become a popular tourist route, but only in one direction: groups are dropped off at the top by bus, then picked up at the bottom by ferry and hauled back to their beach hotels.

Heading up, we were alone. We crested the trail by early afternoon, climbing out of the woods into a freezing mountain wind and a light patter of rain. We took a breather before pushing on to Lakki, a village somewhere on the far side of the grassy Omalos Plateau. As we tore into sardines and chunks of bread from our packs, we watched a man snipping something by the side of the road and shoving it into a blue plastic grocery bag. Pete walked over for a closer look, and discovered one of the special weapons of the Cretan Resistance.

"It's nasturtium," Pete reported back: an orange weed with tasty leaves and flowers. Like most places, Crete has weeds growing in every stony crack; but unlike most places, Cretans devour them. Weeds of all stripe—dandelion, purslane, chicory, sorrel—are picked and braised and tossed together in a peppery mix called *horta.* With a citrusy squirt of lemon and a little olive oil for fat and flavor, *horta* is a nutritional powerhouse of iron, calcium, omega-3 fatty acids, plus an alphabet soup of vitamins. For a man on the run, it was a life saver; superfood fixin's were nearly everywhere, nearly any time, and always fresh and delicious.

Unless you had Paddy's palate, that is. "He *hated* horta," says Artemis Cooper—but he had to respect it.

Oddly, I'd discovered a living handbook of the ancient Cretan eating arts in the form of a ballerina prowling Brooklyn's Prospect Park. When she's not teaching dance in Manhattan or choreographing new pieces, Leda Meredith likes to walk the park in both winter and summer and stuff her backpack with foraged findings: garlic mustard and pepper grass, lemony sorrel and asparagus-like pokeberry shoots, gummy mallow leaf and tangy lamb's-quarter and delectable ginkgo—yes, ginkgo, those horrific gooey globules that litter city sidewalks every spring and stink up the bottom of your shoes.

"I have to race Koreans for the ginkgo," Leda mentioned when we set off into the park one September morning. "If I'm too slow, all I'll find is the remains where they field-dressed a pile. You take the fruit, squeeze off the yellow squishy part, and save the kernels for roasting. Delicious." I figured the early autumn cold snap meant we'd come home empty-handed, but within four feet Leda had already spotted prey. "Lamb's-quarter!" she exulted, easing a leafy clump out of the lawn. She singled out a strand and pointed to the powdery coating on the arrowhead leaves.

"They look dusty, right? That's your identifier."

"I've seen this all over every lawn I've ever mowed," I said. "It's edible?"

"It's like kale and chard," Leda said. "It sells for seven-fifty a pound in the Park Slope Coop, but guess what? It's growing in the sidewalk right out front." Leda squatted and came up with a fistful of another weed I'd seen forever. She pointed out its tiny pink flowers and the dark smudge on a slender droopy leaf which resembles the smudge of an inky thumb. "Lady's Thumb. It's a little bitter, but chop it into a salad with some sorrel and it's wonderful. It's from the buckwheat family, so it's packed with nutrients."

As a girl, Leda learned the art of foraging from her Greek immigrant family in San Francisco. Leda's mother was a ballerina with a Los Angeles ballet company, so Leda was raised mostly by her grandmother. "Every spring, there came a moment when Yia-Yia Lopi, my great-grandmother, stubbed out her Kool menthol cigarette and declared that it was the right day to gather *horta* in the park," Leda explains. "The timing had to be just right: too soon and the leaves would be too small, too late and they'd be too bitter. Yia-Yia was the expert on when to go because she'd grown up picking wild edibles in Greece." Back in the kitchen, the women steamed the greens and mixed them with olive oil and chopped garlic. "Their eyes would gleam," Leda notes. "The first wild greens of spring were better to them than chocolate."

Leda followed her mother into dance, winning a full scholarship to the American Ballet Theatre and later signing with the Manhattan Ballet. But she still kept roaming the parks for feral foods, once shocking prima ballerina Cynthia Gregory by sliding in next to her at a dinner party with her arms covered with raw scratches from reaching between thorny branches. During downtime between dance tours, Leda would spend months harvesting olives with her relatives in Greece or traveling Europe and California as a seasonal fruit picker, happy to be surrounded by fragrant, pluckable, biteable life. She began taking classes in ethnobotany at the New York Botanical Garden and studying with the yup-that's-her-real-name herbalist Susan Weed. Leda would lead her friends and fellow dancers on all-day hunt-and-picks, then bring the famished hikers back to her apartment and teach them how to cook their haul. As her performance career came to an end, Leda realized she'd been working on her new calling since she was six years old.

"The parks department has a limited weed-control budget, which is great for me," she says. Leda now leads foraging tours and teaches classes at both the New York and Brooklyn botanical gardens. "People have no idea what's right here," she adds. Streams and ponds all over the Northeast are thick with watercress, a leafy green "superfood" that outscores spinach and chard as the most nutritionally dense of all vegetables. Often, however, wild watercress is mistaken as a nuisance weed and either discarded or ignored.

"Like this—" Leda points to a cabbagey mess I've grown to hate on sight. As a kid, I scraped my knuckles bloody every summer trying to dig those things out of sidewalk cracks in front of the house. "That's burdock," Leda explains. "It grows in cities where nothing else will, and it's fabulous." Burdock has a long, thick taproot that's a bear to unearth, but take it home and slice into a stir-fry and you've got a plateful of the Japanese delicacy *gobo*.

The challenge for beginners is knowing what you're yanking. Crete alone has more than a hundred varieties of wild edible greens. Many look identical but have different flavors and aromas, not to mention nutritional and medicinal benefits. "Stomach problems, skin disorders, breathing difficulties, even emotional uneasiness—you can treat them all with so-called weeds," Leda explains. "It's too bad we've developed this mentality that if it's free and natural, it can't be good."

Actually, a closer look shows that this Cretan snack stuffed with wild greens packs more nutritional punch than just about any fruit or vegetable you can buy. When scientists from Austria and Greece performed a chemical analysis of a Cretan fried pie in 2006, they were struck by two things: the sheer variety of the filling and the sky-high levels of vitamins, antioxidants, and essential fatty acids. The bite-size crescents, called *kalitsounia*, are typically packed with a combination of fennel, wild leeks, sow thistle, hartwort, corn poppy, sorrel, and Queen Anne's lace, all of it growing wild and calorically dense. "In most cases," the researchers found, "the wild greens had higher micronutrient content than those cultivated."

Even more intriguing: greens keep Cretans in harmony with two million years of human history. For most of our ancestral existence, humans maintained a healthy balance between omega-6 fatty acids— which provide a healthy amount of protective inflammation—and omega-3's, which keep inflammation in check. Overdo it with omega-6 and you become high-risk for heart disease and neurological disorders. Our hunter-gatherer ancestors had a one-to-one ratio. Today, ours is more like *sixteen* to one. Since the proliferation of vegetable and soybean oils in processed foods, omega-6 consumption has been through the roof. Instead of a small fire to warm the house, we've created an inferno that's burning it down.

Except on Crete. "By including daily wild greens in their diet, the population of Crete was able to supplement their diet not only with vitamins and antioxidants but also with essential fatty acids in a ratio similar to that kept by the local Minoan population 4,500 years ago," the researchers found. "The traditional diet of Crete," they add, "is similar to the ratio kept during human evolution."

But for beginners, foraging is bewildering. Books aren't much help: greens all kind of look the same on the page, and they're usually photographed in blossom, when the pictures are prettiest but the prime plucking period has already passed. Luckily, Leda came up with a genius solution: let hatred be your guide.

"Do you have something around your house you can't stand?" she asked.

"Nettles," I immediately replied. "Burn nettles. I can't get rid of it."

"Stop trying. You're lucky. Nettles are free spinach." Cooking or drying neutralizes the sting, and what you're left with is a tasty, leafy green that makes a great lasagna, pesto, soup, or pizza topping.

"If you hate it, you'll recognize it," Leda explains. "Start with two or three things you see all the time—like dandelions and Lady's Thumb—and add things you hate, like nettles, and that's plenty to keep you busy as you expand your visual vocabulary." And like the "Evaders" on Crete, who scrabbled to feed themselves from the harsh stones of the Samaría Gorge, it won't be long before you realize that everything you need to survive—and thrive—is right at your feet.

From the top of the Samaría Gorge, Chris White took aim for the hilltop village of Lakki.

By map it was only a few miles off, but that meant nothing on an island where geography is measured by degree of difficulty rather than distance. We found a faint footpath, but when it climbed into the rocky highlands and disappeared, we seized on a free guide service: goats. Goats head back to the fold as it gets dark, and since there was nothing else between us and Lakki, all we had to do was follow the coppery clong of their bells and they'd lead us right to the village.

"Wait wait WAIT!" Chris threw his arms wide to stop us. He was staring down at a long drop a few inches from his feet and remembering a crucial detail we'd forgotten: goats have a much different approach to risk management. Our guides had bounded right over the edge, hopping along a staircase of tiny perches that was impossible to follow without hooves or ropes. We had to back up and bushwhack a new route; which failed; so we reversed course; tried again; failed again. . . .

By the time we got off the cliff, the bells were long gone. We found a dry creek bed and decided to stick with it, clambering over driftwood jams and rock washes until, just before nightfall, we reached the last hill below Lakki. Thank heaven. Fourteen hours of hard trail were coming to an end.

An hour later, Lakki was no closer.

The village was *right there*. We could see it; we could *smell* it as the woodsmoke from evening fires drifted down. But. We. Could. Not. Get. There. We'd pushed our way through brambles and climbed rock walls, but every route we tried was a dead end or a semicircle, dropping us right back in the creek bed. The stinking hill was bewitched.

To hell with it. Pete dropped to his belly and began to claw his way straight up, kneeing and pulling himself along like a man escaping quicksand. Chris and I watched, knowing he wouldn't get far before he hit an unclimbable cliff and gave up. Then we shrugged, dropped to our bellies, and followed. Stupid movement seemed better than no movement at all. Instead of a cliff, Pete came to an ancient stack of lava rock, wedged nicely into the hill like a climbing wall, and on the far side, a muddy pen behind a lonely farm house. We crawled up and sploshed through and came out to find the road.

You pull any stunts out there, I thought as we trudged under the early-evening moon into the tiny village, *you better know what you're doing*. We were filthy, exhausted, and shivering. It was hard to fathom sleeping a few hours in a cave and setting off to do it again—or racing up that hill, with a hostile German general in tow, to save our own lives.

CHAPTER 22

[Xan] Fielding had a plan to kidnap the GERMAN
commanding officer . . . and hold him as a hostage.

—OFFICIAL BRITISH REPORT OF THE CRETAN RESISTANCE,
1941–1945

LET'S GET THE BUTCHER.

The idea was insane, but once it took hold in Paddy's mind, it
refused to let go.

Let's make the Butcher . . . disappear.

If Paddy could learn what the Clown knew, he might just be able
to pull it off. It would be a masterpiece of street magic, the perfect
crime perpetrated on one of the world's worst criminals—a man protected by five divisions of German troops suddenly vanishing without
a trace. George Psychoundakis liked to tell the British secret agents
he'd teach them the Cretan art of sheep stealing so they could go
home after the war with a practical skill. Well, this was his chance.
They'd bring the rules of the shepherd to the battlefield.

But for a romantic poet, Paddy had a hard-nosed side. He'd lived
by his wits during his years on the road and understood the difference between striving and surviving. Getting the Butcher wasn't the
biggest problem; the biggest problem would be getting away. As far as
Paddy knew, no one had even thought of kidnapping a general before.

Colin Gubbins had written an entire "Art of Guerrilla Warfare" manual for SOE agents after Churchill put him in charge of training, but nothing in there related to sneaking a general through enemy lines and off a fortified island. Nothing, that is, except Gubbins's motto:

> To inflict damage and death on the enemy and to escape scot-free has an irritant and depressing effect. . . . The object must be to strike hard and disappear before the enemy can strike back.

And in a peculiar way, John Pendlebury was proving it. About the time Paddy arrived in June, information was surfacing from Cretans who'd been with Pendlebury during the invasion. Bit by bit, it was beginning to sound as if he'd never made it to the White Mountains at all. In fact, Pendlebury may have been killed while Allied troops were still being evacuated from the island. Fragments of the story were still coming together, but if true, then for nearly a year the Germans had been chasing a dead man. Even in death, Pendlebury was still in the fight.

Maybe that was the best Paddy and George could hope for. "I had read somewhere that the average life of an infantry officer in the First World War was eight weeks, and I had no reason to think that the odds would be much better in the Second," Paddy acknowledged. He was even more at risk as a sabotage agent—and if a mountain-hardened, Crete-savvy outdoorsman like Pendlebury couldn't make it, what chance did Paddy have? Likewise, George knew he was a marked man. German storm troopers had already tried to trap him once in his village. They'd be back. The noose was tightening.

So why not die a hunter, rather than the hunted? When the Germans captured Athens, they ordered the old flag keeper at the Acropolis to lower the Greek flag and replace it with the swastika-emblazoned Reichskriegsflagge. Konstandinos Koukidis obediently took down the Greek flag—then wrapped himself in it and dived headfirst from a battlement. The Germans raised the Reichskriegsflagge over his corpse, but a few nights later, two Greek teenagers snuck behind the guards, cut it down, and ran for it. The Gestapo issued a death order for the two boys and anyone harboring them, but months afterwards, they were still on the loose. At a time when no force on earth seemed powerful enough to defy the Nazis, two boys electrified Europe by honoring an old man's sacrifice and snatching Hitler's flag. Imagine snatching one of his generals.

There was one chance of pulling it off, Paddy figured: they'd have to become as strong and wily as the Clown. They'd have to master the art of survival in those "merciless mountains," as Paddy called them, and rely on whatever it was the Clown did out there—running, climbing, dodging, conniving, foraging on the fly. They'd have to go places the Germans couldn't, and move faster and more nimbly than anyone thought possible.

They'd have to follow in the footsteps of Odysseus, that other inventive and unstoppable Greek—and try to forget that, out of all his crew, only Odysseus made it home alive.

Oddly, both Paddy and Xan had come up with the same idea on their own. Before Paddy told Xan about his plan to snatch the Butcher, Xan was already mulling the possibility of grabbing a general to protect the villagers from German attacks.

We grab the bugger, tie him up, and tell the Jerries whatever they do to a Cretan, we do to him. It was an idea worth considering, but first Xan would have to endure a different ordeal. George led him through the night to a tiny village in the mountains—and there, ready to celebrate Christmas, were Paddy and Tom Dunbabin, another Oxford archeologist, who'd been sent to replace Monty Woodhouse.

The three men were positive the Germans would ease up for the holidays—well, pretty positive—so they threw themselves into the full onslaught of Cretan merrymaking. "We reeled happily from home to home eating and drinking with hosts who seemed as carefree as though no Germans had ever been heard of in Crete," Xan recalled. "We found the same conditions in every village we passed during our slow three-day procession down the valley."

Paddy knew the Germans weren't having this kind of fun, because he'd heard them say so. Shortly before Xan's return, the Firm sent Paddy on a mission to blow up German warships with some magnetic mines. Paddy infiltrated the port and quickly made his assessment: *Not Bloody Likely.* They wanted him to swim across the harbor between the searchlights with those big hunks of metal strapped to his back? The only way he wouldn't get shot was if he drowned first. Which raised another tactical difficulty: the partner he'd been assigned couldn't swim. Paddy decided to abort and beat it out of town. He holed up in a safe house to wait for dark, but suddenly heard German voices. Two German sergeants, he realized, were billeted next door. He tuned in to their conversation and heard something intriguing. *"Weit von der Heimat . . ."* he heard one say. Far from Mother Germany . . .

See? They're homesick. That was the actionable intel Paddy had picked up while Xan was away. *This is the fourth year in a row the Germans have missed Christmas with their families. They're not out drinking and singing with friends like we are. They're scratching lice and eating awful grub and wondering why they haven't heard from their wives. They're lonely and uncertain. We can use that.*

Xan had to marvel at Paddy. Xan's first winter on Crete had left him bony and ragged as a hobo, but this guy—magnificent! Somehow, six months of cave living and mountain scrambling had turned Paddy into a Hollywood pirate. "His moustache always had a dashing twist in it," Xan noted. "His boots, which he wore out at the rate of one pair a month, were beautifully kept until they fell to pieces on his feet; to knot his black turban at the most becoming angle, he took infinite pains; and to complete his operational wardrobe he had just ordered a Cretan waistcoat of royal-blue broadcloth lined with scarlet shot-silk and embroidered with arabesques of black braid." One way or the other, Paddy was coming out of this war in style.

Tom Dunbabin was just as handsome but less of a dandy; when it came to protective coloring, the worse he looked, the better he felt. He was a towering, farm-raised Tasmanian with a mind formidable enough to take him to Oxford and a professorship in Greek classics, so masquerading as a harmless mountain peasant took some serious stagecraft. Xan was quite impressed with the result. "In ragged breeches and black fringed turban, with his overgrown corkscrew moustache coiling and uncoiling in the breeze of his own breath, he looked like a successful local sheep-thief," Xan observed. "He even managed to introduce a characteristic note of hysteria into his high-pitched voice."

Crooks were Tom's favorite mentors, and he recruited as many as he could find. "The best man you can have with you in the hills is a converted sheep thief," Tom explained. "He knows all the paths and pathless ways, and where to lie up and spy out the land. He is a good mover over any country, day or night." You couldn't go wrong with a good murderer, either. "He has probably spent years in the hills avoiding the justice of the state and his victims' kinsmen," Tom pointed out, "and knows every crag and cave." Tom learned so much from his bandit buddies that once, during a recon mission, he came face-to-face with an old acquaintance—a German archeologist turned Wehrmacht officer—who looked Tom dead in the eye without recognizing him inside the shepherd's disguise.

While the outlaws were schooling Tom and Paddy in evasion, shepherds showed them how to forage for survival. "They knew the mountains, knew the paths and hiding places, and most of them had a rifle. If necessary, they could do without the villages and lowlands, and live on their own milk and meat," Tom explained. "They were naturally in fine physical condition, could run up a hill-side most of us would find it hard to get up at all, and were wonderfully light on their feet." Tom and Paddy crested so many mountains during their apprenticeship that they were left with only a single pair of decent boots between them. "I crippled myself over these boots," Tom grimaced, "marching in a pair too small for me while Paddy borrowed the good pair."

But despite all those miles, they were still wrestling with the final test of authenticity: the Cretan Bounce. Paddy once leaped to the top of a stone wall to demonstrate he had it, only to amuse the Clown by toppling back over again. "The quick eyes of the Cretans could generally pick us out by our walk," Tom admitted. "Other details—dress, features, moustache—could pass, but none of us acquired the gait of a Cretan hillman, for all our practice."

The three men had a wonderful Christmas. For four days they wandered about "slightly drunk and unescorted," as Xan put it, calling on friends across the highlands. They sang and danced and feasted, forgetting for a time that they were living under a death sentence. No matter how glib their Greek or how convincing their farmer's cloaks and women's dresses, they knew they couldn't get away with this game for long. Sooner or later they'd meet an ambush, a traitor, or a dark and icy cliff, and Crete would become—as it had for John Pendlebury—their Appointment in Samarra.

Because Paddy was right: down below in the barracks, the Germans weren't having nearly as much fun. They were loading weapons, squeezing informants, and eyeing the weather in the mountains above. Hitler smelled trouble on the Sliver, and he wanted it taken care of *now*.

•   •   •

Defense wasn't Hitler's specialty. He knew how to knock you down; he had no plan for when you got back up. He liked sneak attacks and lightning strikes, the kind of shock tactics that were great when his troops were on the move but useless when they were pushed back and hunkered into trenches. But as Hitler looked at the giant map in his command room during the final weeks of 1942, his eye for a stab in the back came in handy: it told him exactly what Churchill would do next and where he would do it.

Crete *had* to be Churchill's next target; by Christmas, it was already the sweet spot between Hitler's shoulder blades. He'd pushed his troops deep into Africa and Russia, and now they were mired in exactly the nightmare he'd dreaded. Germany's prize panzer corps was gasping for survival in Egypt, while Stalingrad was on the verge of becoming Hitler's bloodiest defeat. The Soviets who'd been surrounded by the Third Reich's Sixth Army had pulled off a miraculous reversal and surrounded them right back, trapping the Germans inside the city and exposing the Führer's inability to counterattack. The German response to the Soviet push was sheer bedlam. Day by day, the German high command second-guessed and dithered while nearly *a quarter-million* German soldiers trapped in Stalingrad were wiped out by bombs, bullets, disease, and starvation.

The last thing Hitler needed now was to wheel around and discover Crete was ablaze. He'd already seen what kind of havoc those lunatic farmers could get up to with their ancient guns and homemade bayonets, and all it would take for them to erupt was the go-ahead from Great Britain that help was on the way. German soldiers were already said to be wary of venturing into the White Mountains because some phantom from New Zealand had taken over for John Pendlebury as the new Lion of Crete.

Rumor had it the Lion was haunting the highlands with his own band of Cretan killers, and the truth wasn't far off. When the war broke out, Dudley Perkins was a university student following in his father's footsteps toward the ministry. He was soon behind barbed wire in a German POW camp after the fall of Crete, but he escaped into the White Mountains and spent a long winter learning to live off the land. Cretan woodsmen taught Dudley to search the riverbanks for eels and snails and freshwater crabs, and how to boil olive-tree fungus and wild mushrooms into a hearty and surprisingly tasty stew. By the time he met Xan Fielding, the aspiring preacher was a new and much deadlier man. The Lion appeared "much like I imagined Lawrence of Arabia must have looked," Xan would comment. "And in character, too, he closely resembled what I had read of the famous Arab leader." After German troops incinerated one village in the high country, Dudley formed the survivors into a fighting force two hundred strong. Not long after, a German patrol entered the Lion's territory; none of them made it out alive. The local German garrison sent eleven soldiers out to commandeer some food; their bodies were found at the bottom of a slot canyon.

This was Hitler's nightmare: invisible agitators who could stir the entire island into revolt. So Hitler decided to beat Churchill to the punch. Soldiers who were desperately needed in Russia were flown to Crete instead, boosting the on-ground strength to a combined German-Italian force of more than eighty thousand. Bunkers were dug, bridges were wired with explosives, access to the southern coast was triple-fortified, and a warning shot was fired from behind the walls of Fortress Crete, the impenetrable garrison in western Chania: "We will in the event of an invasion," German command announced, "defend Crete to the last man and the last round."

Now there was one last thing to do: exterminate the rats in their holes.

Shortly after New Year's Day, George Psychoundakis was hiking toward the village of Alones when he heard the thump of gunfire. "I crept behind a rock, and looking down, saw that the village was full of Germans. Just below me, about ten were climbing up the slope towards my vantage-point," George recounts. "I hid like lightning." Fading into the trees, George circled around Alones until he found someone who could fill him in. The news chilled him.

The Germans went straight to the priest's house and began tearing it apart, a villager told him. *They knew.*

The Germans discovered a British radio battery buried in the priest's garden, and a note to the British radio operator in his son's pocket. If they'd arrived a little sooner, they'd have found the radio operator himself. Luckily, and unbeknownst to the stool pigeon who'd led the Germans there, the Brits had abandoned Alones right after Christmas. But the Germans knew they couldn't be far, and they got right to work. The priest's son, his face battered and bloody, was dragged off to be tortured for information while troops surrounded the valley and began marching uphill in an ever-tightening noose.

Typically, that meant a remarkable number of locals would suddenly be welcoming family. *Our in-laws are arriving*, they'd call out. Others were vexed by livestock problems. *Watch out for your black sheep! They're in the wheatfield again*, they'd complain—loudly and repeatedly.

The alert spread until it reached Paddy, a few miles away. He and four of George's cousins put together a team to spirit away the bulky wireless radio set, hoisting it on their backs along with the big batteries and that brute of a charging engine. "Shifting our base had now become a feat of endurance," Xan explained, since any reasonably walkable trail had to be avoided. Paddy and his gang "had to carry the cumbersome gear piecemeal on their backs over trackless slopes at dead of night."

Freezing rain fell all night, slickening the snowy mountainside and doubling the weight of their packs. It took twelve hours, but by daybreak they'd climbed high enough to stash the radio and cut back to the rendezvous spot with Xan. Paddy's gang was ready to sink down and rest, but first they climbed a nearby peak for a last look around— and spotted dozens of dark helmets trudging through snow straight toward them. "As though they had got wind of our movements," Xan would exclaim, "the Germans had transferred their attention from Alones." Whoever was feeding the Germans information was becoming deadly accurate.

The morning mist gave Paddy's gang just enough of a head start to vanish before being spotted. By the time the sun burned through, most of the Cretans had bolted into slit caves in the cliffs. Xan hid in an old stone hut, while Paddy scrambled into the branches of a big cypress. Tromping boots soon approached . . . paused . . . faded away . . . and then returned, over and over again, as searchers crisscrossed the grove. Paddy was soaked and shivering; he'd barely eaten and hadn't slept, his body was stiff and aching from the all-night radio portage. He forced his body to freeze as the Germans passed back and forth beneath his feet.

And by the time the sun was setting and it was finally safe for him to slide down, one thing was clear: the playboy who'd shown up six months ago could now run and crawl and think and persevere like a Cretan. Maybe he couldn't pass for one just yet—but for what he had in mind, he might just be close enough.

CHAPTER 23

Suddenly the firing stopped, brought to an end not by a
Cease Fire order but by a sound far more blood curdling. . . .

—XAN FIELDING

"BLACK SHEEP!"

A few months after their near miss with the radio, Paddy and his
gang were just settling down for the night when they heard a lookout
calling out a secret warning. Germans were on the move, three hundred or more, still a good way off but coming fast. Paddy grabbed his
rifle and was stunned when it suddenly fired. A few feet away, Yanni
Tsangarakis—Paddy's closest Cretan friend—dropped to the ground,
bleeding. Paddy's bullet had smashed through Yanni's hip and rico-
cheted up through his guts. Paddy and the others desperately shoved
their hands down on the wounds, but it was no use. Yanni whispered
his farewells and died.

Paddy was horrified. He knew what he had to do: as soon as they
were clear of the Germans, he'd go to Yanni's family and put himself
at their mercy.

Terrible idea, Yanni's friend argued. *What good are two corpses? Some
fool will say you did it on purpose, and someone will believe him. Yanni didn't
blame you, but his family will. We've got to say the Germans shot him. It's*

the best thing for Yanni. He'll be remembered as a patriot. You'll get the chance to die like one.

Paddy churned over his dilemma as they slipped Yanni's body off to safety and buried him in the shade of two holly oaks. His gang was right about one thing: island chatter was notorious. "No news? Then tell me a lie" was a favorite Cretan joke. *Okay, then*—Paddy agreed to lie and pretend Yanni had been killed in a firefight. "I want to say that I did not agree to this hateful fiction out of a wish to shirk my responsibilities, but for the sake of Yanni and his family, and our work on Crete," a miserable Paddy would explain. But whether Yanni's clan would believe it was another story. They'd be aching for details; they'd want to know who else was injured, and why was Yanni cornered when he'd escaped so many times. *Tell us again, how many Germans were killed in this fight that killed our Yanni?* The second they smelled something fishy, they'd come looking for answers.

Paddy was still in the dumps over that disaster when he was tapped to perform a bit of street magic. The Allies had invaded Sicily, and the Italians, fed up with Mussolini, had tossed him out of office. Hitler would soon toss Mussolini right back in again, but in the meantime, German command was giving Italian forces two ugly options: they could be folded into the German army or locked up in a German labor gang.

But General Angelo Carta, the Italian commander, was secretly offered a back door. Word was passed by the underground that if he was willing to cooperate with Allied forces, a British operative would find a way to spirit him off the island. Carta agreed, and Paddy got the assignment. Just before setting off, however, Paddy received a strange warning: a band of Cretan Communists threatened to betray Paddy if he got up to any funny business with the Italians. The Communists weren't battling the Germans just so the British could take over, so they wanted Paddy to steer clear of the Italian zone. They were supposed to be fighting the same enemy, but the Communists weren't above a little treachery if they suspected the British and the non-Communist Resistance fighters were gaining too much power.

Paddy's friends, meanwhile, were causing even more trouble than his rivals. Manoli Bandouvas, Crete's most ferocious guerrilla chieftain, was ecstatic when he got news of the Italian pullback and decided it was the time to go for the Germans' throats. Without making sure his allies had his back, Bandouvas and his three-hundred-strong band called for a mass uprising and went on the attack. They wiped out two garrisons and killed more than thirty Germans, which was just enough to infuriate General Müller but not enough to convince Bandouvas that he had a prayer of actually winning. The Butcher lashed out with a spree of retaliation, murdering five hundred civilians and incinerating six entire villages. More than two thousand troops stormed into the mountains with one order: bring back the head of Bandouvas. Somehow, the rebel chief slipped away and showed up at Tom Dunbabin's hideout looking for help. As long as Paddy was taking the Italian general off the island, couldn't he take Bandouvas as well? Just till the heat died down?

Wonderful. Paddy's getaway route was now swarming with fire teams. Instead of one hot target to transport he had two, and instead of one blood enemy, he might be running from three: the Germans, the Communists, and the revenge-seeking clan of poor Yanni. Paddy forged ahead anyway, and emerged from the shadows on September 16 for his rendezvous with General Carta. Just before they left, Paddy was hissed to one side by Lieutenant Franco Tavana, Carta's chief of intelligence.

Don't lose this, Tavana whispered, pushing a satchel into Paddy's hands. *And don't let the general know you have it.* Tavana had stuffed it with classified documents. *Now everything we know about German operations, you know.* Tavana had already won a reputation among his enemies as honorable, brave, and apparently on their side. He had never pulled his trigger on a Cretan; whenever he caught a guerrilla, Tavana would just order him to move along into the German zone. Tavana despised the situation the Germans had gotten him into, and he was about to prove it: given the chance to escape with Carta, he decided to stay and join the Resistance.

Tavana learned very quickly how dangerous that would be. The Butcher was shrewd, and it didn't take him long to connect the dots. Bandouvas wouldn't suddenly go wild on his own; no, he must have spotted an opportunity because he knew the Italians were up to something. The Butcher and an armored security squad raced toward Carta's base but arrived a few hours too late; Paddy and the general had already disappeared into the piney snarls of the snow-capped Dikti Mountains, while Tavana was climbing toward the Resistance's caves with a load of Italian weapons.

No mercy, the Butcher fumed: he wanted Carta dead or alive. To entice the Cretans to turn him in, the Butcher offered a thirty-million-drachma reward, a fortune for a starving farm family. Spotter planes buzzed the mountains, searching for the missing general and scattering reward notices. One leaflet fluttered down at Carta's feet as he and Paddy were slinking through the woods. "Thirty pieces of silver," Carta mused. "A contract of Judas." If he made it to Egypt, he decided, he'd have to send the Butcher a nice letter in return.

Bandouvas and Tom Dunbabin caught up with Paddy during the final push toward the coast, and together they crept down to a hidden cove. A week earlier, General Carta and the rebel chieftain would have shot each other on sight; now, they took a seat on the beach, shuffled a deck, and dealt cards while Paddy and Tom scanned the dark horizon. Long after midnight, a rubber dinghy purred to shore. Tom was going to accompany Bandouvas to Cairo and take some long overdue leave, but first Paddy wanted to ferry Carta out so he could personally put the secret-documents satchel in the skipper's hand. Before Tom could point out that he was just as capable of carrying the bag, Paddy was off.

That'll have to do, the skipper said when Paddy and Carta reached the boat. *Time to go.* The sea was rough and threatening to throw them up on the rocks. Tom and Bandouvas watched in dismay from shore as Paddy—the only one of the four who *wasn't* supposed to leave—remained onboard as the rescue boat faded into the night and headed back to Egypt. Carta settled in for the journey and must have already been composing his reply to the Germans, because shortly after he docked, Crete was hit with a new wave of leaflets wafting down from the sky.

"I am in Egypt," Carta wrote back to the Butcher. "Be sure that there are a great many Cretans who would only be too happy to kill you for no reward at all!"

Once in Cairo, Paddy returned to "Tara," the vacation house nicknamed after the stronghold of ancient Irish kings, that Paddy shared with Xan Fielding and a few other secret agents. Paddy was greeted by Countess Zofia "Sophie" Tarnowksa, a twenty-six-year-old Polish heiress in exile who'd arrived in Egypt with little more than an evening gown, a swimsuit, and two pet mongooses. Sophie became

Tara's live-in hostess, a job that demanded rare skills: at various times, Sophie was called upon to replace chandeliers blown apart as sharp-shooting targets; use the bathtub to brew prune-and-vodka liqueurs; repair furniture smashed during an indoor bullfight; and find a place for the piano stolen from the Egyptian Officers' Club. Tara became such a notorious hot spot, it even attracted royalty: one night, Sophie opened the door to find King Farouk waiting with a case of champagne and an eye for action.

Paddy's nickname at Tara was "Lord Rakehell," and he wasted no time living up to it after his unexpected return from Crete. He found himself in a nightclub with Billy Moss, a Coldstream Guardsman who'd been so eager to enlist at the beginning of the war that he hunted up a private yacht to bring him home from Sweden, across the squally and U-boat-infested North Sea.

Nice work getting Carta off Crete, Billy said when Paddy told him about his scheme to snatch the Butcher. *But could you pull it off with a general who* doesn't *want to go?*

Paddy had two answers. "It could be done," he liked to say, "with stealth and timing in such a way that both bloodshed, and thus reprisals, would be avoided."

Then there was the truth: "I had only a vague idea how."

But in Tara's bathroom, a rough plan began forming. Paddy and Billy ended up there one bleary morning after a long night out, and as they lounged and chatted, a couple of Tara housemates wandered in to find out what was going on. Billy McLean and David Smiley had just pulled off some cracking operations in Albania, so Paddy sketched a map of Crete on the steamy bathroom tiles, and the four men were soon diagramming ambush spots.

Next up: toy shopping. Paddy and Billy Moss went to visit the War Magician in his secret Cairo lab. "He was Jasper Maskelyne, the famous conjurer whose magical transformations, in his theatre in Regent Street, had enchanted me as a child," Paddy would explain. Jasper was a third-generation magician whose father had trained sleight-of-hand spies for Lawrence of Arabia and whose grandfather founded the legendary Magic Circle society. During one of Jasper's shows, he was in the midst of drinking a glass of razor blades when he spotted an army captain working his way down the aisle. Suspecting something was up, Jasper turned a red flower into a puff of smoke, took his bows, and exited to find the officer waiting backstage with a question: Could Jasper work his magic on the battlefield and bewilder enemy soldiers?

Soon, Jasper was head of "The Magic Gang," a band of tricksters who dreamed up everything from button-sized spy gadgets to battalion-strength optical illusions. One of their first triumphs was adapting one of Jasper's grandfather's routines to make an entire harbor disappear. "In a burst of smoke, he'd appear to fly off the stage right up to the great chandelier, where he'd perch and answer questions from the audience," Jasper explained when he first unfolded his scheme. His grandfather's secret, Jasper said, was substitution: a dummy dressed exactly alike was hoisted by wire under cover of the smoke cloud. "I think we can adapt that principle to this situation," Jasper proposed.

The Magic Gang built a replica of Alexandria Harbor in a useless bay a few miles away, then rigged it with gunpowder-packed shacks and floats that would explode like fuel depots and cargo ships. With klieg lights, they cast false moonlight shadows, which threw off the bomber pilots' depth perception and made small-scale models look like full-size warships. As a final touch, the Magic Gang decorated the real Alexandria Harbor with artificial rubble and phony ship wreckage so German recon planes the following day would believe the harbor had really been hit.

Billy and Paddy prowled around Jasper's lab, loading up on exploding goat droppings and fountain-pen guns. "The air of sorcery," Billy marveled, "emanated from every shelf in that dim cell." Even though Jasper was now an army major, he still looked more mystical than military, with his showman's sleeked-back hair and lady-killer's mustache. "Do you want some more toys?" he'd offer, before adding, "I'm terribly glad I'm not going with you."

"GO!" the jump commander shouted.

Paddy was first out of the plane, tumbling into the dark. "The snow-covered ranges of Crete were glittering in the moonlight below, looking aloof, beautiful and dangerous," he noted. It was insanity: this was Paddy's first real parachute drop, and he was attempting to (a) thread a needle between mountaintops, (b) at night, (c) in fierce winds,

(d) between German gun posts. But at least he'd taken some lessons. Billy hadn't bothered, figuring he'd wing it rather than risk injury during training. "I'll be all right on the night," Billy had shrugged.

Paddy pinwheeled toward the ground, "like somersaulting into a very fast stream." Somehow he got his feet under him and yanked the rip cord, hoping for the best. Miraculously, the gusts blew him in perfectly, gliding Paddy between the cliffs and right down toward the target fires in a sheep pasture. Guerrillas came tearing out of their hiding places, helping Paddy yank off his chute and bury it. Then they got ready for Billy. They looked up and . . .

Kept on looking. The plane passed once, twice, then veered over the mountains and disappeared. *Nerves?* Paddy had to wonder. *Or weather?* German patrols must be scrambling by then, so Paddy and the guerrillas slunk off to hide. They returned to the forbidden zone the next night, and the next, but even though a plane buzzed each time, no olive-drab puff ever mushroomed down. *Damn!* What was going on up there? That was Billy's last chance to jump; enemy patrols were now so thick in the mountains, they'd begun popping each other. The guerrillas only got away one night because gunfire erupted ahead of them on the trail: a German squad had walked into a German ambush, killing two in the friendly-fire shooting.

No Billy, no kidnapping. Paddy couldn't see any other way around it. Paddy needed a real fighting man by his side, someone who could be counted on to kill in a pinch and knew soldierly stuff like Morse code; once, Paddy almost botched an escape-boat rendezvous because he couldn't figure out how to signal it in from shore. Billy looked kind of phony in a German uniform—too much like a Brit pretending to be German, Paddy thought—but he was *way* better than Xan. Put short, wiry, sun-browned Xan in a dress, cassock, or shepherd's pantaloons and he was invisible. Put him in anything cut from Wehrmacht field gray and he was begging for a bullet. Xan was back in Cairo at the moment, taking a breather at Tara after a furious few months of sabotage missions, seventy-two-hour escape hikes, and a shootout that killed six Germans and left Xan with a bullet graze across his forehead. But even if he were immediately available, Paddy didn't want him anywhere near the general's headlights. Xan could help the escape, but for the grab, Paddy wanted tall and blond.

Plus . . . well, it was ugly to say but impossible to deny: Billy was expendable. Xan and Tom were now high-value assets: during their months in the mountains, they'd mastered Cretan dialect, disguise, and smugglers' routes, making them hard to replace. Billy, for all his brains and nerve and imagination, was still just another tough guy with a gun. Tom Dunbabin had recently tripped up Rommel with a sharp bit of spying, figuring out from his sources near the airfield when an air convoy was due to leave Crete so British warplanes could shoot it down before it reached North Africa. Rommel was thundering so quickly across Egypt that Allied staff were preparing to flee Cairo in a panic, but without fuel, food, and repair parts, Rommel's tanks were dead in the desert. Tom was up for a Distinguished Service Order medal for that nifty bit of espionage, so there wasn't much appetite for putting him in front of the most dangerous prey on the island.

It had to be Billy. Except there was no Billy.

Paddy spent so many nights watching the sky, he could look at Orion and identify "the starry giant's private parts." Time was running out, fast. Xan had been in a similar situation, Paddy knew, and it cost him his operation. Xan had wanted to grab General Alexander Andrae, commander of the island before the Butcher, but Andrae was replaced before Xan could finalize his plan. A fresh target meant fresh recon; Xan would have to start over, taking weeks to assess the new general's security detail and tracking his travel and work routine. There was no time for that, Cairo decided, not with other sabotage missions pending. Xan's kidnapping was called off.

Finally, word came from Cairo: cloud cover and rough winds kept stymieing Billy's jump, but they weren't giving up: he was on his way, this time by boat. Nearly three months after Paddy's landing, a leaky rubber raft hissed into shore. Billy stepped out and found himself surrounded by "hirsute, piratical faces."

"You friend Paddy?" one of the bearded pirates asked.

Yes, Billy replied.

"Paddy with Germans."

The shock could have stopped Billy's heart. He'd been risking the skies and seas for weeks, only to get there and find Paddy was captured? Then an unmistakable swagger approached through the dark from farther down the beach. Rather than being taken prisoner, Paddy had taken four of his own. Well, deserters, actually, but certainly a tasty little addition to Paddy's witchcraft campaign. Paddy had just finished arranging for them to be ferried off to Cairo on the same boat that brought Billy, leaving the Germans with four more mysterious disappearances to wonder about.

Billy was just as surprised as Xan had been by the change that came over Paddy once he was back on the Sliver. This was the same hungover "Lord Rakehell" last seen slumped in his underwear in a Cairo bathroom? In his place was "a sort o' duke," as Paddy himself put it, giving orders to a bunch of bearded cutthroats and striding around in "a wine-coloured cummerbund into which were thrust an ivory-handled revolver and a silver dagger." Even in the dark, Billy was impressed by Paddy's physique. Whatever he'd been eating in those Cretan caves, whatever he'd been doing, it had turned Paddy into a dynamo. "He was looking extremely fit," Billy marveled. "A little plumper in the face, but radiantly healthy."

That was the good news. Then Paddy delivered the bad:

The Butcher was gone.

CHAPTER 24

With patience first and patience last,
and doggedness all through,
A man can think the wildest thoughts,
and make them all come true.

—GEORGE PSYCHOUNDAKIS,
improvising a *mantinada* poem in Paddy's honor

DURING BILLY'S DELAY, a grocer's kid from West Virginia wandered into the middle of their plot.

Nearly four years prior, Nicholas Alexander had taken his wife and three kids to visit their relatives in Greece. Nicholas immigrated to the United States in 1919, and because he'd been working and scrimping to buy his own grocery store in Wheeling, West Virginia, he hadn't been back since. June 1940 wasn't the best time for a family trip to Europe, but Nicholas realized it could be the last. America was still neutral, and Greece was doing everything possible to stay out of the war, even swallowing hard when an Italian sub fired three torpedoes toward the holy site of Tinos and sank a Greek cruiser sitting peacefully at anchor, so before the world erupted and his children moved on with their own lives, Nicholas wanted to take the chance for a family reunion. The Alexanders set sail for Crete.

Taking that trip was Nicholas's first mistake. Forgetting to register with the U.S. embassy in Athens was his second. Tangling with the Turk was his last.

When the German invasion stranded the Alexanders on Crete, Nicholas and his family holed up in his parents' home in the port city of Rethymno. Nicholas hung an American flag in front of the house and draped another on the roof, hoping that would protect them from bombers and Gestapo. Surprisingly, it seemed to work. So well, in fact, that Nicholas agreed to hide two Australian soldiers left behind by the evacuation. One night, a Gestapo team burst into the house and went directly to the trapdoor hiding a secret room. Nicholas tried to block them, arguing they had no right to search the home of an American citizen. The Turk shot him to death, then dragged the two Australians and Nicholas's seventeen-year-old son, John, off to prison.

A few months earlier, John had been a high school senior looking forward to another slow summer in Wheeling. Now he was scared and starving behind razor wire in a German POW camp on an island in the Mediterranean. Unlike the captured Allied soldiers, John was a skinny kid and no threat to run off, so he was tapped for death detail: hauling decomposing bodies outside camp on a hand-cart and burying them in a mass pit. He and two young Cretans were so harmless-looking, in fact, that only one guard was assigned to accompany them. They smashed him in the back of the head with a shovel, and together the three ran for their lives into the White Mountains.

A rifle in the ribs woke John up on only their second morning of freedom. At gunpoint, the three fugitives crawled from their hiding place—and met George Psychoundakis. The Clown was passing through to deliver a message for the Resistance when friends in a nearby village warned him that three strangers had been spotted in the vicinity. Wanderers in the woods meant trouble; for his own sake, George had to track them down and find out what they were up to in case they attracted German search teams. George shared his food with the fugitives, then veered from his own mission to lead them over the mountains and into the hands of the heroic monks at the Preveli monastery. John wanted to return to Rethymno for his mother and two sisters, but the abbot persuaded him that showing his face would only guarantee their deaths. Instead, on August 20, the

American teenager was led down to the beach and onto a sub bound for Egypt.

John's tenacity, fluency in Greek, and firsthand knowledge of the Cretan mountains made him a natural for Special Forces. He enlisted in the British Army, and after six months of combat training, John was on his way to joining the Firm. The SOE had the perfect assignment: they needed someone to accompany a sabotage squad to Crete on a quick, in-and-out mission to blow up German planes at the Heraklion airfield. The mission was a success, but rather than return to England for a fresh assignment, John remained with the Resistance. Through the guerrilla grapevine, John got news that his mother and sisters were safe in a relative's home deep in the mountains. Then he received another tip: the guerrillas knew a way into the Turk's private residence. Schubert didn't know it, but like many homes built on the waterfront during the Turkish occupation, the one he chose had a secret escape tunnel. John was given a hand-drawn floor plan and shown where the tunnel could be accessed by way of a bamboo screen in the rear garden. Then he was sent off to fulfill the Cretan code and avenge his father's death.

After midnight on a moonless night, John slipped into Rethymno. He found the tunnel's hidden entrance and squirmed inside. Unlike many others that had caved in or were converted to root cellars, this one was still clear. John crawled through the dark until he reached a trapdoor. He pried it open and emerged in an empty bedroom. Down a short hallway, someone was working by lamplight at a desk. John readied his pistol, tiptoed down the hall . . . and discovered he'd stalked the wrong man. With John's pistol in his face, the startled Gestapo officer told him the Turk had just moved. As John would later tell the story, he couldn't bring himself to murder a stranger in cold blood, so he cracked the Gestapo officer across the temple with his pistol and fled back out through the tunnel.

John would later discover that, unlike Rommel, the Turk hadn't needed a tingle of *Fingerspitzengefühl* sixth sense to let him know he was in danger. One of the Turk's own commanders had recently warned him that his brutality was on the verge of igniting a powder keg. Cruelty had to be calibrated; if the Turk and the Butcher pushed the Cretans too far, the entire island could erupt in waves of suicide attacks. Already the Resistance was a handful—imagine it without a shred of survival instinct. Any urge the Turk felt to argue was soon extinguished when eight members of his elite strike force—the Jagd-kommando Schubert—were ambushed and killed by Communist guerrillas near the village of Meskla. So hated were Schubert's men that the entire village dug up its hidden weapons and prepared to fight to the death if the Turk came gunning for retribution.

Instead, he gave up. Schubert must have gotten an inkling that peril was closing in when his commanders decided to leave Meskla be. "The Germans evidently concluded that the gangsters were not worth supporting, and left their deaths unrevenged," British intel-ligence reported. The Jagdkommando Schubert was disbanded, and its leader bolted for the capital, where he hid himself like "a medieval despot," according to British intelligence, "living in a house blocked up like a watch tower and never moving without a bodyguard." In January, soon after John Alexander's assassination attempt, Schubert left Crete for Athens.

Maybe Paddy should have seen the next move coming. After all, there was only one man the Cretans wanted to kill more than the Turk, and nearly every day that man was driven in plain sight down a lonely road to his private residence. A residence, incidentally, that in the eyes of the Cretans belonged to their adored and adopted son, John Pendlebury. If Müller's goal was to choose a house that would equally infuriate all his enemies at once, he couldn't have done better than the Villa Ariadne and its neighboring palace of Knossos. The Cretans revere Knossos as the birthplace of world culture; the British consider it a jewel of national achievement. But on a more heartfelt level, stealing Ariadne was like robbing the grave of Pendlebury—"a golden man," as the Cretans called him, whose final words were pure Greek battle cry.

An eyewitness who'd seen him die was finally discovered. Pendle-bury had been wounded fighting his way out of Heraklion, and two women had cared for him in their home. He was discovered by Ger-man paratroopers, who dragged the women off to prison. A neighbor, Calliope Karatatsanos, saw the paratroopers bring Pendlebury out-side and order him to attention. Three times, the Germans shouted a question at him; Calliope believed it was about the location of English forces. Three times, while facing men who would decide if he'd live or die, Pendlebury shouted the reply that had been a Greek anthem since the beginning of the war:

"No!"

Bullets ripped into his chest and stomach. The paratroopers buried Crete's golden man in a pit by the side of the road, then returned later to carve the glass eye from his skull.

"For the Cretans, it was the loss of an ally and a friend with a status close to that of Ares or Apollo," Paddy would reflect. "John Pendlebury had spent 12 years in Crete. In this time he had become a mythical figure on the island, famous for his energy and enthusiasm, his dedication and his toughness."

Now the Butcher was sleeping in his bed. Until suddenly, he wasn't.

"One item of news, late in March, came as a shock," Paddy would report: Müller had abruptly abandoned the isolated Villa Ariadne. The SOE thought the Butcher had left the island for good, just like the Turk, but then discovered he was still there; he'd transferred his base to the safety of "Fortress Crete," the German coastal stronghold.

Paddy was staggered. There was no way they could get Müller out of the Fortress, and a roadside abduction would be impossible on Chania's narrow and hectic streets. Paddy had to face it: at the last moment, the Butcher had slipped out of their grasp. Taking the Butcher's place in Heraklion was a new commander, an unknown officer whose only offenses so far were wearing an Iron Cross around his neck and moving into the Villa Ariadne:

Major General Heinrich Kreipe, fresh from the Russian front.

So what are we going to do? Billy asked.

Paddy had been on Crete long enough to know that sometimes you just had to grab a hunk of hair. One of the island's special gods is Kairos, the speedy little sprite who was Zeus's last-born child. Kairos was young and wing-footed and forever gorgeous, despite having no hair except a single shock over his forehead. Kairos is the god of golden opportunities and guardian of outlaws, and he could work wonders for you if you were quick enough to grab him by the forelock. But once he flashes past, he's gone for good. Naturally, the god of grabbing-what-you-can-when-you-can was beloved on an island where tyrants had created generations of outlaws. Kairos is the inspiration for the Cretan chestnut "Opportunity makes thieves." What matters is the *timing*, not the target—seize any opportunity, even if it's not the one you planned.

Paddy put it more bluntly: one general is as good as another. But they'd have to move fast; any more delays and the operation could be called off, same as it had been for Xan. Even extra recon put them at tremendous risk; Paddy had to disperse his first team of guerrilla accomplices because locals spotted them slipping in and out of the hideout and began gossiping about what the armed strangers were up to. They'd need a quick and easy plan, something that didn't depend on heavy manpower or tricky timing. Paddy had just the ticket. All they had to do was hop over the wall at Villa Ariadne, grab Kreipe in his bedroom, bundle him into his staff car, and blaze off to the coast. Rendezvous with a sub and they're on their way.

Paddy ran it by his band. The Cretans came from a rich tradition of body snatching—grabbing sheep, Turks, and elope-able girlfriends have long been honored island pastimes—so it was easy for them to assess Paddy's proposition and recognize it as *autoktonia:* suicide. The moment they were in Ariadne's courtyard, all it would take was an alert watchdog or a muffled sneeze and they'd be cornered. "The triple barriers of wire, one of which was said to be electrified, the size of the guard and the frequency of patrols offered too many chances for mishap," Paddy had to concede. "Besides, to avoid all excuse or pretext for reprisals on the Cretans, I was determined the operation should be performed without bloodshed." Paddy was firm on that point: any plan with the possibility of a shoot-out was off the table.

Even if they did figure out how to disappear the general from under the nose of his bodyguards, they'd need a sizable head start to stand any chance of getting him off the island. There were too many warships in the harbor and too many rocks near the capital to bring any kind of escape craft close to the northern coast. That meant heading south, on foot, up and over the toughest natural obstacle in southern Europe, with seventy thousand soldiers in hot pursuit. Paddy had also lost the one advantage he'd counted on from the start: instead of being in their clutches, the Butcher would be on their heels.

There was only one way to pull this off, in other words: the hard way.

CHAPTER 25

As I write now we are still in the cave,
and dare not move for fear of being seen.

—BILLY MOSS, scrawling in his diary before zero hour

A FEW HOURS before midnight on April 26, 1944, Paddy scrunched into a ditch by the side of the road and began scouring the darkness for a stab of light. He was dressed in the field-gray uniform of a German military policeman, pinched for him by a Cretan tailor who lived near the German base. By his side, also in a stolen uniform, was Billy Moss, who was about to discover if he could impersonate a German soldier without speaking any German.

There! In the distance, Paddy's confederate began blinking out a flashlight code.

Blink: "General's car."

Blink blink: "Unescorted."

Blink blink blink: "Action!"

"Here we go," Paddy whispered. He and Billy scrambled out of the ditch as a black Opel sedan, each mudguard emblazoned with the generals' Wehrmacht eagle insignia, swept around a bend and sped toward them down the dark road.

Paddy switched on a red signal lantern, and Billy held up a small stop sign. They took their positions at a hard-banking turn where the general's car would have to slow to merge onto the main road. Were their disguises convincing? Was the general surrounded by edgy guards with cocked machine guns? Paddy had no idea.

Paddy raised his lantern and stepped into the full glare of the speeding headlights.

"*Halt!*" Paddy shouted.

The black car roared straight at them, then slowed. Paddy and Billy cocked the pistols hidden behind their backs, then split up to approach the side windows.

"*Ist dies das Generals Wagen?*" Paddy barked into the darkness of the passenger window.

"*Ja, ja.*"

Paddy could just make out a jutting chin, gold braid, a black Iron Cross. Kreipe was in the front passenger seat.

"*Papier, bitte schön,*" Paddy demanded. Papers, please.

Before the general could snap at these idiot soldiers to get out of his way, Paddy jammed his pistol into his chest.

"*Hände hoch!*" Paddy shouted. Hands up!

Paddy heard the general gasp. The chauffeur's eyes were terrified but his right hand, Billy noticed, was sliding toward his automatic. Billy quickly cracked him across the head with his blackjack. A gang of Cretans burst from the brush alongside the road and yanked open the doors. The backseat was empty; instead of traveling with bodyguards, the general and his driver were alone. Billy and the Cretans pulled the stunned chauffeur into the road, but the general came out swinging, staggering Paddy with a sharp kick and a sock in the face. The Cretans quickly nixed that nonsense; one jammed a dagger under Kreipe's chin while another snapped handcuffs on his wrists.

"*Was wollen Sie in Kreta?*" one of the Cretans screamed in Kreipe's face. What are you doing in Crete?

Paddy pleaded with him to shush. Fury right then would get them killed.

"This was the critical moment," Billy realized. "If any other traffic had come along the road we could have been caught." Paddy could barely drive, so Billy slid behind the wheel, hoping he could figure out how to start the unfamiliar German sedan and get it into gear. Good news: "The engine of the car was still ticking over, the handbrake was on, everything was perfect." There was even a full tank of gas. Three Cretans shoved the general into the backseat and climbed in beside him while Paddy, straightening the general's hat upon his own head, slipped into the front. Two Cretans dragged the slumped and bloody chauffeur off with them into the brush.

Let's go, Paddy said.

Headlights blasted their eyes. "A convoy was bearing down on us," Paddy realized. "Two trucks full of soldiers sitting with their rifles between their knees, some in steel helmets, some in field caps." A minute earlier and it would have been game over. But the truck squads rumbled past, oblivious, and Billy hit the gas.

"Where is my hat?" the General kept asking. My hat. Where is it?

Keep quiet, the Cretans in the backseat hissed. Then to Paddy: What's he saying?

The chatter! Paddy had to snip it, quick. They were fast approaching the Villa Ariadne. Two sentries had already spotted them and snapped to attention. A third was opening the striped crossbar blocking the Villa's entrance. Any commotion now and the sentries would shoot the tires out from under them.

I've got your hat, Paddy told General Kreipe. Paddy froze as they whizzed past the bewildered sentries, then wheeled around to face the general. If any of them were going to survive, including the general, he had to get something straight. "Herr General," Paddy said. "I am a British major. Beside me is a British captain. The men beside you are Greek patriots. They are good men. I am in command of this unit, and you are an honorable prisoner of war. We are taking you away from Crete to Egypt. For you the war is over. I am sorry we had to be so rough. Do everything I say and all will be well."

"You are really a British major?" General Kreipe said.

"Yes, really. You have nothing to fear."

Then can I have my hat back?

"Checkpoint ahead," Billy warned. Two German soldiers were in the road, waving a red stoplight.

I need your hat right now, Paddy said. You'll get it back later.

Billy throttled back but kept driving straight at the soldiers. "*HALT!*" one shouted. Suddenly they leaped back and saluted, apparently catching sight of the general's flags. Billy accelerated and sped past.

"This is marvelous," Billy said, jamming his foot down on the gas.

"Herr Major," General Kreipe asked. "Where are you taking me?"

Good Lord. Was he going to ask about the damned hat again, too? "To Cairo," Paddy repeated.

"No, but now?"

"To Heraklion," Paddy said.

"To *HERAKLION*?"

Yes, that was actually Paddy's plan: to drive the general away from the safety of the mountains and straight into a city bustling with Germans.

A few weeks earlier, Paddy had ridden the bus into Heraklion, disguising himself as a farmer heading to market. Rather inconveniently, the best abduction route ran right from the general's residence through the heart of Heraklion and into the hills beyond. But street access, Paddy discovered, was awful: every road was thicketed with checkpoints. There was only one way in and out, and all the side streets were dead-ended with razor wire and antitank blocks or guarded by troops. It was madness; no matter how well they forged their travel documents and drugged the general, driving directly past the front door of Gestapo headquarters with a conked-out German officer in the boot and standing up to the scrutiny of more than twenty-two armed control posts was far too risky.

As he walked around town, Paddy found himself repeatedly passing the Gestapo building, morbidly attracted to the torture den, "which," he reflected, "had meant the doom of many friends." These were the stakes he was playing for: if the abduction went sour, those doors would shut behind him and he'd never come out. Paddy pulled himself away and made his way south, heading three miles down the road to the Villa Ariadne. By sheer luck, Paddy's best Cretan spy lived right next door. Micky Akoumianakis was the son of Villa Ariadne's former caretaker, and he was still allowed to live in his father's old quarters. And it was there, while Paddy and Mickey were pretending to chat with a shepherd tending his flock by the side of the road but really scoping out the security, that Paddy and General Kreipe first locked eyes.

The general's sedan suddenly appeared, barreling toward them down the road. Through the windshield, Paddy spotted blue eyes and a chestful of medals. Without thinking, Paddy popped up his hand and gave the general a friendly wave. Startled, the general responded, gravely raising a gloved hand toward his . . . his . . .

Paddy had a flash of inspiration. *The general's hat!* It was the one thing that made sentries stand down and roadblocks disappear. Who would bother to check the face beneath it? Who even *knew* what that face looked like? General Kreipe had been on Crete for barely five weeks, after two years on the Russian front. Few of his troops would recognize him, but they would instantly recognize—and respect— the gold-braided oak cluster and rampant eagle.

It was perfect. Rather than making the general vanish, they'd use him as their passport to a short cut right through the guts of German headquarters. "The results of a mishap in the town were too disastrous to contemplate," Paddy knew, "but a plunge straight into the enemy stronghold with their captured commander would be the last idea to occur to them."

Three generations of Maskelynes would have applauded. If Jasper and his *Magic Gang* could impersonate an entire harbor, Paddy was sure he could impersonate one man. Especially at night.

Unless that night was Saturday.

"It was truly unfortunate that we arrived in town at the moment," Billy discovered. Billy tooted the horn, grinding through the mob clogging the street. The weekend movie had just gotten out, and Heraklion was jammed with idling troop buses and strolling soldiers. Paddy sank back into his seat while the three Cretans behind him pulled the general down on the floor. One clamped a hand over the General's mouth and kept the dagger at his throat while the other two pointed their Marlin submachine guns up at the windows.

Paddy had put together a superb team, all of them icy under pressure. Manoli Paterakis was a goatherd and high-mountain hunter who'd been mentoring Paddy for much of the past year. George Tyrakis was a younger version of Manoli who'd instantly bonded with Billy even though they could communicate only with "grins and gestures," as Paddy put it. Paddy's last recruit, Stratis Saviolakis, was born and bred for this kind of operation: in regular life, Stratis was a cop from the southern rebel enclave of Sphakia, so he knew how to keep peace *and* raise hell.

German faces crowded around, passing just inches from the windows. Billy inched along, praying the car wouldn't overheat or stall. "Tension," Paddy noted dryly, "rose several degrees." After what seemed like hours, they circled the central market roundabout and began the straight descent to the Canae Gate. Once past that thick stone arch, it was open road—but that's when Billy knew they'd been discovered. Ahead of them, a sentry was standing fast in the middle of the road, red lantern held high. Behind him, extra manpower had massed. "There were not only the normal sentries and guards, but a large number of other soldiers in the gateway as well," Paddy realized. "The one wielding the red torch failed to budge; it looked as though they were going to stop us." Could they smash through? Doubtful; the passage had been narrowed with cement blocks and blocked with a thick wood barricade.

Paddy readied himself to kick open the door and run for it. They were outgunned and outnumbered, true, but they'd also been trained in the Cretan mountains. "There was a maze of alleyways, walls one could jump, drainpipes to climb, skylights, flat roofs leading from one to another, cellars and drains and culverts," Paddy was thinking, "of which the Germans knew nothing." Billy cocked his automatic and put it in his lap. Paddy's pistol was already in his hand. Three Marlin guns clicked back behind them. Billy crawled the car forward, waiting for the signal to floor it. Paddy rolled down his window.

"*Generals Wagen!*" he shouted. No general would ever shout like that but, well . . . "*GENERALS WAGEN!*"

Billy hit the gas. The sentry leaped out of the way. The soldiers scattered, barely dodging the Opel's bumper. Billy braced for gunfire but instead heard Paddy. "*Gute Nacht,*" Paddy was hollering. Billy couldn't resist a quick glance back. All the soldiers and sentries were saluting.

They left Heraklion behind and drove on into the countryside, rolling up and down the dark coastal foothills. Billy lit a cigarette, "the best I had ever smoked in my life." He handed the pack around to Paddy and the Cretans and—

Wait, stop! Stratis blurted. Wrong way. Billy had veered off the road to Rethymno and was instead barreling along to Rogdia—a dead end with a German garrison in the middle. Billy wrenched the Opel around in a U-turn and began driving right back toward the city they'd just escaped, praying the alarm hadn't been raised and a pursuit team wasn't coming at them. After a few nail-biting minutes, Stratis spotted the cutoff and got them back on the right road.

They hummed along in solitude, the snowcap of Mount Ida glowing above in the moonlight. Billy and Paddy burst into "The Party's Over." The three Cretans sang along, joyfully and nonsensically. The general got up off the floor. Paddy handed him back his hat.

Twenty miles past Heraklion, Billy pulled over and got out. Manoli and Stratis pulled General Kreipe out of the backseat. Paddy and George remained in the car, Paddy at the wheel. Paddy fought with the hand brake and accidentally blew the horn instead of pressing the starter, but eventually he figured out how to grind the car into bottom gear. Paddy and George pulled away, swerving uncertainly down the road, while Billy and the Cretans began marching the general into the mountains.

When Paddy reached the shoreline, he and George parked the car on the beach. They littered it with a British Raiding Forces beret, a handful of Player's cigarette butts, and an Agatha Christie novel, then chucked a Cadbury milk chocolate wrapper on the ground, going a little overboard in their attempt to make it look like a solo operation by Great Britain's messiest commandos.

Paddy checked the time. Already past 11 P.M. Time to move.

Off we go, George said. *Anthropoi tou Skotous!* Men of Darkness! German propaganda coined the term to blacken the name of the sneaky Cretans, not realizing the sneaky Cretans loved it and began singing it out as a rallying cry before night missions. Paddy had one thing left to do. The night before, he and Billy had written a letter and marked it in hot wax with their signet rings. Paddy pulled it out and pinned it to the front seat:

To the German Authorities in Crete, April 23, 1944
Gentlemen,

Your Divisional Commander, General Kreipe, was captured
a short time ago by a BRITISH Raiding Force under our
command. By the time you read this both he and we will
be on our way to Cairo. We would like to point out most
emphatically that this operation has been carried out without
the help of CRETANS or CRETAN partisans and the

only guides used were serving soldiers of HIS HELLENIC MAJESTY'S FORCES in the Middle East, who came with us.

Your General is an honourable prisoner of war and will be treated with all the consideration owing to his rank. Any reprisals against the local population will thus be wholly unwarranted and unjust.

Auf baldiges wiedersehen!

P. M. Leigh Fermor
Maj., O.C. Commando

C. W. Stanley Moss
Capt. 2/i.c.

P.S. We are very sorry to have to leave this beautiful motor car behind.

Paddy and George yanked the general's flags off the hood as souvenirs—"We couldn't resist it," Paddy would say—and together they began the lung-aching climb to catch up with the rest of their team. Maybe the Butcher would fall for it. Maybe he'd believe a sub had already come and gotten them and they were now long gone.

Maybe. Because if not, at dawn all hell would break loose.

CHAPTER 26

We lost the general.

—GERMAN RADIO TRANSMISSION, MAY 1944,
intercepted by British intelligence

CHRIS WHITE was true to his word: a few months after refusing to show me Paddy's escape route, he agreed to show me Paddy's escape route.

"You think I can handle it?" I asked.

"I'm sure Paddy wondered the same thing," Chris replied, or something to that effect; I didn't jot it down because I was already hurriedly clicking through the calendar to see how much prep time I had. On the one hand I was relieved; it meant I must have passed the White Brothers' selection process during our first hike across the island three months earlier. On the other, I knew we'd be pushing into tougher and more remote terrain than anyplace they'd taken me before. That was Paddy's game plan from the start; his only hope of pulling off the abduction was to run and hide through no-man's-land, going places where German troops, even Alpine forces, wouldn't think to follow.

Chris was eager to get back on Paddy's trail, because he was starting to believe he knew where Paddy went better than Paddy did. That actually made sense. Paddy and Billy were fleeing through the dark, led by outlaws to places only outlaws knew. It would have been tricky enough if the escape had gone well, but from the moment the general stepped out of his car, things began going wrong. From that point on, every day was an exercise in improvisation. Any route Paddy had in mind had to be scrapped and reinvented, instantly and on the fly, to dodge the Butcher's pursuit. Paddy once got so turned around that later, when he described peeking out of a cave as sunrise lit a mountain, he named the wrong mountain. It wasn't surprising; when you're being chased by seventy thousand armed men and a war criminal nicknamed the Butcher, you're more worried about who's behind than what's ahead.

Chris had done an extraordinary job of connecting the lost dots, thanks in no small part to help from Tim Todd, the retired Oxford detective turned Sherlockian war historian, and two adventurers with a unique hobby: Christopher Paul, a London attorney, and Alun Davies, a retired Welsh Regiment major, who specialize in retracing wartime escapes. One winter, they churned across the North Sea to follow in the footsteps of Jan Baalsrud, the Norwegian commando of *We Die Alone* who swam through Arctic waters, cut off nine of his own gangrenous toes, and survived snowblindness, frostbite, and starvation to finally escape the Germans and make it to freedom in Sweden. In 2003, Christopher and Alun were on a similar re-creation in Iran when an avalanche swept them hundreds of meters down the mountain. Battered and freezing, they survived the night by breaking into a hut for shelter. The following year they were hit by another avalanche, this time in Turkey on Mount Ararat. Alun and his climbing partner disappeared beneath tons of snow. Their teammates began frantically probing and digging. After twenty minutes, they managed to locate Alun and pull him out alive. His Scottish expedition mate, Alasdair Ross, wasn't so lucky.

"We decided that if we went anywhere else, it would have to be warm," Alun told me when I met him and Christopher one evening in London. They took me to Paddy's old club, the Travelers, and showed me the map over the fireplace of Paddy's walk across Europe as a teenager, signed with Paddy's trademark doodle of a flock of flying birds. Tracking Paddy across Crete, they said, turned out to be more than they'd reckoned on. "You look at the maps that are available.

They're not accurate at all," Christopher said. "And even if you're shown where to go, it's quite hard to find your way. We went looking for a particular cave and were told we were right in front of it. For the life of us, we couldn't find it."

They also learned to tread lightly around the Cretans: *xenía* still ruled, except when loyalty was at stake. "When the police went to arrest someone in Anogia while we were there, they were stopped on the edge of town by machine-gun fire and had to turn back," Christopher Paul said. The entire village was ready to go to war—including the clergy—if the police tried arresting a local boy. "We met a Greek priest with a Glock under his cassock," Christopher added. "He pulled it out of his sock."

Alun and Christopher had battled through plenty of rough stuff before, but they'd never dealt with the rocks that ripped the boots off one of their teammate's feet in their first six hours on the ground. They arrived lean, fit, and well-provisioned (unlike Paddy and Xan, who survived on local forage), but still found themselves burning weight to the tune of nearly twenty pounds in two weeks. "Anytime you're on an expedition like this, the unexpected will find you," Alun advised. "That's the question that's always intrigued me: How strong does your character have to be to deal with disaster?"

Fortunately, I had two advantages before seeing what Chris and I would find—or what would find us—on Paddy's route: I had a six-month head start, and access to my own Hero School.

The school I had in mind was born, as Alun Davies would have expected, from one man's reaction to a nightmare. During the first week of May 1902, a twenty-seven-year-old French naval officer named Georges Hébert was stationed on the warship *Suchet* off the coast of Martinique, "the Paris of the Caribbean." For days, Martinique's Mount Pelée had been spraying up bursts of sparks, but no one was really concerned. The volcano had been dormant for more than a century, and both the island's governor and the mayor of the capital city, Saint-Pierre, insisted there was nothing to worry about. Posters were nailed up all over Saint-Pierre encouraging everyone to rest easy and enjoy the free fireworks. Even when the sparks were joined by a plume of dark smoke and the stench of sulfur, Martinique remained unevacuated and largely unconcerned.

By May 7, everything was calm again. "The sun was now shining out nice and bright," steamship captain Ellery Scott noted in his ship's journal, "and everything appeared to be pleasant and favorable." So pleasant, in fact, that there were plenty of seats available on the last steam ferry of the day; it left the island barely one-third full. The sparks had died down and the volcano had gone back to sleep. . . .

Until early the following morning, when pent-up gases tore the top off the mountain. Two explosions boomed—one seven miles straight up in the air, the other a cannon of burning gas and fiery rock pointed right at Saint-Pierre. Sizzling lava gushed down the slope, launching swarms of fleeing vipers and crazed animals. People ran from their homes, only to be pelted by red-hot boulders, choked by ash and smoke, slashed by venomous snakes, and buffeted by 120-mile-per-hour winds. Darkness descended; superheated volcanic gas blanketed the city in a dark cloud broken only by flames and blasts of lightning. Rain fell, scalding hot. Screams, explosions, earth-shaking crashes, a riot of agony and panic . . .

And into this nightmare plunged Georges Hébert. The *Suchet* tried to approach port on a rescue mission, but blistering heat and furious winds churned the sea and threatened to crash the ship into the rocks. Hébert helped lower a launch and set off with a small band of seamen. While everyone else in Saint-Pierre was running away from the horror, Hébert and his crew were fighting their way toward it. They'd be among the very few who looked straight at the nightmare and lived to remember. For hours, Hébert and his crew fought to stay afloat while pulling scorched survivors from the water and rowing them to safety on the *Suchet*. More than thirty thousand people were in the city. More than twenty-nine thousand died.

"One of the greatest calamities in history has fallen upon our neighboring island of Martinique," President Theodore Roosevelt would lament. Beyond the body count, the tragedy had a morbid fascination: it seemed so puzzlingly *avoidable*. How much warning do people need to outrun a volcano? Have our survival instincts decayed so badly that even when fire flares into the sky, we don't pay attention? But one question in particular needled Georges Hébert: how many people were betrayed by their own bodies? They weren't killed—they died, frozen and uncertain, when they could have been running, crawling, jumping, and swimming for their lives.

Years later, a young British writer would reflect on Martinique in the same way. Paddy Leigh Fermor was so fascinated by the eruption, he made it the subject of his first and only novel, *The Violins of Saint-Jacques*. In Paddy's depiction, Martinique has two types of survivors: a few dumb-but-lucky Europeans, and canny natives saved by their own strength and skill. "They were the descendants of the cannibal savages that inhabited the archipelago long before the whites or blacks arrived," Paddy writes. "Some unconscious or atavistic wisdom had prompted them to escape, just as it had prompted the iguanas and snakes and armadillos, while the black and the white intruders had received, or at least, had taken, no hint of the disasters ahead. These primitive men had an inborn knack of survival when dealing with their ancestral problems which was lacking in everybody else."

The Caribs' "inborn knack" was really nothing special; it was just the same familiarity with their bodies and the natural world that humans have relied on for most of our existence. The Caribs were quick enough to get to the water and strong enough to stay afloat when their dugout canoes were capsized by scorching chunks of flying rock. The Caribs are what Homer had in mind when he created Odysseus, his ultimate unsinkable hero: not superstrong, just smart and sinewy enough to adapt to any jam. "Once the heaving sea has shaken my raft to pieces," Odysseus declares, "then I will swim."

Can that inborn knack be reborn? Georges Hébert chewed the problem over during the journey home to France. He was greeted as a hero, but he felt his real rescue operation had yet to begin. We've been living a lethal fantasy, Hébert realized. We've lulled ourselves into believing that in an emergency, someone else will always come along to rescue us. We've stopped relying on our own wonderfully adaptable bodies; we've forgotten that we can think, climb, leap, run, throw, swim, and fight with more versatility than any other creature on the planet. But how many of his fellow Parisians, Hébert wondered, could pull themselves up on a ledge, leap a three-foot chasm, carry a child to safety? Could *he*? He couldn't remember the last time he saw any grown-up crawl, climb a tree, somersault to cushion a fall, or even sprint.

Which was strange, because until recently you weren't an adult until you *could* rescue someone. Rites of passage for most cultures were based on sheer physical usefulness: you counted as a person only when you showed you could be counted on. Some proved it in blood, like the Spartans and the Zulu *impi*; the *impi* had to stomp barefoot on thornbushes to demonstrate they were ready to race into any situation without flinching, while Spartan teenagers were handed a dagger and sent off into the countryside to secretly stalk and murder the boldest local peasants "in such a way," according to Thucydides, "that no man was able to say, either then or afterwards, how they came to their deaths." By ruthless Spartan logic, this *krypteia* was the perfect multipurpose path to citizenship: it kept insurrection at bay and turned young Spartans into masters of stealth and survival.

Speed and strength weren't just a young man's game. The Navajo *kinaaldá* and Apache *na'ii'ees* were coming-of-age ceremonies for young women that focused on speed, endurance, and a lifetime of muscular fitness. The young women set off on daily morning runs into the rising sun and had their arms and backs massaged in hopes they'd always be strong and supple. The stronger the women, both tribes believed, the stronger the community. "Throughout most of *na'ii'ees*, the girl's power is used to benefit herself," one anthropologist notes. "However, immediately after the ceremony, it becomes public property and is available to everyone."

So Georges Hébert had to wonder: What went wrong? Why did we turn our backs on this tradition of strength and allow ourselves to become so helpless? But even as he was asking the question, a machine-shop worker in Philadelphia already had the answer.

Edwin Checkley was born in England in 1855, right at the teeter point when the Industrial Revolution was shifting from radical innovation into unstoppable juggernaut. It was the end of the era of the amateur, a time when everyone had to be a bit of everything. You helped your neighbors build their homes, fight their fires, raise and butcher and preserve their own food. You knew how to repair a weapon, pull a tooth, hammer a horseshoe, and deliver a child. But industrialization fostered specialization—and it was fantastic. Trained pros were better than self-taught amateurs, and their expertise allowed them to demand and develop better tools for their crafts—tools that only they knew how to operate. Over time, a subtle cancer spread: where you have more experts, you create more bystanders. Professionals did all the fighting and fixing we used to handle ourselves; they even took over our fun, playing our sports while we sat back and watched.

Checkley straddled the two worlds: he landed a factory job as a machinist but soon left to travel with his own tumbling act. He was nineteen when he immigrated to the United States, in 1874, and spent the next few years as a human tornado: he studied medicine at Long Island College Hospital, trained and taught at a gym in Brooklyn, and moonlighted weekends at a machinist's shop in Philadelphia. It was all propelling him toward a masterpiece: in 1890, Checkley released an explosive little book titled *A Natural Method of Physical Training: Making Muscle and Reducing Flesh Without Dieting or Apparatus.*

Critics' reactions were weird and rather frenzied: everyone loved it, without knowing exactly what it was. Science reviews excerpted it; so did literary journals, women's magazines, fitness publications, even coffee-table flip-throughs like *Ladies' Home Journal*. The only people who hated Checkley's book, it seemed, were the ones he was writing about: gym owners and exercise scientists. Because the one thing wrong with the fitness industry, Checkley proclaimed, was everything.

Barbells? Forget it.

Weight machines? Waste of time.

Women are sweet, men are sweaty? Ridiculous.

Diets, exercise circuits, resistance training? Hopeless, useless, and unnatural.

Look at every other creature on the planet, Checkley urged. They don't binge and starve, or heave and strain to make one part of their body bulge. They don't sit on a bench and lift a weight to their nose over and over again. Why *would* they? You'd never do that in the real world, so why do you do it in training? All you're creating is "hard muscle" and "stiff strength," as he put it—the exact opposite of true fitness.

"You pull this and push that so many times a day and you get to be a little amateur Samson," Checkley wrote. "You already feel the muscles expanding. Those biceps especially draw attention, as if they were the synonyms of health and strength. The strength of the man so trained has no reliance on itself. It is superficial—only skin deep, as it were—and will not 'stay put.' The truth is that there can be no proper training that does not educate the whole system of the man."

Wait—make that the whole system of the *human*. This idea that women were fragile little flowers was a farce that Checkley wanted to end. "The 'weaker' sex would occupy no such position of relative weakness if natural laws were followed," Checkley argued. "If women must, as is so freely complained, remain physically short of man's strength, there is no reason why the disparity should remain so great as it often is. Where women lead an active life their strength and endurance comes remarkably close to the strength and endurance of the other sex, and in the control of their own systems may readily under development excel the other sex. In other words, tradition has more to do with the 'weakness' of women than has nature."

Conventional exercise advice was so bad, Checkley believed, you were better off doing nothing at all. At least you'd know you were doing nothing—instead of being duped into thinking that feeling bored, sore, and swollen was the same as being fit—and with luck you'd eventually get disgusted and do the right thing.

And the right thing was?

Natural training.

Natural training, as one of Checkley's disciples testified, gave him everything: "shape, speed, strength, suppleness, endurance, abounding health, and every blessed physical advantage a man can have." Checkley's method involved no repetitions, no weights, and no fussy food restrictions. It was based on fun and play, and was apparently remarkably effective: business was booming at the Edwin Checkley Gymnasium, in Philadelphia, and even well into his fifties Checkley himself looked carved from marble. After studying under Checkley, the founder of a barbell company publicly declared he'd been wrong all along about weights.

So what exactly was "natural training"? Well, you wouldn't find the details in Checkley's book, which was more manifesto than manual and gave only the raw basics. Checkley was trained as both a performer and a businessman, so he knew how to build an audience and control trade secrets. First, he'd whet appetites and win converts; then, over time, he'd feed the faithful with future books. It was an excellent marketing plan, taking into account all but one thing: the leaky gas pipe in his home. Before Checkley could write a second book, he died in 1921 from gas poisoning.

When Georges Hébert set out to create his own French version of natural training, he picked up where Edwin Checkley had fallen short. Hébert wouldn't just make people healthy. He'd make them heroes. Because if you do it right, Hébert suspected, they're the same thing. That's the math at the foundation of every heroic tale from the *Odyssey* to the Old Testament to *Xena: Warrior Princess:*

Health = heroism.
Heroism = health.

Heroes are protectors, and being a protector means having strength enough for two. Being strong enough to save yourself isn't good enough; you have to be better, *always*, than you'd be on your own. The ancient Greeks loved that little interlocking contradiction, the idea that you're only your strongest when you have a weakness for other people. They saw health and compassion as the two of the chemical components of a hero's power: unremarkable alone, but awe-inspiring when combined.

What you're aiming for is the hero's holy trinity: *paideia, arete,* and *xenía:* skill, strength, and desire. Mind, body, and soul. Overload on any one of the three, and you'll unbalance the other two. You can charge into action with the noblest *xenía* intentions, but you'll get nowhere without the know-how of *paideia* and the raw *arete* arsenal of fists, agility, and endurance. That's what made Odysseus, trickster and semi-scoundrel though he was, the greatest Greek hero. Odysseus wasn't the best fighter: he was actually a draft-dodger who tried avoiding the invasion of Troy by pretending he'd gone loopy and was too addled to leave home. One of his fellow warriors saw through that scheme, however, because Odysseus was well known for slipping out of a scrap if he didn't like the odds and only using his spear if he couldn't deploy guile instead.

But as a hero he was one of a kind, as even a superstar warrior like Achilles would admit. When Odysseus visits the underworld during his journey home from Troy, the ghost of Achilles tells him enviously, "I would rather be a paid servant in a poor man's house and above ground than king of kings among the dead." Achilles went down in battle, but Odysseus remained alive and scrapping. And why? Because his *paideia* and *arete* were balanced by *xenía*—his loyal heart. Nothing will stop Odysseus from getting home to protect his wife and son—not storms, not vanity, not a Cyclops, not even a magical sex goddess. Mind, body, and soul: that's what made Odysseus "the best of the Acheans."

Georges Hébert grasped that, which is why he could see what was missing from Edwin Checkley's notion of "the whole system of the man." Checkley's natural training was dynamite when it came to strength and skills, but where was the higher purpose?

"Exercise only with the intention to carry out a physical gain or to triumph over competitors," Hébert believed, "is brutally egoistic." And brutal egoism, Hébert believed, just isn't human. We like to think of ourselves as masters of our own destinies, as lone wolves in a dog-eat-dog world, but guess what: Dogs don't eat dogs. They work together. As do most species. As do we. In fact, when it comes to wolf-pack tactics, humans are even better than wolves. We're the most communicative, helpful species that's ever existed. If anything, we *over*share. We share every idea, every tool, every belief. Even when we fight, we do it as a team; in war, we unite in fantastic numbers.

So forget brutal egoism, Hébert argued. That's not our real strength. The single greatest moment of his own life came when he plunged that little boat into the seething cauldron off Martinique and began pulling burned, frightened survivors into his arms. Young Georges Hébert wasn't out there because of ego. He was out there because it was *natural;* because being a god on earth is a natural human desire, and saving someone else is the closest we'll ever come to achieving it. All Greek mythology and every major religion that followed has really been devoted to that single premise: the hero who leads the way is half god and half human, fueled as much by pity as by power.

Hébert, consequently, came up with the strangest mission statement ever devised for getting in shape. He called it Méthode Naturelle— the Natural Method—and it would be ruled by a five-word credo that had zero to do with getting ripped, getting thin, or going for the gold. In fact, it had zero to do with "getting" anything; Hébert was heading the opposite direction.

"*Être fort pour être utile,*" Hébert declared. "Be fit to be useful." It was brilliant, really. In those final two words, Hébert came up with a complete philosophy of life. No matter who you are, no matter what you're seeking or hope to leave behind after your time on the planet—is there any better approach than simply to be useful? "Here is the great duty of man to himself, to his family, his homeland and to humanity," Hébert wrote. "Only the strong will prove useful in difficult circumstances of life."

Now that he had his purpose, Hébert needed a method. Luckily, he had the perfect case studies right under foot: his kids. When children play, he realized, they're really role-playing disaster scenarios. Turn them loose and they'll run, wrestle, hide, roll around, kick-fight with their feet, and leap off anything they can climb—exactly the skills that could keep them alive in a real emergency. Natural training should spring from nature, Hébert decided, so kids' play would be his starting point. It didn't take long to realize that most roughhousing is a selection from three basic menus:

Pursuit—walk, run, crawl.
Escape—climb, balance, jump, swim.
Attack—throw, lift, fight.

With his list of "10 natural utilities" in hand, Hébert went looking for guinea pigs. The French navy stepped up and agreed to let him experiment with a class of new recruits. Hébert began by testing the young seamen in basic rescue and evasion maneuvers. Could they climb a tree, a rope, a pole leaning against a wall? Lift a slippery log, a lumpy human body, a heavy stone? Throw with range and accuracy with either hand? Hold their breath, tiptoe along a narrow ledge, fend off two attackers throwing punches?

Next, Hébert set to work on an outdoor training facility. Gyms, he believed, are a joke. What's invigorating about being cooped up in a room full of foul air and clanking metal? What's the point of practicing real-life skills with artificial equipment? Gyms benefitted one person, Hébert believed: the gym owner. No, the Natural Method should be open-air all the time, "in rain and dark and beating snow."

Hébert created a giant adult playground, equipping it with climbing towers, vaulting horses, sandpits, and ponds. Scattered about were rocks and logs and long poles to be used for throwing, vaulting, balancing, shinnying up, passing from hand-to-hand while running, or anything else an athlete dreamed up at the moment. All you had to do was pick a combination of challenges, combine them into an obstacle course–like sequence, and have at it. "One can select a few exercises from each group, ideally all of them if time permits," Hébert said. "There should be little or no rest between exercises."

Hébert had one firm rule: No Competing. *Ever.* That meant no championships, no world records, no races. You didn't get belts, medals, or rankings. To be honest, Hébert had little regard for competitive sports, which he dismissed as artificial "entertainments."

"An individual who is satisfied with performing in exercises or sports of entertainment such as these games—soccer, tennis—but ignores the art of swimming, self-defense, or fears vertigo, is not strong in an useful manner," he argued. "A weightlifter or a wrestler who cannot run nor climb, or a runner or a boxer who doesn't know how to swim, or cannot climb, is not strong in a complete manner."

Competition perverts true fitness, Hébert believed. It tempts you to cheat; to overdevelop some talents while ignoring others; to keep tips for yourself that could be useful to everyone. It's a short cut; all you have to do is beat the other guy and you're done, but the Natural Method is a never-ending challenge for self-improvement. Besides, competitive sports focus on rivalry and class divisions. The Natural Method was all about collaboration; every teacher was a student, every student was a teacher, bringing fresh ideas and new challenges. Raise the bar, but help the next guy over it—*paideia* and *arete*.

What's most fascinating about Hébert's theory is that it extends far beyond fitness and into every aspect of life. Hébert believed natural training would make people more noble, intelligent, resourceful, generous, successful, and happy. Why? Because every day, you practice problem-solving under extreme conditions, and once you've figured out how to carry a hunk of timber through a swamp in your bare feet, nothing at work will stress you. Natural training makes you introspective, not combative; you see conflict as something to be resolved with force and dexterity, not violence and its brother, fear.

In 1913, Hébert astounded the International Congress of Physical Education with the results of tests performed on 350 navy recruits who'd been trained in Méthode Naturelle. On a rating system that scored performance according to strength, speed, agility, and endurance, French sailors were performing on a scale with world-class decathletes. The French Ministry of War assigned a team of colonels to study under Hébert, and Natural Method "playgrounds" were soon being installed at eight military bases across the country.

Unlike Edwin Checkley, Georges Hébert was eager to opensource everything he'd discovered. He published a monumental work—*L'Éducation Physique, ou, L'Entraînement Complet Par la Méthode Naturelle*—that crammed together more than five hundred pages of theory, practice, photos, training sequences, and muscular anatomy. But the whole thick stack, Hébert admitted, could be summed up in a single sentence: "Teach your boys to walk, to run, to jump, to box, and to swim, and leave those artificial extension movements, which mean nothing, alone!"

The time had come to take Méthode Naturelle to the world. Hébert handpicked an elite team of trainers and prepared to deploy them throughout Europe, Asia, and America. Right before they scattered, Hébert captured the moment on film; in the photo, he and his Natural Method team are stripped down to rather alarmingly loinclothy shorts, and they look fantastic. They're of all ages and sizes, but they share the same body; to a man, they're lean and carved, looking lithe and powerful as a pride of lions. None of them are flexing, because none of them have to; their true strength, they know, lies beneath their muscles, in the knowledge that whatever challenge arises, they're ready.

That photo was snapped in late 1913. Months later, German troops were tromping through Belgium and Luxembourg on the way to France. The men of Méthode Naturelle joined the fight, and because of their superb physical conditioning and dedication to service, many were leading front-line charges in the Great War. Four years later, every one of them—along with nine million other combatants—was gone.

Georges Hébert was heartbroken, but not surprised. He was a realist, and he understood that no matter how skilled you were, being useful could sometimes be lethal. The Natural Method was never about trying to live forever; the goal was to make a difference before you died. Hébert barely survived his own wounds; he'd spend the rest of his life struggling to regain the ability to walk and talk. He'd be honored as a Commander of the Legion of Honor, but it was like laying a wreath over a sinking ship; Hébert's noble dream of heroic health was swept away by a world that was sick of danger and wanted to pretend that it was gone forever.

The Natural Method was all but forgotten. Until many years later, when a guy selling glow-stick bracelets on a Corsican beach came across an old paperback and began to read. . . .

CHAPTER 27

When I became Governor, the champion middleweight
wrestler of America happened to be in Albany, and I got him
to come round three or four afternoons a week. . . . While
President I used to box with some of the aides.

—THEODORE ROOSEVELT,
the only U.S. president who swam naked in the Potomac
in winter, went blind in one eye from boxing in the
White House, gave a speech immediately after taking
a bullet in the chest, and nearly died mapping
an uncharted river in the Amazon

NEARLY ONE HUNDRED YEARS after the Natural Method disappeared,
I witnessed its rebirth in the form of a half-naked man vaulting
through my second-floor window.

"Ready to play in the jungle?" he says. "You're not afraid of heights,
are you?"

"I'm not wild about them."

"That's because you never learned how to climb. Let's get started."
He vanishes back through the window, which is about three feet from
an unlocked and perfectly functioning door. For a man pushing forty,
his energy and suppleness are off the scale; it's not even 6 A.M. and
Erwan Le Corre is already straining to go. His last name sounds like

the French word for "the body"—*le corps*—and he certainly lives up to the billing: Erwan is tall, sun-bronzed, muscular as a puma, usually barefoot, and rarely in anything more than surf shorts.

I'd arrived the day before at Erwan's base in Itacaré, a tiny village squeezed between the Brazilian rain forest and the Atlantic Ocean. Itacaré is ordinarily a sleepy outpost of fishermen and roving surfers, but it has lately become a rambling outdoor training camp for a bizarre collection of adventurers who are trying to pick up the Natural Method that the Great War cut short.

Wild as he looks, Erwan is dead serious about one thing: he's convinced the entire multi-billion-dollar health club industry is based on a lie. And judging by raw numbers and results, he's probably right: fitness clubs are the only business that depends on customers *not* showing up. It's an amazing financial success story, especially since it's based on such a defective product. Health clubs, by their own metric, just don't work: the more gyms we join, the fatter we get. In fact, the rise in obesity tracks right alongside the rise in health club revenues, with both climbing steadily at about 2 percent a year.

"For most people, the gym is broken," agreed Raj Kapoor, the well-known tech entrepreneur who cofounded Snapfish and was quoted in an interview about his new focus on American health. "Globally, it's a $75 billion business, and more than 60 percent of people don't go, even though they're paying." Here's how it works: Every January, gym enrollments skyrocket. Gold's typically doubles its membership, while other clubs report increases of up to 300 percent. At the maximum rate, that means *four times* the number of bodies are squeezing into the same amount of space. No facility can handle a stampede like that without the walls bulging.

"It's like a damn cattle call" when the doors to exercise classes open, one regular complained to the *Wall Street Journal*. But no worries. Gym owners know they can pocket the cash without bothering to expand, because within a few weeks a fresh cycle takes over: by spring, fewer than half of any gym's members turn up anymore. Ordinarily, that would mean death for an operation that counts on repeat business, but shame and magical thinking are powerful marketing tools: by the following January, the majority of the dropouts— roughly 60 percent—will feel guilty and decide once more to open their wallets and get in shape. No wonder the fitness mill keeps booming while other businesses are folding: during the recession's darkest days, health club memberships increased by 10 percent.

So what went wrong? How did the modern health club, with all its whiz-bang machinery and calorie-crunching digital technology, prove so ineffective at actually improving health? With total revenue exceeding fifty billion dollars a *year*, you should expect at least some visible effect on overall health. It's a staggering investment in a demonstrably failed approach, and it's not as if people aren't trying. We go to gyms; we just don't stay. You can blame the public for not forcing themselves, but that's like a restaurant blaming customers who don't like the food; ultimately, you're responsible for what's on the menu.

And by 1980, the health club menu had undergone a radical overhaul. Until then, the standards for American gyms were set by the country's best-conditioned athletes: boxers. Fighting is the art of perpetual motion—"Move or die," as mixed martial artists like to say—so old-time trainers kept you on the hop with true functional movement. If you went to, say, Wood's Gymnasium on East Twenty-eighth Street in Manhattan, the way young Teddy Roosevelt did, you were trained by prizefighters. When Teddy first came through Wood's door, he was a wheezing, short-sighted teenager who was constantly getting roughed up by other kids. His father sat him down and explained that without *arete*, there is no *paideia*. "Theodore, you have the mind but not the body," his father said. "And without the help of the body the mind cannot go as far as it should. You have to *make* your body."

So Teddy got to work. "Professor" John Wood didn't stick him on a padded seat and tell him to push a bar back and forth fifteen times, or plunk him on a stationary bike to crank the pedals. Wood partnered Teddy up with pro fighter John Long, and together they attacked Wood's "beautiful and effective combined exercises": skipping rope, swinging on parallel bars, vaulting over gymnastics horses, shuttle running with a medicine ball, hitting the heavy bag, shadow sparring with Indian clubs. One of Wood's specialties was the lost art of strength rings: two circles of steel that a pair of partners grip between them, each grabbing an end in their hands. Then they go at it, pulling and resisting, each trying to make the other lose his grip or footing. The rings were a combat art as intricate as fencing; John

Wood could diagram at least thirty-eight combinations of lunges, thrusts, and body twists.

"These certainly may be classed among the movements that are most generally useful," one of Wood's protégés remarked, "for they bring into play every joint and muscle of the body, secure geniality and generous emulation, and afford a great deal of exercise in a brief space of time." Proficiency and power—*paideia* and *arete*.

But at the end of the 1970s, the curtain suddenly dropped on fight training. Ordinarily, it's rare to pinpoint the Patient Zero who starts an epidemic, but in this case, it happened right on camera. In 1977, a womanizing, pot-smoking, cigar-puffing, steroid-injecting, gay-magazine pinup model suddenly became the poster boy for American fitness. *Pumping Iron* was released and, thanks to Arnold Schwarzenegger's swaggering charisma and chemically-enhanced physique, bodybuilding was transformed from underground entertainment into a worldwide phenomenon. Arnold would become Hollywood's most bankable star, and bodybuilding—a form of male modeling that has nothing to do with agility, endurance, range of motion, or functional skill—became the new gold standard for gym training. Just like that, the best-conditioned athletes in the world were being replaced by some of the worst.

From a fitness standpoint, it was a step backwards. But economically, it was genius. Fight training takes up lots of room, but bodybuilding is about staying in one spot. It requires remarkably little floor space; if you're not sitting or lying down, you're standing or squatting. The idea is to isolate one muscle group at a time and blast it to the point of tearing, repeating the same movement over and over until you approach muscle failure. Like any other damaged tissue, the stressed spot will swell. That's an emergency reaction, blood rushing in to immobilize the area and initiate healing. Oddly, that discomfort became a selling point: because bodybuilding is about appearance, not skill, sore and swollen muscles began taking over as a sign of strength.

And just as bodybuilding was becoming the new fitness model, a new device came along that made it as tidy and efficient as an assembly line. In 1970, a bizarre character from Florida showed up at the Mr. America competition with a product to sell. Arthur Jones was a chain-smoking high school dropout turned big-game hunter whose hobby was trying to overfeed his fourteen-foot alligator to Guinness

World Record size. He was also a self-taught mechanic who'd built an exercise machine he called the Blue Monster. Jones's brainstorm was a kidney-shaped cam that evenly distributed resistance as the weight was pushed higher. Because the gear also resembled a seashell, Jones renamed his creation the Nautilus.

Finally, gym owners could offer one thing your basement bench press couldn't: a specialty machine that made you feel like a pro. Nautilus was compact and quiet and safe, allowing gyms to herd many more customers through much less space. Even during the New Year's rush, you didn't have to worry about members smacking one another with medicine balls or turning the joint into a full-combat mosh pit as they careened around with strength rings and Indian clubs. There were no dumbbells to rack or techniques to teach; no spotters were even needed for the bench press. Expertise wasn't required, so neither was an expert staff: you only had to look pretty, take money, and wipe down the equipment.

"The idea of a health club really changed. It became big business. It was Arthur Jones that started that," one of Jones's designers would later tell the *New York Times.* "Mr. Jones' invention led to the 'machine environment' that is prevalent today in health clubs," the *Times* article continued. "The machines helped to transform dank gyms filled with free weights and hulking men into fashionable fitness clubs popular with recreational athletes."

But the Rise of the Machines came at a cost. The goal became to create bodies that looked as much alike as possible, and you accomplish that by insisting on exact repetitions of the same motion, over and over. Even the vocabulary changed to fit the factory-floor mentality: our parents exercised, but we "work out." And like any other factory, progress isn't measured by whether you mastered a new skill; it's measured by whether you hit your numbers—in this case, pounds and inches. The Greek ideal of a supple, balanced, *useful* physique was out. Massive McBodies were in.

And why? Because along with the Rise of the Machines came the Dawn of the Super-Males.

"With the advent of anabolic steroids in the last 30 to 40 years, it has become possible for men to become much more muscular than is possible by natural means," notes Dr. Harrison Pope, M.D., a psychiatry professor at Harvard, who coined the term "bigorexia nervosa" to describe our dangerously misguided idea that bigger = sexier. Pope knows plenty about fitness; at age sixty-six, he could still shuck his suit jacket and tear off a half-dozen one-armed pull-ups on his office door. He can glance at a magazine cover or a movie trailer and instantly spot who's juiced; sadly, more of those famous bodies are syringe-pumped than you'd think. But then again, was anyone really surprised when Sylvester Stallone was caught in Australia with nearly fifty vials of human growth hormone in his baggage?

Even kids' toys and comic books were infected; action figures soon became as artificially overmuscled as the Italian Stallion. Take *Star Wars:* do you remember spotting any tank-tread abs or veiny biceps among the Rebel Alliance? Luke Skywalker and Han Solo barely take off their shirts in the films, and when they do, they're amazingly . . . average. Just a couple of skinny guys who get by on dexterity, not Dianabol. But over the past thirty years, their plastic doppelgängers have gotten crazy huge. Same with G.I. Joe and Batman: their toy biceps have nearly tripled in size.

"Our grandfathers were rarely, if ever, exposed to the 'super-male' images," Pope notes. "They didn't do bench presses or abdominal exercises three days a week." Their grandkids, however, are caught in an endless self-image onslaught. "A young man is subjected to thousands and thousands of these super-male images," Pope complains. "Each image links appearance to success—social, financial, and sexual. But these images have steadily grown leaner and more muscular, and thus more and more remote from what any ordinary man can actually attain." The payoff from all those gym reps is supposed to be a Hollywood bod, but once you discover that the road from Rambo I to Rambo II is paved with injectables, you face the same deflating choice pro cyclists had when they sniffed out Lance Armstrong's secret: go dirty or go home.

"There's a fairly sharp limit to the degree of muscularity that a man can attain without drugs," Pope explains. "Most boys and men who exceed this limit, and who claim they did so without drugs, are lying." Before the Rise of the Machines and the Dawn of the Super-Males, you went to the gym to become an athlete. Teddy Roosevelt focused on performance, not appearance, and it made him an athlete for life. Like all self-made men, he was afraid of backsliding, so even after he became president, Roosevelt stuck with what he learned at Wood's:

he boxed with soldiers, swam naked late at night in the Potomac, and squared off with his buddy, an army general, for bruising battles with wooden cudgels.

Some evenings, Roosevelt would slip out of the White House, pick a spot miles in the distance, and head straight for it. The challenge was to reach the goal no matter what obstacles were in the way. "On several occasions we thus swam Rock Creek in the early spring when the ice was floating thick upon it. If we swam the Potomac, we usually took off our clothes," Roosevelt would recall. "We liked Rock Creek for these walks because we could do so much scrambling and climbing along the cliffs . . . Of course under such circumstances we had to arrange that our return to Washington should be when it was dark, so that our appearance might scandalize no one."

Decades later, Roosevelt's midnight rambles inspired one of the strangest fads of the Kennedy administration. After becoming president, John F. Kennedy was appalled to discover that half the young men called up for the draft were rejected as unfit. Americans were becoming dangerously soft and therefore, in Kennedy's eyes, stupid. "Intelligence and skill can only function at the peak of their capacity when the body is healthy and strong," Kennedy declared. "In this sense, physical fitness is the basis of all the activities of our society." JFK was interested in true fitness, not bench presses or beach muscle, so he zeroed in on the two factors that matter most: endurance and elastic strength.

Thus began America's weird, brief love affair with ultradistance. JFK found an old order from Teddy Roosevelt that required U.S. Marines to hike fifty miles or ride one hundred in less than seventy-two hours. (Teddy, naturally, led the way by doing the ride himself during a winter rainstorm.) Some of Teddy's troops finished the hike in a single day, so JFK made that his challenge: Could modern Marines cover fifty miles of wild terrain in twenty-four hours? But before the military could give the command, civilians—including Kennedy's own kid brother—beat them to it. At 5 A.M. one freezing Sunday in February, Bobby Kennedy set off with four Justice Department aides to hike the C&O towpath from D.C. to Harpers Ferry. All four aides dropped out, but by midnight Bobby had hiked fifty miles in less than eighteen hours.

The race was *on*. College frats, Boy Scout troops, high school classes, postmen and policemen, "pretty secretaries" and "beautiful girls" (as *U.S. News & World Report* put it) all tackled the "Kennedy Challenge." Congressional staffers marched off in mobs, and a pub in Massachusetts offered free beer at the finish of its own fifty-miler. "The 50-mile hike verges on insanity," warned the National Recreation Association, and the doom prediction was seconded by the American Medical Association: "We get distressed when people go out and strain themselves." News photographers fanned out to capture the carnage—and instead found the same expression on faces across the country: grins of pride. People who'd never moved their legs for more than an hour at a stretch were thrilled to discover that just by heading out the door, they could keep on going. Speed records tumbled: Bobby Kennedy was beaten by a high school girl in California, who was edged out by a fifty-eight-year-old postman in New Jersey, who was bested by a Marine who smoked it home in under ten hours.

Kennedy's murder brought the armies of Challengers to a halt—except in one small town in Maryland, where the same shock of personal discovery has been playing out every year since 1963. Only four people finished the first race. Seven the next. Eighteen after that. But while all the other Kennedy Challenges died away, Boonsboro kept getting stronger. It's a tough race; the JFK 50 sends you up the steep and rocky Appalachian Trail and then down long switchbacks to the C&O towpath to follow in Bobby Kennedy's footsteps. A half-century later, Boonsboro is still holding fast to Kennedy's vision. Now, nearly a thousand entrants set off on the Saturday before Thanksgiving to discover for themselves what Kennedy suspected from the beginning: if we have the confidence to start, we'll find what we need to finish.

The JFK 50 is no longer the country's longest race, and it's never been the sexiest. Big-city marathons have rock bands and movie stars; Tough Mudders have Arctic Enema ice-water plunges and mud scrambles and electric-shock hazards; while the JFK has . . . silence. For long, lonely stretches, it's just you and your doubts. No cheering, no glimpses of Pamela Anderson and Will Ferrell, no victory lap through Central Park. But like one of those old family diners dwarfed by new sky-rises, JFK survives for a reason: it's where soldiers and Marines are honored as elites, and a thirteen-year-old girl who's told she's too young for the New York City Marathon can run a double through the mountains instead. It's where Zach Miller, an unknown cruise-ship worker who trains on a treadmill at sea, could shock even himself in 2012 by uncorking one of the greatest performances in the race's history. The JFK could have been designed by Teddy Roosevelt and Georges Hébert; it's the kind of enduring testament to the spirit of natural movement—to proficiency and purpose—that you rarely find anymore.

Unless, of course, you're in Brazil. Down here, another route to excellence has been dusted off from the past. It's been lost for so long, it now sounds exotic and oddly stirring. And one of the few who still know how it's done—how to be fit to be useful—has just jumped out my window and is waiting impatiently below to lead me into the jungle.

CHAPTER 28

The athlete that you remember is the
beautiful dancing athlete.

—EDWARD VILLELLA,
undefeated welterweight boxer and lead dancer
in the New York City Ballet

ERWAN LE CORRE and I are staying in a small cabana hotel in the
woods, built by a French hippie couple who came to Itacaré twenty
years ago to explore the jungle and never left. From behind the
cabanas, a smooth dirt trail wanders over the forested hills and down
to the beach, about three miles away. As much for his mind as for his
body, Erwan likes to run it barefoot. Awareness of the world begins
with your feet, he believes.

"Do you know why you get stressed after staring at your com-
puter for a half-hour?" Erwan asks after I join him outside. "Because
humans evolved to always be aware of threats around them. That
stress you feel building up is your body's reminder to get up and take
a look at the landscape. Same with your feet—if you're not letting
them do their job and tell your back and knees when they can relax,
then your body stays stiff, giving you knee problems and backaches."
Your bare feet can sense when you're balanced and on solid terrain, in
other words, so they can signal to the rest of your body that it's safe
and can loosen up a little.

We set off at an easy jog, winding through the trees until we emerge on a serene half-moon of beach just as the first slants of morning sun slash across the waves. We have it all to ourselves—until a gang of men emerges from the trees behind us.

"Mais uma vítima!" shouts a tattooed bruiser who looks like he just escaped a prison yard. "Another victim!"

Erwan glances around. He spots a bowling-ball-size rock on the sand. With a quick crouch, he scoops it up and snaps it with a sharp, two-handed throw straight at the bruiser's chest. Instead of diving out of the way, the guy catches the rock like it was a basketball, tosses it aside, and comes right at Erwan, raising his fist and growling like a grizzly. They lock arms around each other's necks, then break apart, grinning.

"He's no victim," Erwan says in Portuguese, jerking his head toward me. "He's a work in progress. Like you." Erwan introduces me to his buddy Serginho, a burly jiu-jitsu instructor who moonlights as a spearfisherman. The other seven guys are stripping off shirts and kicking off flip-flops, ready to get down to business.

Erwan wandered here from his home near Paris more than a year ago and quickly realized Itacaré had all the natural training apparatus that Georges Hébert would have loved, plus the perfect band of collaborators: a small community of Brazilian fighters who support themselves by moonlighting as surfing instructors and spearfishing guides. It's an ideal alliance: the fighters help sharpen Erwan's grappling and swimming skills, while Erwan dreams up new ways to frustrate the hell out of them.

Zuqueto can attest to that. Zuqueto is a two-time jiu-jitsu world champion and a free diver who once killed a shark using only a scuba knife and a lungful of air. But the afternoon before, Zuqueto had met his match. Erwan had lashed a long bamboo pole between two trees, forming a bouncy balance beam about eight feet long and as high as my head. Erwan swung himself up, then beckoned Zuqueto to join him.

"What are you waiting for?" Erwan taunted. Zuqueto grabbed the pole with two meaty fists, muscled himself up like a swimmer getting out of a pool, and . . . lost his balance and fell back to the ground. He leaped again and again, while Erwan amused himself by hopping from foot to foot. When Zuqueto finally stepped back, his chest heaving in fatigue and frustration, Erwan hopped down. He grabbed Zuqueto by both shoulders and gave him a friendly, tousling shake.

"This guy is in amazing shape," Erwan said. "He's strong and has great endurance. But what happened here? All he had to do was get on top of this pole, and he couldn't. I can do it. Zuqueto's great-grandfather could probably do it. At one point in time, just about every man alive could do it. But Zuqueto can't. And why? Because his body isn't smart enough."

A "smart body," Erwan explains, knows how to convert force and speed into an almost endless menu of practical movements. Hoisting yourself atop a pole may seem trivial, but if you're ever caught in a flood or fleeing an attacking dog, elevating your body five feet off the ground can make all the difference. "I meet men all the time who can bench four hundred pounds but can't climb up through a window to get someone out of a burning building," he continued. "I know guys who can run marathons but can't sprint to anyone's rescue until they put their shoes on first. Lots of swimmers do laps every morning but can't dive deep enough to save a friend, or know how to carry him over rocks to get him out of the surf."

Erwan was talking with his back to the pole. Without warning, he pivoted and launched himself into the air. He caught the pole on the fly, arched under it to gain momentum, and then, just before his mount, he slowed enough for us to follow his moves. He twisted his hips and knees, rising like a surfer catching a wave. He hopped down, light as a cat, and mounted the pole two . . . three . . . six more times, using his elbows, ankles, shoulders, and neck to create new climbing combinations.

"Being fit isn't about being able to lift a steel bar or finish an Iron-man," Erwan said. "It's about rediscovering our biological nature and releasing the wild human animal inside." He stepped back so Zuqueto could try again, and grinned with satisfaction as Zuqueto maneuvered himself up and found his balance, pumping his fist in the air like he'd won his third world championship.

This is what I came to find: the Natural Method in its natural habitat. Georges Hébert had made some pretty powerful promises about what it could do, and if he was right, it might just explain how Paddy and the other Brits on Crete accomplished something that most of the other dirty tricksters couldn't: seeing their next birthday.

In the operation's first year alone, more than half of Xan and Paddy's fellow members of the Special Operations Executive on the Continent were killed, captured, or otherwise eliminated. One SOE agent was assigned to infiltrate the Riviera's casinos but mysteriously vanished—along with a briefcase full of cash—before he could lay a bet. In Holland, an SOE radioman was captured by the Gestapo and forced at gunpoint to send messages that lured other agents to their death. In Austria, one of the SOE's top men—Alfgar Hesketh-Prichard, the best "mathematical brain of his age in England" and son of a legendary army sniper—hiked into the mountains and never hiked out. "This is no place for a gentleman," he messaged before disappearing. In France, Gus March-Phillipps revealed a spectacular talent for sneaking up on solitary German soldiers and hauling them back to Britain as prisoners. "There comes out of the sea from time to time a hand of steel which plucks the German sentries from their posts with growing efficiency," Churchill raved in a radio broadcast—but said nothing when, soon after, the Hand of Steel met a blaze of bullets.

Yet on Crete, a man trap prowled by subs and crawling with enemy troops and informants, British undercover ops hadn't lost a single man since John Pendlebury was killed during the invasion. You can't chalk it up to their training, woeful as it was, or their raw ability; with their taste for sword-sticks and poetry, with their tendency to describe German harbor mines as "about the size of a jeroboam of champagne," the Cretan crew seemed more at home with cocktails than combat. At best they had, as Antony Beevor put it, "a rather dashing and eccentric amateurism, what might be expected from a mixture of romantics and archeologists."

But once on the Sliver, they didn't just learn; they learned *fast*. Georges Hébert knew the reason, though maybe not the modern term: it's likely they were aided by biophilia, or "rewilding the psyche." We're all familiar with the way the human body evolved, the way our backs straightened and our limbs lengthened as our ancestors left the trees and adapted to life on the ground as long-range hunter-gatherers. But natural selection didn't just affect the way we look; it also shaped the way we *think*. We're living proof that our ancestors—those puny, furless, fangless wimps—developed a superb ability to read the trees, air, and ground. They lived or died by the element of surprise, which meant they had to detect danger before danger detected them, and track their prey by interpreting the faintest scents, scuffs, and rustles.

That's why we're still attracted to what eco-psychologists call the "soft fascinations" of the natural world—moonlight, autumnal forests, whispering meadows—and aren't too surprised when we hear that certain prime ministers and ex-presidents feel the compulsion to paint, over and over, mountain ranges and grazing horses. Winston Churchill began painting during World War I and relied on it the rest of his life to keep the "black dog" of depression at bay, while George W. Bush picked up the brushes immediately after his two-war presidency and has been turning out a stream of landscapes and kitten and puppy portraits ever since.

Because nature is so soothing, right? So relaxing? No—because it's Red Bull for the brain.

Or so University of Michigan researchers found when they ran a series of tests in 2008 pitting, essentially, *Your Brain In The Woods vs. Your Brain On Asphalt.* Student volunteers were given a series of numbers and asked to recite them in reverse order. Then they were split up and sent on a roughly one-hour walk: half of the volunteers strolled Huron Street, in downtown Ann Arbor, while the other half meandered the Arboretum. When they got back to the lab, they were tested again. This time, Arboretum crew didn't just outscore the street walkers; they outscored *themselves.* "Performance on backwards digit-span significantly improved when participants walked in nature, but not when they walked downtown," the researchers found. "In addition, these results were not driven by changes in mood, nor were they affected by different weather conditions."

But maybe it was a matter of noise? Maybe the city walkers were temporarily frazzled from all that traffic clatter. So the researchers came up with a new experiment, and that's when things got really interesting. Volunteers were given the same test, but instead of going for a walk afterward, they were shown pictures of either urban or woodland scenes. Then they were retested. Once again, City lost to Nature—and not just to nature but *fake* nature. So if you think sunsets and seacoasts are just pretty views, the researchers concluded, you're making a big mistake. "Simple and brief interactions with nature can produce marked increases in cognitive control," they explain in a paper for *Psychological Science* called "The Cognitive Benefits of Interacting with Nature." Treating that oceanfront hotel room "as merely an amenity," they add, "fails to recognize the vital importance of nature in effective cognitive functioning."

That's all it takes, just a reminder of our ancestral past can be enough to flip a switch in the brain that focuses attention and shuts out distractions. You slip back into hunter-gatherer mode—and when you do, you're capable of remarkable things. You can close your eyes and track by nose like a bloodhound, and even ride a mountain bike down a trail blindfolded and never miss a turn or hit a tree. Journalist Michael Finkel learned about human echolocation—the ability to "see" by sound, like bats—when he met Daniel Kish, a blind adventurer. Kish had his eyeballs removed when he was one year old because of a degenerative disease, but he grew up to become a skilled cyclist and solo backcountry hiker by relying on the echoes from sound waves he creates by clicking his tongue.

"He is so accomplished at echolocation that he's able to pedal his mountain bike through streets heavy with traffic and on precipitous dirt trails," Finkel reports. "He climbs trees. He camps out, by himself, deep in the wilderness. He's lived for weeks at a time in a tiny cabin a two-mile hike from the nearest road. He travels around the globe. He's a skilled cook, an avid swimmer, a fluid dance partner."

Kish says his hearing isn't special, just his *listening*. As proof, he holds up a pot lid. When Finkel closes his eyes and clucks, he's surprised to find he can instantly detect the difference when Kish moves the lid closer and farther from his face. You've actually got more raw ability to echolocate than a bat: our mouths aren't as suited for squeaking, but we've got a big advantage when it comes to interpreting echoes. "Just the auditory cortex of a human brain is many times larger than the entire brain of a bat," Finkel points out. "This means that humans can likely process more complex auditory information than bats."

For years, Kish has been teaching other blind students how to move in real-life ways. He sent two of them off to mountain-bike with Finkel in California's Santa Ana Mountains. "To determine where the trail is going, and where the bushes and rocks and fence posts and trees are, the boys rely on echolocation," Finkel notes. The riders slap their tongues against the bottom of their mouths, listen for the echoes, and form a mental image of the trail ahead—all at full speed. One "flies down the dirt trail in aerodynamic form, hands off the brakes, clicking as fast and as loud as he can," an awestruck Finkel finds. "I try and warn them when the trail presents a serious consequence, like a long drop-off on one side or a cactus jutting out. But mostly I'm just along for the ride. It's difficult to believe, even though it's happening right in front of me. It's incredible." The only crash, in fact, is Finkel's fault, when he hits the brakes in front of one of the blind riders and turns himself into an instant tree.

Your nose, which can detect more than a *trillion* distinct odors, has as much untapped ancestral power as your ears. A research team at the University of California, Berkeley, was curious to see whether humans can mimic bloodhounds and track by scent. So they blindfolded thirty-two student volunteers and had them put on earmuffs, thick gloves, and kneepads to eliminate any sensory input except smell. Then they laid out a thirty-foot trail of chocolate essence in a grassy field and turned them loose. "Two-thirds of the subjects successfully followed the scent, zigzagging back and forth across the path like a dog tracking a pheasant," the researchers reported in *Nature Neuroscience*. With zero training, most of them did well; with a little practice, they were great. Their tracking speed more than doubled after a few days, and that was just the tip of their potential. "Longer-term training would lead to further increases in tracking velocity," the researchers noted.

Yale University neuroscientist Dr. Gordon Shepherd had the money quote when he learned of the experiment: "If we go back on our four legs and get down on the ground, we may be able to do things we had no idea we could do." Seeing in the dark, tracking prey by nose—today they sound like superpowers, but for two million years, they were just survival. We haven't lost the natural strengths that made us the most formidable creatures on the planet. We might just need the Natural Method to wake them up.

On Itacaré's beach that morning, Erwan Le Corre hoists a rock about the size of a watermelon and passes it to Serginho, who pivots and hands it to me. I swing it into the hands of the guy beside me as Erwan hands Serginho another rock, then another, until there are five in play and it's all I can do to get one rock out of my hands before the next is shoved into my gut. Unlike medicine balls, which always have the same, easily graspable shape, the unpredictable size and weight of rocks forces you to focus intensely on grip and balance. Even though the rocks are slickening with sweat and my arms are burning, I'm desperate not to be the first to let one slip. Luckily, just when I'm in danger of smashing my toes, Erwan raises a hand for us to stop. I drop my rock, relieved—until I find out what's up next.

He pairs us off for Erwan-style wind sprints: Each of us has to hoist another guy across our shoulders in a rescue hold and race in and out of the knee-high surf. If there's a more nerve-racking workout than preventing a 220-pound Thai fighter from falling on your head while you're sprinting through churning water, I don't want to know about it. Humans are heavy and lumpy and oddly balanced, forcing you to constantly adjust your posture, footing, handholds, and core. Keeping control of a body on your back, as I soon learn, demands intense concentration.

Next Erwan has a pile of six-foot-long driftwood poles at the ready. The other guys know what to expect and start trotting down the beach. As they pass Erwan, he tosses some of them a pole. He tosses the last one to me, then takes off on a run with his hands outstretched. I toss it back, and he immediately flips it toward me again, this time a little ahead so I have to accelerate. We cross the entire beach this way, mixing up our throws, totally absorbed in our run-'n'-gun until I notice we're about to crash into the rocks. Without breaking stride, Erwan flips the stick around, plants it in the sand, and pole-vaults up onto the boulders.

By the time I climb up after him, he's twenty yards away, scuttling to the top of a giant rock overhanging the sand. "The secret to a good jump," he says, "is a good second jump. Remember your springs—" And with that, he's sailing through the air. He lands ten feet below with a deep knee bend, but instead of rolling or dropping to his knees, he bounces right up with a hop and tears off at a sprint. "You never see an animal stick a jump by flopping all over the ground," he calls up as he loops back around. "Cats are running the second they land. If you do it the same way, you'll decrease impact and be ready to flow into your next move."

All that empty air below makes Zuqueto pause. *"Caralho! Esse gajo e forte,*" Zuqueto mutters. Damn! That guy is *strong.* Then he surrenders to trust and sails off over the rocks.

For Erwan, finding Itacaré was lucky, but no accident. He'd grown up in Étréchy, an old-worldish city in northern France that's only twenty-five miles from Paris but still surrounded by tumbling rivers and old-growth forest. Erwan's father worked in a bank during the week and loved to plunge into the woods on the weekends, taking his son on long, rambling hikes. "He would climb a boulder that was too hard for me," Erwan recalls. "I'd ask him for help. He'd just shake his head and go like this"—Erwan lets his face go stony and crooks a beckoning finger.

Any soccer coach would have drooled over this tall, fearless, cat-quick kid, but those woodsy weekend boot camps with his silent father squelched any interest Erwan might have had in team sports. Instead he went the solitary route: first martial arts, earning his karate black belt by the time he was eighteen, then Olympic-style weight lifting, then triathlons. Oddly, the better he did, the worse he felt; he worried constantly that he wasn't training hard enough and became enraged whenever he lost in competition. Erwan was still a teenager, but already his fun was making him miserable.

He needed a way out, and the werewolf of Paris just might have it. For some time, Erwan had been hearing rumors about a mysterious inner-city savage who roamed the rooftops at night and called himself Hors Humain—"Beyond Human." Erwan asked around and eventually was led to Don Jean Habrey, the Fagin of a secret gang of young men who turned the city into their own wilderness park. Don Jean was pushing forty at the time, but Erwan couldn't tell by his fight-ready physique and mane of thick black hair held back by a sensei's headband. Soon Erwan was part of the tribe, learning a kind of urban guerrilla training that Don Jean called Combat Vital.

"It was like a 'Fight Club' of natural movement," Erwan explained. "We would train most of the time at night so as not to be seen, climbing bridges, balancing on the top of scaffoldings, kicking walls to toughen our bare feet, moving on all fours, dropping off bridges into the Seine in the freezing cold of winter." Combat Vital was equal parts hardcore conditioning and high-wire performance art, both without a net. Don Jean's gang would hang by their legs from a pedestrian over-pass and do upside-down crunches over speeding traffic, and climb to the top of apartment buildings to leap barefoot from roof to roof.

"There is no 'try' for this kind of practice," Erwan says. "If you miss, you die."

But Don Jean seemed unkillable. Over time, he graduated from secret midnight stunts into full-on spectacles, leaping from a heli-copter in nothing but a bathing suit to swim around an iceberg off Greenland and, at age sixty, serenading the Loch Ness Monster with a one-man kettledrum sonata before free-diving into the freezing lake to look for it. For seven years, Erwan roamed Paris and dodged police by night with Don Jean and the Combat Vital crew. He spent his summers working the beaches of Corsica, selling toys and junk jewelry and stick-on tattoos to sunbathing tourists, eventually figur-ing out a way to become his own middleman; he designed his own plastic refrigerator magnets and found a factory in Shanghai to man-ufacture them. Soon he was earning enough in royalties to live on the rest of the year.

As Don Jean drifted toward showmanship, his student got serious about scholarship. Erwan's eyes first opened to Combat Vital's roots when he was prowling the secondhand-book stalls along the Seine and happened across an old copy of Georges Hébert's *L'Éducation Physique*. He'd vaguely heard of it—there was talk among the Combat Vital disciples that Don Jean, and even the Yamakasi creators of Par-kour, had gotten some of their ideas from Hébert. Erwan dug in and was electrified.

"Be useful"—genius! It wasn't just a motto, Erwan realized; it was a law of nature, a first principle that explains how human history formed the human body. Suddenly it made sense: we're weird-looking for a reason. Strip us naked and humans look more like insects than ani-mals, what with our spindly legs and gangly arms and fat, round heads swiveling on top of peculiarly inflexible spines. We're slow and weak and can barely climb to save our lives, and we lack all the really good stuff like tails and hooves and fangs. We'd be helpless if we couldn't do three things: hunt, gather, and share.

Period. That's it. Those three occupations have been the human career path since the dawn of time, and we're still at it today. Shake-spearean sonnets, Google, the Super Bowl, NASA—strip all human achievement down to basics and they're essentially the same thing: we look for stuff, we hit it with a rock, we share the goodies and the info with the clan. We're far from the baddest cats in the jungle, but we don't have to be; for those three jobs, our bodies are the perfect tool. We can stand tall and pivot, allowing us to throw with deadly accuracy. We've got multi-jointed arms and awesome thumbs, ideal for gripping and toting. We've got language and literature because our necks are long, our lips are nimble, and our thoracic control is off the charts, all of it combining to allow the power of speech. We're Mother Nature's problem child, the species that can't sit still, because our upright posture and rubbery legs give us fantastic running range. We are what we do, and what we do is *move*—up mountains, across rivers, through the snakiest rock-face wormholes. We can't even stay put on our own planet.

Hébert didn't invent this stuff, Erwan knew. Well before witnessing the Martinique volcano, Hébert had been intrigued by the ocean-going gymnastics of the *gabiers*, deckhands who wrestled sailcloth and scaled masts and wet rigging in wind and surging seas. *Those guys must have been really impressive and great athletes*, Erwan thought. Hébert also spent time in French colonies and found his ideal athletes in Montagnard mountain tribesmen in Vietnam and African hunter-gatherers. "Their bodies were splendid, flexible, nimble, skillful, enduring, resistant and yet they had no other tutor in Gymnastics but their lives in Nature," Hébert observed.

Hébert wasn't an inventor; he was an observer. That's what made him so fiery about things like female strength, because he knew the truth was right under the nose of anyone willing to open their eyes and minds. "Young black African woman, where the magnificent development of the torso stands comparison with Venus," Hébert argued. "What a marvelous ideal for the French mother!" Renoir's paintings of bathing beauties drove Hébert *nuts*—why pretend women are nothing more than animated cream puffs? Men and women don't have the same bodies, but they have the same motor skills. "The natural doctrine applies as much to girls' education as it does to boys'," Hébert insisted.

Wait, put gender aside for a sec. What about age? If Hébert was right, Erwan thought, he wasn't just promoting good health—he was freezing time. How did Hébert put it? *Their bodies were resistant.* Exactly. There's no margin for error in the wilderness, so our survival depended on long-lasting suppleness and sinew. When that volcano blows, when the clan needs your help, when the moment comes to *move*, you can't be icing your sore knee on the sofa or excusing yourself as too old, young, or girly. Méthode Naturelle could make you not only powerful, Erwan realized, but also age resistant. You'd get strong and *stay* strong, deep into old age.

Erwan was on fire. He went on a research pilgrimage to Reims, site of Georges Hébert's first training playground, which was destroyed during frontline fighting in World War I. The Marquis Melchior de Polignac, owner of Champagne Pommery, was a big fan of Hébert's work, so he made sure it was later restored to Hébert's original specifications. While Erwan was in Reims, he knocked up at Pommery headquarters to see if maybe they had some old Georges Hébert stuff lying around? Journals, possibly. Or photos?

They had something even better: a phone number.

In the suburbs of Paris, Hébert's son was still alive. Régis Hébert agreed to let this intense young disciple visit . . . and keep on visiting. Every time Erwan returned to the Hébert house, he was hungrier than before. "I came back with a big list of questions—questions I couldn't find any answer to in Hébert's book, about Hébert, his personal lifestyle, how he educated his children."

Régis said his father had lived what he preached, including the revolutionary step of deploying his wife and other women as Méthode Naturelle instructors. Just before the war began, Georges felt he was close to connecting true health with heroism. "It was the great time of MN," Erwan says. "Hébert believed that if everyone was practicing MN with its altruistic goal, with its moral education benefits, there would be no wars anymore, no reasons for people to be in conflict with each other."

Hébert didn't live to see his dream come true, but Erwan could. *Someone* had to remind the world what Méthode Naturelle had to offer. Erwan went to get Régis's blessing—and the old man erupted. How *dare* Erwan think he could follow in the great man's footsteps? If Erwan tried, Régis warned him, he'd regret it. Erwan was stung and mystified. *What the hell just happened?* A few weeks earlier, Régis had been all smiles and encouragement. Now he was sputtering and threatening.

·   ·   ·

Erwan couldn't figure out what went wrong, until he tracked down some other MN old-timers who wised him up. "Hébert's son is the gravedigger of his father's work," they told Erwan. Régis can't revive Méthode Naturelle himself but is afraid someone else will, they said. So he just clutches his father's legacy to his chest and monitors anything said or written about it "like some kind of censor."

So the old man never really wanted to meet me in the first place, Erwan thought. *He just wanted to find out what I was up to. Okay*, Erwan decided; *so that's how we'll play.* Erwan knew Georges Hébert had sucked up information from all over—not just from native islanders but also from thinkers like Edwin Checkley; Dr. Paul Carton, the pioneering French physician; Francisco Amorós, the Spanish military instructor; and Johann Heinrich Pestalozzi, the Swiss education innovator. From their ideas, Hébert fashioned his own.

"Did Hébert just replicate the path Amorós had designed?" Erwan asks. "Nope. He followed it but retooled it, improved it, redesigned it."

So to hell with Régis. Now it was Erwan's turn.

Serginho and the guys have to scoot, and only then does it hit me that we've been working out nonstop for nearly two hours. I'm wiped out, but exhilarated. Erwan suggests we cool off by practicing one more skill—open-water deep dives—but before we reach the surf, we're approached by a young woman who'd been watching from under a coconut tree.

So, she asks, what's with all the rock jumping and stick throwing?

Instead of explaining, Erwan grabs a driftwood pole. He plants one end in the sand and rests the other on his shoulder. He bends into a squat. "What's your name?" he asks.

"Sandra."

"Sandra, if you can get to the top of this pole, I have a surprise for you."

Sandra studies his face for hints of a prank. Then she *sprints*, straight up the pole and over the top of Erwan's head. She's on the ground before she realizes she really did it.

"Bravo!" Erwan says, delighted. Then he removes the pole from his shoulder and places it on hers. "Surprise!"

Erwan barely gives her a chance to protest before he's off, quick-footing up the pole like a tightrope walker. Sandra's face flashes through four emotional peaks in four seconds: surprise, fear, resolve, and—as Erwan reaches her shoulder and hops off—triumph.

"Did you know you were that strong?" Erwan asks.

Sandra shakes her head.

"Now you do. Don't get into trouble!"

Sandra smiles and starts to head back to her tree. But Erwan has another question.

"Are you doing . . . *yoga*?"

Uh-oh.

"Yes, I'm an instructor and—"

"You *teach* that?" Erwan says. "Have you ever used yoga for anything useful?"

"It's very use—"

"No, in real life. In an emergency. Has anyone ever shouted, *Quick! Sun-salute for your life!* Of course not. But you hear *Run for your life! Climb for your life! Don't worry, I'll carry you out of here!* all the time. Humans made yoga up for recreation, not for survival. No animal would ever do it. Changing postures in the same place with your head down? Forget it! In the wild, that's death. You need the luxury of a no-danger environment for yoga. Everything is controlled—the soft mat, the temperature, some guru telling you what to do. It's not instinctive or natural. It's make-believe."

Yoga isn't about emergencies, Sandra argues. It's about finding balance and a mind-body connection.

"Your body will never be more connected to your mind than when something is at stake," Erwan retorts. "That's how you measure the value of a movement: by its consequences. Climb a tree, throw a rock, balance on the edge of a cliff—you lose focus for a fraction of a second, you're screwed. It takes a very affluent and indulged culture to convince itself that standing around in weird poses is exercise."

Despite Erwan's rat-a-tat-tat attack, it's obvious he wants to win Sandra over, not beat her down. That's enough to make her step once more into the buzz saw.

You're forgetting flexibility, she offers. Yoga makes you more limber.

"If your muscles resist a movement, it's because the movement is unnatural. So why change the muscle? Change the movement!" Erwan drops down in the sand and juts a leg out in a hurdler's pose. "If your hamstring won't let you stretch like this," he says, bending forward with his head over his knee "then move like *this*." Swiftly, he jackknifes the leg back so it folds under his butt. He's able to reach much farther forward, and he's much better balanced.

"Now, which one is a real mind-body connection?"

"I think he's really onto something," says Lee Saxby, a physical therapist and technical director of Wildfitness, a London-based exercise program built around an evolutionary model of human performance. Saxby is convinced that true human health has nothing to do with exercise machines and everything do to with hunter-gatherer movements, and when he stumbled across a remarkable video by Erwan, he found Exhibit A in the flesh.

As declarations of war go, it's unique: in a magical three and a half minutes called "The Workout the World Forgot," Erwan makes a devastating case for ancestral fitness—and he does it without saying a single word. It opens with Erwan carrying a log across a tumbling river, then rockets along as he charges across a savage landscape, instantly molding his body under and around everything in his path. He sprints straight at a stone tower . . . crashing waves . . . a breathtakingly high ledge . . . a mixed martial-arts fighter who appears out of nowhere . . . and Erwan never slows, instead twisting, sprinting, swimming, climbing, fighting, and vaulting past them all. He's utterly serene and terribly powerful, a human animal in command of his body and everything it meets.

"What impresses me most about that video is his athleticism," Saxby says. "It drives me crazy that women think being in shape is being skinny and men think it's being big. But the best athletes don't look like models or bodybuilders. They're lean and quick and mobile. That's what I like about Erwan's video. It's a demonstration of real functional fitness, the opposite of the bulking-up stuff they teach you in the gym."

Erwan, in fact, could be one of the best living examples of what our bodies were originally designed to do. "Versatility was absolutely the key to survival, because early humans had to be ready for anything at any time," explains E. Paul Zehr, Ph.D., a neuroscience and kine-siology professor at the University of Victoria who examined human biomechanical potential in his book *Becoming Batman: The Possibility of a Superhero.* "When early *Homo sapiens* set off in the morning, he never knew what he'd encounter. If your daily life is hunting and being hunted, at a moment's notice you might have to sprint, jog, throw a spear, scramble up a tree, hunker down and dig. The specialization we enjoy today, be it as a marathoner, tennis player, even a triathlete, is a luxury of modern society. It doesn't have great survival value for *Homo sapiens* in the wild."

But Erwan's most important throwback could be the way he's welded purpose and playfulness, function and fun. When he jumps and tumbles and chucks stuff around, he looks just like a kid goofing around in the backyard, which Dr. Zehr believes could be our true ancestral workout. "You never see your dog running nonstop around and around in a circle for an hour," Zehr points out. "If he did, you'd think there's something really wrong with him. Instead, he'll chase something, roll around, sprint, rest, mix things up. Animal play has a purpose, and it's not hard to surmise that human play should as well."

"Most people see exercise as punishment for being fat," adds Saxby. "So instead of being a release for stress, it's one more mental burden. That's why I think what this guy Erwan is up to is bang on. If you can reverse the idea that exercise is punishment, that's a great gift."

Reverse the idea . . . maybe by creating giant adult playgrounds? With mud pits and flaming straw bales and wacky electrical shock hazards that look like jellyfish tentacles? In 2010, one of the least likely voices in fitness (a Harvard Business School student) traveled to the least likely place to launch a trend (Allentown, Pennsylvania) and rigged together some big-kid toys on a backwater ski resort. Five years later, "Tough Mudders" and other obstacle-course challenges, like Warrior Dashes and Spartan Races, are sonic-booming. Jogging is even in danger of losing its crown as Most Popular Participation Sport, because this year more people are likely to splash through a freezing pond en route to a wall climb than run a half-marathon. Granted, these mass muck-athons are more about thrills than skills; few Spartan Racers do anything more to prepare for the cargo-net scrambles and water-tower leaps than paint their faces and pay the fee. Still, there's a good bit about these events that would warm Georges

Hébert's heart. Tough Mudder has no winners or finishing times, focusing instead on camaraderie over competition. And all of them at least *champion* the idea of functional fitness: by the time you finish, you'll know lots about what you can't do. As far as doing it, that's where the Box comes in.

In the early 2000s, word began to spread among California police officers and local Navy SEALs that the best place to find a real-world workout was the vacant lot behind a FedEx depot in Santa Cruz. There, a former competitive gymnast named Greg Glassman was leading the faithful through sprints, dead lifts, and his holy trinity of functional fitness: squats, pull-ups, and burpees (a push-up that explodes into a hop). Those three maneuvers—getting up off your butt, up off your belly, and up off the ground—are basic for animal survival, yet Glassman found that many people couldn't handle them. And isn't that the whole point of exercise, just mastering your body weight? He called his approach CrossFit, and the cops he trained said it felt less like a conventional workout and more like "a foot race that turns into a fight." CrossFit remains so wedded to pure and simple movement that if Teddy Roosevelt were to rise from the dead, the one place he'd feel at home after ninety-six years would be a CrossFit "Box" (so dubbed because an early training facility was a storage unit in a San Francisco parking lot).

But on Crete, there weren't any boxes. For Xan and Paddy to survive, they'd have to rely on something even more urgent and ancestral, something that could prepare them for a fugitive's life in the mountains. Something like what Erwan is getting up to in the branches overhead.

"Ready?" Erwan asks from his perch twenty feet up in a tree.

"Sure you are," he answers himself before we can speak. "Let's do it!"

After three days of double-sessions training, it's time for my combination going-away present/final exam. Erwan has fashioned an obstacle course that will both test my jungle-man skills and give me a model to reconstruct back home in Pennsylvania. In keeping with his gospel of group dynamics, he asked Zuqueto and Fábio, another Brazilian fighter, to join me.

"The test," Erwan says, "is to finish the course twice in less than twenty minutes." He drops his hand—*GO!*—and we're off, chasing hard on each other's heels. Erwan's course has about twelve stations, all of them sequenced into a natural flow through the forest. We're springing up into trees, contorting through the branches, and shinnying down fifteen-foot poles. He has us hoisting heavy *curdurú* logs up on an end and flipping them, bottom over top, up a hill. Then we're crawling around stakes in the ground and snaking on our bellies through an overturned dugout canoe mounted a few inches off the ground. Even a small cabin comes into play: we're vaulting through one window and out the other.

The most ingenious thing about Erwan's course, I realize as I finish the first lap, is how universal it is. Sure, it's a blast to horse around in trees in the middle of the Brazilian rain forest, but there isn't anything here that can't be duplicated in a suburban backyard—or even a suburban street, if you're blessed with Erwan's total disregard for arched eyebrows. The day before, I'd watched him stroll down Itacaré's main street and treat it like his personal rec center. He monkeywalked up a staircase on all fours, tightrope-walked along a railing, and vaulted back and forth down the length of a fence. By the time we'd walked five blocks, he'd knocked out a healthy workout and was ready for pizza.

I have three minutes left and only two obstacles to go—a leap from the porch, then a quick climb up a twenty-foot pole braced between the ground and a branch high in a tree. I'm trying not to show it, but through the sweat and grime on my face, I'm beaming. Two days ago, my heart was in my throat before every jump. Now, after just seventy-two hours, I feel unstoppable. All I need to do is push a little harder and I'll be right on Fábio's heels.

Naturally, that's when disaster strikes.

When I stick the landing off the porch, a red-hot knife jabs me in the spine. My back is seizing so badly, I can't even stand up straight. I should have known I was pushing my luck—fourteen-hour plane trips always leave me tight as a banjo string. So that's it, I'm done. Until I remember Erwan's motto.

Smart body, I remind myself. *Use your smart body.*

I take hold of the long pole that extends on a forty-five-degree angle up into the tree. Gingerly, I hook one foot up, then the other, until I'm hanging upside down from the pole like a pig on a spit. I tighten my grip and wonder what the hell to do next.

"Any ideas?" I ask Erwan.

"Claro," he responds. "Sure. Lots of them." It's an excellent teaching moment, the perfect opportunity to dig into his mental archives and pull out a few of the innovations he's compiled over the years. I've seen them in his notes, pages and pages of stick-figure drawings dating back to Georges Hébert's original field experiments. Erwan has a lot of wisdom to pass on—but instead he just stands there, arms folded across his chest. He doesn't give me a clue, or even a smile.

Neither do Zuqueto or Fábio. They've become hardcore converts to the essence of Erwan's philosophy: when that volcano blows, you've got to be ready to go on your own. You won't have any lifting partner to ease the bar off your chest, no volunteer handing you Gatorade at the twenty-mile mark. A group dynamic may be our natural impulse, but in a pinch, count on being a lonely man. The only thing you can always rely on is the ingenuity and raw mobility preprogrammed into your system by two million years of hope and fear.

My hands are slick with sweat and starting to slip off the pole. Just to get a better grip till I can think of something, I slowly start swinging from side to side, building up momentum. At the top of every swing, my body is suspended for a sec in midair. That's when I move my hands and feet farther up the pole, gliding higher and higher with almost no pain or effort.

"Ahhh, you learned my secret!" Erwan calls from down below as I approach the top of the pole. "The best secret of all—your body always has another trick up its sleeve."

CHAPTER 29

May God deliver you into the hands of the Greeks.

—A CORSICAN CURSE PADDY LIKED TO QUOTE

PADDY HAD A FEW TRICKS up his own sleeve. He had a pretty good notion of what to expect from the Butcher, and so he'd schemed accordingly. The Butcher was vicious but cautious, preferring to hit a target he knew wouldn't hit back. He wouldn't storm into the mountains after he discovered General Kreipe was missing; no, he'd make a move only when he knew what was going on. So first he'd fan out his spies and ransack the coastal villages, and that would lead him right to General Kreipe's staff car, with the note inside and the phony British commando clues scattered around.

And by that point, Paddy's last two bits of Magic Gang trickery would be in play: as soon as SOE headquarters got word they'd made the snatch, BBC Radio would broadcast a news flash saying the general was off the island and en route to Cairo. At the same time, British planes would letter-bomb Crete with leaflets saying British commandos had delivered the general to Egypt.

The Butcher would be furious, but he wasn't crazy. With no blood on the ground, he wouldn't launch a manhunt if there was no man to hunt. He'd probably triple-down his attempts to root out rebel nests, but those attacks would be localized and concentrated on specific targets; unless he absolutely had to, there's no way he'd risk any more abductions by scattering his men across the mountains. That would take the heat off a little, giving Paddy and his gang enough breathing space to dart out in the open and get the general up and over stony Mount Ida and then down to the real embarkation point, on the southern coast.

All around, it was a lovely plan. For about six hours.

Paddy had split his band into three teams. Billy was up front, leading the general to the first rendezvous point. Paddy was catching up from the west after ditching the car on the beach. Andoni Zoidakis and his crew were coming from the east with Alfred Fenske, the general's driver. Fenske was really slowing them down; he was still so wobbly from that crack across the skull Billy Moss gave him that he could barely walk. With sunup approaching, Zoidakis decided to take cover and let Fenske rest until dark. They wouldn't have to worry about search parties until noon, maybe midafter—

Zoidakis froze. He poked his head out for a look, then yanked it back. Impossible. The Germans were on the hunt already? It was still night. How could they even know the general was gone? But there they were, fanned out in a search sweep just three hundred yards or so behind them. Zoidakis had to decide, fast, if they could slip away, with Fenske stumbling all over the place. Zoidakis must have looked worried, because the German driver got curious and stood up to see what was going on. Zoidakis slashed Fenske's throat before he could open his mouth.

Almost immediately, Zoidakis regretted it. Fenske hadn't actually done anything wrong. And Paddy was going to be *so* upset. . . .

Which reminded him: they had to get word to Paddy right away. For some reason, the hunt was already on.

Destination 1 was a cave just outside the village of Anogia. The closer Billy and his team got, the more trouble they had with the general. As soon as Kreipe felt confident he wouldn't be executed, he slowed down to a grumbling trudge. He was thirsty and really hungry, he complained; they'd grabbed him on his way home for supper. And his leg was killing him. Why'd they have to drag him out of the car like that? And where was his Knight's Cross? Had anyone seen his medal? Billy kept pushing him along, finally making it to the cave in a cliff face. They pushed the general up, one handhold at a time, then slipped inside and disguised the mouth with torn branches. One of the gang slipped off to Anogia to rustle up some food and ask around for news.

Paddy and George Tyrakis weren't far behind. But instead of going directly to the rendezvous, Paddy slipped into Anogia. He needed to get a messenger to Tom Dunbabin right away, and then sit tight for Tom's reply. Tom was the last, crucial part of Paddy's Magic Gang plan: Paddy was counting on him to make radio contact with Cairo and coordinate the letter bombing, the BBC broadcast, and the pickup boat.

As Paddy and George entered Anogia, doors and windows slammed shut around them. "All talk and laughter died at the washing troughs, women turned their backs and thumped their laundry with noisy vehemence; cloaked shepherds, in answer to greeting, gazed past us in silence," Paddy observed. "In a moment we could hear women's voices wailing into the hills: 'The black cattle have strayed into the wheat!' and 'Our in-laws have come!'"

So this is what it's like for the Germans, Paddy realized. *Good!* Many of the most effective Cretan freedom fighters—the *andartes*—were sons of Anogia. So deep was the villagers' loathing for the Germans that even though Paddy was a well-known friend, all they could see was the uniform he was wearing. Even when he knocked up at the house of his good friend, the rebel priest Father Charetis, he wasn't allowed through the door.

"It's me, Pappadia!" he whispered to the priest's wife. He gave her his code name: "It's me: Mihali!"

"What Mihali?" she replied innocently. "I don't know any Mihali." Then she took a closer look. Only when she recognized the familiar gap between Paddy's teeth did she let him inside. Paddy didn't explain what he was doing there or why he was dressed like a German corporal, and everyone knew better than to ask. Father Charetis simply sent a boy off with Paddy's message to Tom Dunbabin, then laid out food.

Paddy was still resting and waiting for Tom's reply when leaflets began fluttering down over the village. Excellent! The runner must have made it to Tom's hideout in record time. Paddy got one and read:

TO ALL CRETANS:
LAST NIGHT THE GERMAN GENERAL KREIPE WAS ABDUCTED
BY BANDITS. HE IS NOW BEING CONCEALED IN THE CRETAN
MOUNTAINS. HIS WHEREABOUTS CANNOT BE UNKNOWN
TO THE POPULACE . . .

Wait. What happened to Paddy's leaflets?

IF THE GENERAL IS NOT RETURNED WITHIN THREE DAYS, ALL
VILLAGES IN THE HERAKLION DISTRICT WILL BE BURNED TO
THE GROUND. THE SEVEREST MEASURES OF REPRISAL WILL BE
BROUGHT TO BEAR ON THE CIVILIAN POPULATION.

Damn. Either way you looked at it, it didn't make sense. If the Germans had found the car already, how did they know the general was in the mountains and not on a boat? And if they *hadn't* found the car, why were they searching?

Paddy's calculations turned out to be very right and very wrong. As he expected, the Butcher didn't tear off in a rage and start burning villages. He was taking his time, asking questions, and circling the trail. But instead of falling for Paddy's ruse, the Butcher was getting dangerously close to the truth.

The Butcher first became suspicious after one of the sentries radioed the fortress to ask about the general's whereabouts. The Butcher always ranted that the Cretans were brutes and the Brits were harmless pests, but privately, he suspected there was a lot more going on in the mountains than he could see. Air convoys were swarmed within moments of leaving Crete, German sergeants left their rooms for an hour and returned to find them ransacked, an Italian general vanished from under the Butcher's nose and popped up in Cairo . . . and now a commanding general goes on a nighttime joyride? No, something was up.

So this time the Butcher went to the maps and began thinking like a bandit. If General Kreipe were dead, they'd know it by now. His corpse was too valuable as a shock tactic, and attacking German morale was a key Resistance tactic; the Butcher couldn't prove it, but he had to suspect it was bandits, not German soldiers, who were chalking walls with graffiti-like *scheisse Hitler* ("Hitler is a shit") and *Wir wollen nach haus!* ("We want to go home!").

So where do you hide a German officer on an island full of Germans? The general's car was definitely spotted in Heraklion; it never arrived in Chania; the northern shore was too exposed for boats; the coastal villages had too many turncoats. That left . . .

Anogia. High in the hills, bristling with patriotic fever, gateway to Mount Ida and a single night's hike from the road to Heraklion. That had to be it. They'd kidnapped him and fled to Anogia. The Butcher sent out the order: by first light he wanted thirty thousand troops on the march and plane crews ready to scramble. *Search the hills around Heraklion*, he commanded. *Get aerial photos of all the footpaths leading out of Heraklion. But our priority is Anogia.*

By dawn, the Butcher had seized back the advantage. The kidnappers wouldn't expect anyone to confirm the general's disappearance until morning. By then, they'd be surrounded.

Paddy expected a pretty hot response at Father Charetis's house when they discovered what kind of a jam he'd gotten them into, and he was right. "The room was convulsed with incredulity, then excitement and finally by an excess of triumphant hilarity," Paddy observed. "We could hear feet running in the street, and shouts and laughter." The entire village was facing destruction, but instead of cowering, they were erupting with joy.

"Eh!" Paddy heard one old man say. "They'll burn them all down one day. And what then? My house was burnt down four times by the Turks; let the Germans burn it down for a fifth! And they killed scores of my family, scores of them, my child. Yet here I am! We're at war, and war has all these things. You can't have a wedding feast without meat. Fill up the glasses, Pappadia."

They loved Paddy's plot because it was more than an act of war: it was a tribute to them, personally, as Cretans. Nothing is more Cretan—or more Greek—than pulling off an impossible hustle. Greek heroes were always stealing stuff, the bigger and weirder and more impossible the better. Sticky fingers are so important to Greek theology, it's hard to find a myth that doesn't involve someone pulling a fast one. Half of Hercules' Twelve Labors were heists, including snatching an Amazon's girdle and a team of man-eating horses. Prometheus made off with the gods' fire; Jason grabbed the Golden Fleece; Theseus was constantly dragging off women who caught his eye, namely a warrior queen and a Cretan princess. The *Iliad* and the *Odyssey* are a pair of true-crime classics; nothing gets done in either one until someone gets sneaky.

And that someone is usually Odysseus, whose rogue's eye made him the greatest of the Greek heroes. Breaking into Troy by hiding inside a hollow horse was Odysseus's idea, and he warmed up for it by first sneaking behind enemy lines and making off with a rival king's armor and prized warhorses. Odysseus was a born thief, the descendant of a long line of light-fingers: his dad was Laertes, one of the Fleece-seizing Argonauts, although his true biological father was rumored to be Sisyphus, famous for robbing houseguests. His granddad was the Thief Lord, Autolycus, and his great-granddad was Hermes, god of thieves.

But for all their shenanigans, you don't see the heroes piling up a mountain of loot. They're not in it for gold; given a choice, Odysseus would be happier farming at home with his wife. Stealing wasn't his job; it was a calling, an art, a way of making the impossible possible and the imaginary real. Pulling off a clever heist is as close as humans can come to magic, allowing something in your mind's eye to suddenly appear in your hand. Other religions condemn thieves as sinners and outcasts, but the ancient Greeks shrugged and decided, *Eh, let's give 'em their own god.* Because who else will teach us that our stuff doesn't really matter? That our possessions are fleeting, forgettable, and that anything you have someone else can take? What you'll be remembered for isn't your wealth and power, but your creative imagination—your *mêtis*.

The brazen *mêtis* of a thief—that was the animating spirit of ancient Greek, and it sparked an explosion of creativity unrivaled in intellectual history. The Olympics, the Acropolis, democratic government, trial by jury, the dramatic rules of comedy and tragedy, Pythagorean and Archimedean geometry, Aristotelian and Platonic philosophy, the predictive cycles of astronomy and the humanitarian principles of medicine—it all came careening out of a tiny island nation so small and thinly populated, it was as if the dominant force on Western thought for more than three thousand years was the state of Alabama.

What fueled it all was a kind of Outlaw Outlook: *Instead of relying on laws passed down from some god or a king, let's think like outlaws. Let's think for ourselves.* An outlaw outlook calls on every citizen to create, not conform; to decide what is right and wrong and act on it, not just *baa* along with the rest of the herd. Outlaws have to be poised, smart, and independent; they have to cultivate allies, assess risk, and keep their antennae fine-tuned to everyone and everything around them. Outlaws focus on what people *can* do, not what they shouldn't. In Athens, the outlaw outlook worked so beautifully, it became a civic responsibility. The Athenians still had laws, but they were proposed by average citizens, not imperial rulers. Anyone who started acting too bossy—who thought he knew what was best for everyone else—was marched to the border and sent into exile under Athens's steely "No Tyrants" policy.

Not even gods had the final say: instead of one Almighty there were a dozen, all divvying up the work and jockeying for position. Zeus was the big dog, but he was constantly being one-upped and second-guessed. One of his biggest worries was being outsmarted by his first wife—whose name, of course, was Mêtis. She was an alluring Titan known for her "magical cunning" and close friendship with that master thief Prometheus. Zeus managed to muster a little cunning of his own and con Mêtis into briefly transforming herself into a fly, giving him a chance to grab and swallow her—forever uniting, in the eyes of the ancient Greeks, the bond between imagination and immortality: the spirit of resourcefulness was now buzzing inside a god who would never die.

Not that everyone was on board. An outlaw outlook meant freedom, which put it at odds with *biê*—"brute force." *Biê* was for kings and conquerors, the mighty and the muscle-bound; *mêtis* was power to the people, especially the weak and poor who had no other options. Achilles was bursting with *biê* and sneered at the schemes of Odysseus, who was "equal to Zeus in *mêtis.*" Too late, Achilles discovered that even a golden warrior can be taken out by a nobody with a good idea; an idea like, say, infuriating your enemy so much he forgets to cover his vulnerable heel. Achilles' cousin, Ajax, was just as much of a raging bull and learned the same lesson: when he wrestled Odysseus, he was twisted around and thumped down on his back before he saw it coming.

"It is with *mêtis* rather than *biê* that a woodcutter is better," the ancient warrior Nestor coaches his son in the *Iliad.* "It is *mêtis* that lets a pilot on the wine-dark sea keep a swift ship on course when a gale strikes. And *mêtis* makes one charioteer better than another."

For young Brits like Xan and Paddy, brute force was everything they were trying to escape. *Biê* was boarding school beatings, Victorian prudishness, the blind obedience to the dogma of "Theirs not to make reply, / Theirs not to reason why, / Theirs but to do and die" that sent their fathers and brothers marching into machine-gun fire during the Great War. Weirdly, religion had a lot to do with it. Once the Greek myths were replaced by Christianity, the raucous tribe of Olympians were replaced by just one God. Instead of becoming our own heroes, we were given a list of commandments and told to follow the rules, bend our knees, and wait for a savior.

Not on Crete, though. The Island of Heroes still followed the ancient code, and when Xan and Paddy and Billy Moss arrived, they discovered a whole new level of outlaw thinking.

"*Klepsi-klepsi*—translatable into English as 'swiping' or 'pinching' but hardly stealing—is something of a Cretan sport," Billy learned after being awakened with a cold splash of outlaw thinking when his bedroll and warm clothes were nicked by a fellow rebel. "Sympathy is usually on the side of the 'pincher' rather than of the loser. If you allow someone to steal from you, it is you who are the mug, he the clever fellow."

Crete had been under the heel of invaders for so long that stealing had become the job of patriots. Sheep rustling was the only way for Resistance fighters to survive during the Turkish occupation, so heroic struggle became synonymous with banditry. They're even the same word: in Cretan dialect, rebels and robbers are both *klephts*. "It's one of the most important Greek lessons you could learn," George Psychoundakis told a new SOE recruit, urging him to steal some grapes. "As your teacher, I insist on it!" To survive on Crete, you had to think and act like an old-time hero.

Which is exactly what Paddy had done. He'd gone into the Minotaur's lair and not only defeated the monster but snuck it out on a leash.

The roar of trucks brought an end to the merriment. A German convoy was grinding up the mountain road and pouring into the Anogia town square. Within minutes, soldiers were hopping down and scurrying into formation.

Up, up, the Cretans told Paddy. *You've got to get out of here.* The Germans could surround the village at any moment and begin the house-to-house ransack. Paddy and George scrambled their gear and headed toward the door. Could someone guide them to Billy's hideout? And was there a donkey they could bring along for the general?

Yes, yes, their host replied. *Whatever you need. But hurry.*

"You'll see!" Paddy promised as he went out the door. "Those three days will go by and there won't be any villages burnt or even shooting!" Privately, however, he wasn't feeling so bully. "I prayed that urgency would lend wings to the messengers' heels," he thought to himself, "and scatter our counter leaflets and the BBC News of the General's departure from the island."

The town square was teeming with troops as Paddy and George cautiously worked their way through the streets. Paddy couldn't figure out how the Butcher got his men to Anogia so quickly, but he was even more perplexed by why they were still standing around. The Butcher had the drop on them, so why didn't he snap shut the trap? If the Germans had circled Anogia as soon as they arrived, Paddy and Billy might be in chains by now. So what were they waiting for?

The Butcher was frozen by a chilling thought: *What if it's a feint?*

The bandits were smart, so smart that the Butcher hadn't managed to lay his hands on a single Brit the entire time he'd been on Crete. Every time he got close, they were one jump ahead. So could trapping them really be so easy this time? Or did they *want* to be chased? The bandits had to know that nothing would outrage the Germans more than kidnapping a general from right under the nose of the Gestapo. Thousands of German foot soldiers would be hot on their trail, racing into the mountains and drawing fleets of fighter planes into the backcountry . . . *leaving Fortress Crete and the capital exposed!*

So that was their game. *Maybe,* the Butcher thought, *Kreipe's abduction was an Allied ploy to make him move large forces towards the mountains, thereby allowing them to land on the plains while the* andartes *and commandos attacked from the rear.* He wasn't going to fall for it. The Butcher sent word to Anogia: *Bring one company back to Heraklion immediately.* He ordered the reconnaissance planes back to base and the leafleting postponed till further notice. Before scattering his troops all over the mountains, the Butcher needed to be ready for invasion.

By nightfall, the coast was secure. The hunt for General Kreipe was ready to resume at full force—but Paddy and his crew had already slipped back into the wilderness.

CHAPTER 30

Where danger is,
Deliverance also beckons.

—FRIEDRICH HÖLDERLIN, "Patmos"

CHRIS WHITE AND I began hunting Paddy's trail as soon as the sun rose high enough for us to see the ground. We'd set off before daybreak from Heraklion, hopping a bus to the exact spot along the shore where, according to Chris' calculations, Paddy had ditched the general's car. Chris checked his bearings: Mount Ida straight ahead, rocky thumbnail of beach dead behind. Yup, we'd found the right meadow. But there was no hint of a path, nothing except a snarl of brambles leading straight to an unclimbable cliff.

"Brilliant, isn't it?" Chris said. "It would have been just as wild when Paddy came through. You can just imagine the Germans looking at this and thinking, *Well, they certainly didn't go* that *way.*"

Chris had been exploring on foot over the past two years with his brother, Pete, and exchanging notes with his fellow escape sleuths, Alun Davies and Christopher Paul and Tim Todd, so he was pretty sure he could now connect all the dots of the escape route. Except, that is, Dot #1. Pete would have been a huge help; his years of work in the New Forest had given him a flair for backcountry navigation, as I'd learned on our previous expedition, but he couldn't make it this time. It was just Chris and I, and we were lost before we began.

Chris was unfazed. He scanned the thorny mess slowly, walking as far into the brambles as he could and dropping to a crawl when he couldn't, working his way back and forth until his hand shot into the air and we were on our way. We followed the faint goat track high into the hills, climbing in and out of gullies until we emerged, just before noon, on a bluff overlooking a weird oasis: far below was a small cluster of stone buildings surrounded by tidy gardens.

We picked our way down and entered a silent cobblestone courtyard. Chris reached for the bell rope over the entrance, but before he could pull, a little Hobbit's door creaked open.

"*Kalos orisate*," we heard from somewhere in the darkness. "Welcome."

We ducked inside the low door and found ourselves in a small, stone-floored kitchen. A monk with a chest-length black beard pressed a hand over his heart and gave a slight bow. He was Father Timothy Stavros, curator of the tiny Vossakou Monastery. How, he asked in halting English, could he be of service? Chris pulled out his letter, the one in Greek and English that explained our interest in the Kreipe kidnapping.

Father Timothy nodded. "Yes. They were here."

He led us through the kitchen and outside to a porch overlooking the valley. Clay bowls full of foraged greens and spinach covered a shelf along the wall; hanging from nails in the beams overhead were mesh bags full of snails, airing for a few days as they purged themselves for cooking. Snails were freedom fighters' food; you could harvest them on the run and they'd go dormant and keep fresh in your pockets until you were in the clear to cook. The Germans didn't eat them, so villagers could gather them by the bushel without worrying they'd be seized and sneak them to guerrillas without fearing their food supplies would look suspiciously low. *Kohli me stari* has become one of my favorite meals on Crete—snails stewed in a broth of garlic and tomatoes and olive oil, with maybe an onion and some torn mint thrown in and a fistful of coarse cracked wheat added to thicken it into a paella-like porridge.

We sat down as another monk silently appeared with a pitcher of cold water and a plate of small, hard biscuits sprinkled with sesame seeds. Vossakou was built more than four hundred years ago, Father Timothy explained, but had been repeatedly destroyed by generations of invaders. "Eighteen of us were killed by the Turks," he said. "Two of us were

executed here"—he pointed a few yards away to a spot in the garden—
"by the Germans. People who needed food came for help, so we helped.
The Germans didn't like that." Father Timothy wasn't here at the time;
he's only about fifty and had originally been a florist in Rethymno.
For the past eight years, he's been mostly alone at Vossakou. The
older members of the order have all died off, leaving Father Timothy
as one of the last living custodians of the monastery's stormy history.

"The general spent about an hour here that night," Father Timothy
said, which baffled us until suddenly it made perfect sense. Billy and
his prisoner had gotten out of the car *past* Vossakou, not behind, so it
must have been Paddy in his German uniform the monks had seen.
Paddy and George Tyrakis would have been parched and ravenous
when they arrived here long after midnight; they'd had nothing to eat
or drink since early in the evening and had been on a roller coaster
of fighting and fleeing ever since. Their best hope for a place to refill
their tanks was the monastery, so George would have banged on the
door while Paddy lurked in the shadows. An hour was a long time to
linger, but Paddy and George had to play it smart. They needed to
gather their strength for the long climb to Anogia, and they wouldn't
want to carry anything that could be traced back to the monks if they
were caught. They'd have taken the time to finish their biscuits and
mutton. Then they were off.

Father Timothy pushed a bag of his hard, homemade biscuits into
our hands as we got up to go. Chris and I trundled down the long
slope into the valley, then followed a creek that knifed through a gorge
with rolling foothills along both banks. By late afternoon, the monk's
biscuits were gone, my water pack had an ominously empty-sounding
swish, and the foothills on our side of the gorge had sharpened into
a sheer cliff. Across the creek, we faced a choice: pull ourselves up
a long staircase of crop terraces carved into the mountain face, or
gamble on a dirt road that might spiral all the way to Anogia if it
didn't dead-end in a pasture. The sun had sunk behind the mountain,
leaving us only an hour of good light, but the terraces and dirt road
were good signs that Anogia was right above us.

Chris pointed to the cliff rising at our backs. Only a Japanese
painter could have loved that thing. It was snarled with prickly oak
and so sheer it could have been cut from the mountain with a cleaver.
"Somewhere in that mess, Billy stashed the general the first night,"
Chris said. He and Pete had punished themselves searching for the

cave on their last trip, but I could see why they'd gotten nowhere. Even if you knew where to go, you'd be at the mercy of prickers and dodgy handholds. Billy Moss described the cave as so painfully small and hard to reach that they only pushed inside as a last resort.

"Germans coming!" one of the guerrillas had warned him. "Plenty Germans in village!" Billy and his crew were right out in the open, taking a breather along the banks of the stream because Paddy had told them Anogia would be safe. "We hurriedly threw our kit on to our backs and made off along the bank of the stream," Billy would recall. "Five minutes later, we reached a steep cliff face and up it we scrambled, heaving the General from foothold to foothold until we found ourselves at the entrance of a tiny cave." All four squeezed into a space barely big enough for two, then screened the entrance with branches. They huddled there, listening to the rasp of their own breathing as a German search plane growled by so low that Billy could peek out and see one of the rear crewmen searching the valley through binoculars.

That evening, Billy and his crew led the general back down to the creek to meet up with Paddy. It was here, roughly where Chris and I were standing, that Paddy and Billy discovered that the man they were counting on most—Tom Dunbabin—might already have been captured.

How is it going? Paddy asked. Is the General putting up a fuss?

"Quite a pleasant catch" was Billy's assessment. "Not the raving Nazi he might well have been."

Have you heard anything from Tom? Paddy asked.

Nothing, Billy replied. His messenger had returned from Tom's hideout dumbfounded. "He said he had searched the entire area for Tom, but had found no trace of him, nor had anyone in the district a notion of his whereabouts." This was sad news. Tom's radio operator turned up, but with a broken radio and no more idea than anyone else what happened to his boss. Tom Dunbabin wasn't just their link to the outside world. He was supposed to be spearheading all clandestine ops on the island. That meant one man and one man alone knew the secret locations of the last two remaining wireless operators: Tom.

"He was the only Open Sesame to the other two stations," Paddy realized. Without him, they could send messages only through a series of human firewalls, with each guerrilla knowing only the identity of the next man in the chain. Xan Fielding had as much credibility on Crete as "O Tom," as Dunbabin was known, and could possibly tighten up communications, but Xan hadn't made it back from Egypt yet. Were the Germans tightening the noose so quickly that Tom had to go into hiding? Or was he already in their hands? Paddy and Billy had both taken the precaution of using the human relay to send news of the kidnapping to another radio operator, but predictably, it arrived disastrously garbled: at that moment, the BBC was reporting that General Kreipe *would be* taken off the island, not *was* off.

What about our leaflet drop? Paddy asked.

Canceled, Billy replied. Too much cloud cover for our planes to get through.

Billy and Paddy were still absorbing the bad news when worse arrived. The guerrillas escorting the general's driver showed up—without the driver. Germans are *everywhere*, the guerrillas reported. There were full-scale drives, the Cretans told Paddy, launched in every direction, and they themselves had only just escaped capture.

Okay. But where's the driver?

Andoni sliced a finger across his throat.

Paddy was heartsick. Their chances for escape had just plummeted, and his dream of a bloodless, Magic Gang–style triumph was over. As soon as the driver's body was discovered, the Butcher would go berserk. He'd have to assume General Kreipe was dead as well, which meant he no longer had to worry about getting a hostage back alive. Instead of a rescue operation, it would be total war. The Butcher's only objective now would be vengeance for the murder of a brother officer.

Time to get moving. Ahead lay Mount Ida, sprawling across a quarter of the island and climbing to over eight thousand feet. The general was still complaining about his injured leg, so they helped him up on the donkey and moved out, following a nearly invisible goat track into the woods. "It was vital for us to get into the mountains and among friends," Paddy decided, "away from the enemy-infested plain and in the right direction for escape by sea, at high speed."

Wait. By sea? The guerrillas were doubtful. *Why don't we fly him out, Wolf style?*

Ugh. Wasn't the sky already dark enough without that name coming up? Otto Skorzeny: "Hitler's Wolf." The evil genius with a dueling scar down his cheek and a specialty in killing anyone, anywhere, and disappearing without a trace. Whenever a job seemed impossible,

the Wolf was called in. He led a special force of *Jagdkommandos*—
"Hunting Warriors"—who were said to "live off the land, think for
themselves and never be daunted by the disastrous mess they often
found themselves in." A year earlier, Skorzeny and his Hunters had
snuck into a fortified Italian castle high on a mountain and broken
Benito Mussolini out of prison. Mussolini had been overthrown in a
coup, but Hitler was determined to rescue "Italy's greatest son, our
dear friend and close ally," and restore him to power. Skorzeny landed
by glider at night with a small attack squad, then forced the two-
hundred-man guard detail to surrender. Skorzeny spirited Mussolini
to an escape plane in a nearby field, and before long Il Duce was back
in command. To prevent Hungary's leader, Admiral Miklós Horthy,
from surrendering to the Soviets, Skorzeny kidnapped Horthy's son,
rolled him into a carpet, and snuck him off to a concentration camp,
where he was held hostage until the end of the war.

A few months later, as the story goes, the Wolf parachuted into Iran
intent on assassinating Churchill, Stalin, and Roosevelt with a single
blow. The Wolf and his Hunters crept closer as the Big Three Allied
leaders were meeting in Tehran to discuss war strategy. Just in time, a
Russian spy exposed Operation Long Jump and many of the Hunters
were captured. But Skorzeny got away, reemerging in an American
uniform and jeep far behind enemy lines as he atomized from place
to place, sabotaging Allied troops and getting so close to Supreme
Headquarters that for days at a time, General Dwight Eisenhower
had to be hidden in a guarded location. Skorzeny is "the most dangerous man in Europe," Eisenhower fumed. "Public Enemy No. 1."

"We couldn't evacuate our prisoners by air, in Skorzeny style,"
Paddy told the disappointed Cretans. "The Germans had put all the
big mountain plateaux out of action for long-range aircraft by forcing
labour-gangs to litter them with cairns of stones." But the burning
question wasn't whether they could follow in the Wolf's footsteps; it
was whether the Wolf was following theirs. Rather than flail around in
pursuit of the kidnappers, why wouldn't the Butcher call in Skorzeny
and put the Hunters on their trail? It made perfect sense. As an outlaw himself, Skorzeny would know exactly what Paddy was planning.
Instead of chasing the kidnappers, he'd think ten moves ahead and be
waiting in ambush.

So the faster Paddy and his crew ran, the closer they could be getting to the Wolf.

CHAPTER 31

It makes people rub their eyes in amazement that this
proverbial home of individuality, lawlessness and revolt should
unite, when the need came, in this durable harmony.
But so it was.

—PATRICK LEIGH FERMOR

CHRIS AND I ARRIVED in Anogia about the time of day Paddy would
have been slipping out, pulling ourselves up the last terrace as the sun
went down. At the entrance to town was an iron signpost so ominous,
it looked more like a warning than a welcome. When we got closer,
we discovered why: once the Butcher discovered his suspicions about
Anogia were true, he erupted in a Hitler-like fury. What he did next
was engraved on that grim memorial:

> *Order of the German Commander of the Garrison of Crete:*
>   Since the town of Anogia is a centre of the English
> espionage in Crete, since the Anogians carried out the murder
> of the sergeant of the Yeni-Gavé garrison, since the Anogians
> carried out the sabotage at Damasta, since the *andartes* of
> various Resistance bands find asylum and protection in
> Anogia, and since the abductors of General Kreipe passed

through Anogia, using Anogia as a stopping place when transporting him, we order its RAZING to the ground and the execution of every male Anogian who is found within the village and within an area of one kilometre round it.

Chania, 13-8-44.

The Commander of the Garrison of Crete
H. Müller

The Butcher's troops surrounded the village and penned every-one inside. More than a hundred people were dragged to the town square and murdered. The survivors fled into the mountains while everything they had—their homes, their food, their clothing and blankets—went up in flames behind them. Two elderly sisters were too afraid to leave their home; they were burned to death inside. The Butcher was unrelenting; for three weeks, his men pounded away at the little town, dynamiting buildings and searching the hills for any Anogian men who escaped the dragnet. By the time the Butcher's rage subsided, there was nothing left of the nine-hundred-year-old city on the hill except rotting corpses and smoldering rubble.

Chris and I got a glimpse of the aftermath in a taverna off the town square. A mural filled the entire side wall, and depicted the valley Chris and I had just climbed up from. Two German soldiers have their hands in the air, and a third has dropped to his knees. They're surrounded by Anogian freedom fighters about to open fire. It's a strange and awful image to stare at over a glass of raki and a plate of spanakopita, but it explains why Anogia exists again today. Guerrilla sniping became so common that for the rest of the war and afterwards, the area around Anogia would be known as "the Devil's Triangle." "I saw Germans crying," one Anogian would recall. "I saw it when they shuffled into our ambush like sheep and didn't stand a ghost of a chance."

Strategically, the Butcher's massacre was a terrible mistake. Stripped of everything they had to live for, the Anogians were ready to fight to the death. They dug in, determined to out-endure the invaders. And they did: Anogia was eventually rebuilt with such pride and charm, it feels like it was never gone. The streets are steep and narrow, sloping naturally into the side of the mountain. Small, whitewashed houses cluster around a pleasant town square ringed by shady trees and family cafés. Looming overhead by daylight and moonlight is the majestic, snowy presence of mighty Mount Ida—symbolic birthplace of the rebel lord Zeus and gateway to bandit country and the freedom of the sea.

But as gateways go, it's a punisher. By foot, the fastest route out of Anogia is the trail created by and for goats. It starts with a climb steep enough to make you pump your knees with your hands, then plunges you through acres of the same kind of knife-edge lava rock that left Paddy barefoot the day he arrived. One look was enough for the general to insist his leg was so injured he needed to ride the whole way. "Seen in silhouette upon his mule, the General looked for all the world like Napoleon on his retreat from Moscow," Billy observed. "And we, as jaded-looking a rabble as ever fought an enemy, must have perfectly suited this picture."

By two in the morning, the kidnap party had been hiking for more than six hours. Through the darkness, they followed the clonging of sheep bells to a small hut with the smell of wood smoke wafting from the roof hole. "The shepherd, a dear old man with white whiskers and almost no teeth, was delighted to see us and immediately asked us into his hut so we could rest and warm ourselves in front of the fire," Billy would relate. Even though the old man had been rousted from sleep and opened his door to find a band of armed thugs leading a German general on a donkey, he obeyed the Cretan hospitality code of *xenía:* He offered food. He offered shelter. He asked no questions.

"The shepherd gave us some cheese to eat, and with it some rock bread which was first left to soak in a stone jug," Billy noted. Once the general had thawed out and the starving kidnappers had shared portions of the shepherd's prison-style rations, it was time to be off. "We gave him a fond farewell and were soon on our way again." Giving an enemy who'd terrorized his island a bite to eat and a place by the fire was the last kindness the old man would ever perform; soon after, Billy later found out, a German foraging patrol in search of food shot the shepherd in the back of the head and stole his flock.

The kidnappers had to pick up the pace. Dawn was coming fast, and the most treacherous obstacle still lay ahead: the Nida Plateau, a nearly half-mile stretch of pasture as smooth and open as a football field. Nida is one of the marvels of the Cretan mountains: it's treeless and almost supernaturally flat, leading like a royal carpet straight to the base of Mount Ida. It would be an ideal airstrip if it weren't such a death trap; it's perfect for landing planes, but the surrounding hills make it a sniper's dream. Nida could only be crossed by night; by day, the Germans would be watching it from the air with search planes growling around and around the perimeter.

Except the more the kidnappers walked, the farther away Nida got. The Lasithi range, south of Anogia, is bewitched; it's a masterpiece of deceptive topography, with hills so steep and tightly packed together that when you see one in the distance, you won't notice the other three in between. Every time you pull yourself up a peak and expect to see Nida waiting below, you're sure to find another climb awaiting. You won't find it any easier on the descents, either; the gorges are so clotted with tumble-down stone from the mountaintops, the kidnappers could only avoid tripping by lifting their tired legs as high on the way down as they did on the way up.

Just as the sky was turning pink, the band made it to the grassy plain and hurried the general across. In the gray morning light, they could see the dark outlines of rebel watchmen all across the hilltops. The general was shocked—the Butcher's propaganda had made him believe rebel manpower was nothing more than a few scared Brits and a handful of bandits. "Kreipe was very impressed," noted the rebel fighter Giorgios Phrangoulitakis, known as "Scuttle George," "by our guerrillas posted all along the southern heights, watching over us without coming down. He must have thought the whole mountain was full of them." When one of the band wanted to slip into town past German sentries, several others offered him their German travel passes.

"Have they *all* got our identity papers?" Kreipe asked Paddy.

"You would never be able to escape from the men you see all around you," replied Paddy. Angry elf eyes backed him up: whenever the general glanced back, he found a little old man glaring daggers at him. Manolis Tsikritsis "was very small and wore a sort of fez like a deacon's cap," as Scuttle George put it. "He didn't care for the General either and stared at him fiercely throughout the journey."

Tough talk didn't come naturally to Paddy, but as they pushed into a damp cave at the foot of Mount Ida to hide out for the day, the time had come to make the general believe this was checkmate and his last chance for rescue was gone. Because the following night, they'd be fully exposed as they summited the barren moonscape of Mount Ida. Even if there were someplace up there to hide, their footprints in the snow would give them away. It was a vampire's mission: either get off the mountain and under cover by sunrise or you're dead.

And if the general figured out they were making it up as they went along, he could outfox them with the slow drip of subtle sabotage. All he had to do was drop items from his pockets in the dark for search teams to follow. Or detour the escape route by pretending he knew German outposts were up ahead. Or simply clutch his chest and fall down. Paddy couldn't let that happen; he had to persuade the general he was in the grip of a clockwork operation run by skilled and deadly masterminds, and not, in reality, a seat-of-the-pants scheme cooked up in a bathroom after an all-night party by a military school reject who spent the past five years freeloading across Europe as a wandering playboy poet. So when the general sighed one morning as the sun was rising over Mount Ida and recalled Horace's ode to Mount Soracte, Paddy seized the chance to take his rook:

"Vides ut alta stet nive candidum Soracte," the general murmured. You see Soracte standing white and deep with snow . . .

Nec jam sustineant onus, Paddy blurted.

Silvae laborantes geluque,

Flumina constiterint acuto. The woods in trouble, hardly able to carry their burden, and the rivers halted by sharp ice.

"One of the few odes of Horace I know by heart," Paddy would reveal. "I was in luck." He kept reeling off verses until he reached the end.

The general sat in silence.

"Well remembered," he finally muttered.

While the general dozed inside the cave, Paddy and Billy sat outside in the morning sun and got the morning's bad news. Tom Dunbabin was still missing, which meant their communication with Cairo was getting worse by the mile: the farther they fled, the farther behind they left the two remaining wireless operators. "In both cases," Billy realized, "the journey would take the fleetest of runners at least two days to reach his destination, a further day to await Cairo's reply, and another two days in which to return to us."

Five days round-trip for a single message. So instead of a few days, it would now take a few weeks to coordinate a pickup to get the general off the island. Food was dangerously thin and about to get thinner; for the past two days, they'd hiked twelve hours each night on little more than bread crusts and water. Now they were facing two more weeks on the same starvation diet. "It was impossible for our friends to help," Scuttle George reported. "The villages that would have helped us were all surrounded."

They were exhausted and hungry, but they couldn't give themselves more than a few hours to rest. Every day they spent in the same location increased the risk of getting trapped inside a German dragnet or tracked to their hideout if Hitler's Wolf showed up. Troops were already mobilizing to cut off their escape route on the far side of Mount Ida. "Large numbers of Germans are concentrating around the foothills of this mountain and there is every reason to believe a full-scale drive over the area is imminent," the guerrillas told Billy.

Paddy saw only one way out: *Solvitur Ambulando*. When in doubt, walk. Billy agreed: "We have decided that the best course for us is to make the long climb over Ida's crest and the descent down its southern slopes before the German action has time to develop." They'd wait until nightfall, then do their best to get over Ida and into a fresh hideout before daybreak. If they were caught, it would be on the run.

Paddy and Billy leaned back under a jagged crack running alongside the cave mouth and snatched a few moments of morning sun before going back undercover. Even though it was a top-secret operation, someone fished out a camera and snapped a shot, capturing one last image of the two tired men on what would likely be the last day of their lives.

"That's the crack," Chris White said. "Drop down and I'll show you."

I took a seat in the dirt and leaned back against the rock. Chris snapped a photo, then held it next to one he'd scanned from 1944. The details were identical: my head was right under the same crack, resting exactly where Paddy was before trying to get over Ida. Chris and I had just finished the trek from Anogia, and we'd accidentally put ourselves in a similar situation. We'd set off before dawn with no food, expecting to eat at an inn at the base of the mountain. But the inn was closed, the sun was going down, and the snow-capped peak loomed eight thousand feet overhead.

There was only one way they could have pulled it off. Paddy and his gang must have been tapping into an ancient source of energy to power their way up Ida: they must have figured out how to use their own body fat as performance fuel. It's a technique as old as human existence and the secret of some of the greatest athletic performances in endurance sports, as a broken-down Ironman was surprised to discover.

CHAPTER 32

I would argue that many of the ways in which we
get sick today have a corporate, almost capitalist origin.
We've also got this bizarre notion that finally came
true, that our bodies don't really matter.

—DR. DANIEL LIEBERMAN,
Harvard biologist and author of *The Story of the Human Body*

IN 1983, Stu Mittleman was suffering from a vicious knot on his foot
that baffled every specialist he'd seen.

Until then, he'd been having a spectacular year. "I was now enter-
ing a new phase of my career that placed me among the top endurance
athletes in the world," he'd recall. In the span of just a few months,
he'd smashed his own American one-hundred-mile record, finished
second in the Ultraman World Championships (a double Ironman),
and averaged nearly a hundred miles a day to set a new national mark
for the six-day run. Stu's ultradistance heroics and lady-killer's grin
made him such a media sweetheart that Gatorade named him its first
national spokesman and Ted Koppel featured him on *Nightline* every
evening during the six-day race.

Stu was surfing a wave he couldn't have even dreamed of a few
years earlier. For extreme endurance studs, the eighties were a weird

and wonderful time. Megadistance events were suddenly back in fashion after a century in hibernation, and TV was eating it up. Multiday races used to be all the rage back in the 1870s, not least because they added a dash of drama and cruelty to the typical test of speed: when you lined up at the start, you had no idea how far you'd have to run. *You* were the one who decided when you'd reached the finish, and how much rest—if any—you got in between. Superstars like Edward Payson Weston captivated the crowds by dreaming up new ways to challenge the clock and one another. In 1876, seventy *thousand* fans turned out to watch Weston go head-to-head in a six-day challenge against Daniel O'Leary, an Irish door-to-door book salesman who beat the champ and set a world's best of 520 miles. But it wasn't easy to keep selling tickets to see two guys repeat the same motion over and over again for a week, and eventually long-distance loping was pushed aside by more action-packed, bleacher-friendly games like football— until, in 1982, an exhausted college student named Julie Moss fell to her knees and changed everything.

Julie was on the verge of winning her first Ironman when she collapsed a few yards shy of the tape. Another woman passed her, but Julie kept crawling. Instantly an anthem was born: "Just Finishing Is Winning." Julie the Unbreakable arrived right when America needed her most; she showed she had the sand to stick it out when most of us were wondering, privately, how many of us did. The seventies had left a raw nerve in the national psyche: had we betrayed Plymouth Rock and Valley Forge and turned into a nation of quitters? The evidence was pretty depressing. In quick succession, we'd watched Richard Nixon cheat his way to an easy win, then cut and run rather than face the music. "I would have preferred to carry through to the finish, whatever the personal agony it would have involved. My family unanimously urged me to do so," Nixon said, right before skedaddling. We scrambled onto a rooftop helicopter to get out of Vietnam while the Vietcong stuck it out in the jungle, then cringed as Jimmy Carter wobbled in the face of the Ayatollah's stony resolve during the Iran hostage crisis and fainted less than halfway into a six-mile fun run. "If you get in it," press secretary Jody Powell had warned the president before the race, "then you'd darn well better finish." Well . . .

No wonder "go da distance," as Rocky Balboa put it, became the message of the seventies. You didn't have to win, the Italian Stallion declared; you just had to not wimp out. That was 1976, and it was as if a Bat-Signal had flashed across the sky. Within a few years, all kinds of strange, Not Wimping Out events had popped up, like Alaska's 1,112-mile Iditarod, California's 100-mile Western States trail race, and Hawaii's Ironman triathlon—dreamed up, not coincidentally, by Navy officers just three years out of Vietnam. At first these contests were treated as Battles of the Freaks, until Julie Moss—twenty-four years old, still in college, and One of Us—jolted our eyes from the winners in the front of the pack toward the heroes in the back. TV was soon zooming in to cover these gritty Everymen, as well as a new creation by Fred Lebow, the master showman who started the New York City Marathon: on July 4, 1983, Lebow revived the Six-Day Race and soon made a star out of a Queens college instructor named Stu Mittleman.

A few years earlier, Stu was in Boulder, Colorado, for New Year's when he decided to see if he could run to the top of Flagstaff Mountain. It was only about a two-mile climb, but he was so psyched when he reached the peak that he turned around and ran right back down to the center of town and into Frank Shorter's running store.

"How do I get into this year's Boston Marathon?" he asked.

You don't, he was told. The race was in less than four months, and he'd first have to qualify by running another marathon in under three hours. Fine—two weeks later, Stu averaged a smokin' 6:20 a mile to finish San Diego's Mission Bay Marathon in 2:46. Raw speed he obviously had, but as he began to experiment with longer distances, he discovered his true talent was staying power. Soon he was cranking out more than a half-marathon a day, seven days a week, and leaving the standard Ironman behind to take on twice the distance: nearly five miles in the water, 224 by bike, and 52 and change on foot.

But *damn*. That right foot! Just when he was reaching his peak, a sore spot behind Stu's little toe kept swelling until it was big as a Ping-Pong ball and made his entire leg throb like an abscessed tooth. Stu was supposed to be boarding a flight for France in a few weeks for another six-day race, this time as the only American invited to a showdown of international all-stars, but after shuffling from one specialist to another, his foot wasn't any better. Stu's last tune-up before the event was a triathlon in Long Island. He postponed the inevitable as long as he could and even showed up at registration, but he finally had to limp up to the race director and break the news that he was bowing out.

Please, the race director pleaded, *first do me a favor.* Long Island triathlons don't get many TV sensations in their lineups, least of all model-handsome men of steel fresh off the *Today* show and a week-long spot on *Nightline*. Before you make up your mind, the race director urged, see Dr. Phil Maffetone.

Stu sighed. *I have already seen nearly a dozen medical doctors, chiropractors, and body workers and have basically given up hope that my injury can be healed*, he thought. Still, he decided to humor the guy and hear what Dr. Phil had to say. That way, at least, he could drop out with a clear conscience while satisfying his own curiosity. For some time, he'd been hearing stories that were too good to be true about this healer of last resort who not only fixed the unfixable but coaxed astonishing performances out of slumping runners and triathletes. "Phil has a reputation for getting broken-down, over-trained, world-class athletes back up and running," Stu would recall.

Luckily, Dr. Phil Maffetone was right at hand. He'd come to watch one of his reconstruction projects compete, and he agreed to take a look at Stu right there on the lawn outside the VFW hall. As they chatted, Stu discovered Phil wasn't even an M.D.; he was a chiropractor with such severe attention-deficiency that he'd barely squeaked through high school and still couldn't stand to read books. Granted, Phil was a former track athlete, but otherwise there was no outward reason he should know anything other doctors didn't. Maybe Stu's friends were only impressed because Phil treated them like real patients and not high-functioning psychotics. Phil didn't lecture them that "all that pounding is bad for the body" or answer with a shrug and "What do you expect?" when they described how their heels ached after a two-hour run. Phil wasn't shocked by big miles and didn't smirk at the adventurers who tackled them; as far as he was concerned, a properly fueled and maintained body could click along forever. He took their pain—and their potential—seriously.

Phil had Stu lie down on the grass. He began pushing Stu's arms and legs to assess muscle resistance. "Relax," he said. He grasped Stu's foot and gave it a yank. Angels sang.

"Suddenly," Stu says, "the lump disappears!" He can't believe it. He jogs around gingerly, and for the first time in months he can run without pain. He's so thrilled, he gets stupid; instead of playing it safe and seeing if the miracle lasts until lunch, Stu decides to jump right into the triathlon. He storms along to a top-twenty finish and his foot feels fantastic.

"This is just first aid," Phil warns him. He'd found a dislodged bone in Stu's foot and managed to snap it into place, but worse breakdowns lay ahead unless Stu made some serious changes.

Stu was all ears. Sure. What's my problem—running technique? Weak arches?

Sugar.

Sug—*really?*

And not only sweets and sodas, Phil explained. Pasta, power bars, pancakes, pizza, orange juice, rice, bread, cereal, granola, oatmeal— all the processed carbohydrates that Stu had been told were the ideal runner's diet. They're just sugar in disguise, Phil believed. Humans are superb endurance athletes who've roamed farther across this planet than any other species, and we didn't do it on Gatorade and bagels. We did it by relying on a much richer and cleaner burning fuel: our own body fat.

"The point of your training isn't to see how fast you can get your feet to move," Phil said. "The point is to get your body to change the way it gets energy. You want it to burn more fat and less sugar." And as it stood now, Stu's body was "a sugar-burning, fat-storing monstrosity."

Stu was baffled. Okay. But how does food hurt your foot?

Think of your body as a furnace, Phil explained. Fill it with slow-burning logs and it will run smooth and strong for hours. But fill it with paper and gas-soaked rags and it will burn hot, rattle the pipes, and die out until it's fed again. That's what you did, Phil said. You shook yourself into an injury by stuffing your furnace with garbage. If you want to stay healthy *and* perform your best, you need to teach your body to use fat as fuel. Immediately.

Stu saw three major difficulties. The first problem with Phil's plan, of course, was Phil. The man was—and there's no way to sugarcoat it—a stone-cold hippie. He had long hair and a dangly ponytail and used words that made Stu's stomach heave: "holistic" and "hormones" and "walk before you run." Literally: *walk*. Phil wanted Stu to start his next race by *walking*. Good Lord. The second problem with Phil's plan was Stu: he had a major international championship in three weeks, and Rule #1 for all sports is *Don't Experiment Before Game Day*. Phil wasn't even proposing an overhaul; he wanted Stu to completely reverse his diet, training, and race strategy and do it all in less than twenty days.

But the biggest problem was Everyone Else in the World. Everyone Else in the World thought the "Maffetone Method" was nuts. Carbs were warrior food; everybody knew that. Stu was an academic by training, and right from the beginning he'd made himself a student of his sport. "I cut back my work hours, lived like an ascetic monk, trained like a maniac, ate only what *Runner's World* told me I should, and did a carbohydrate depletion followed by a carbo load in the last few days before the event," Stu would recall. So now what? *Runner's World* was dead wrong? All those pre-race pasta dinners were poison? Carbohydrates were hurting, not helping?

The Maffetone Method even defied the greatest voice of all: Dr. Tim Noakes, author of *Lore of Running* and one of the world's most respected sports scientists. Dr. Noakes was both a medical doctor and the head of Exercise and Sports Science research at the University of Cape Town, and so trusted an authority that he served as expedition doctor for Lewis Pugh's North Pole swim and spearheaded reforms that dramatically reduced South African rugby injuries. Moreover, Noakes was his own space monkey; by age sixty-four he'd run South Africa's fifty-six-mile Comrades ultramarathon seven times and had another seventy marathons under his belt. With more than four hundred scientific papers and two thousand competitive miles to his name, Noakes knew more about runners, living and dead, than the runners themselves. He'd not only written the eight-hundred-page *Lore*, but he kept *re*writing it; every few years, Noakes updated his bible with fresh science. The best in the world listened to Dr. Tim Noakes, and Dr. Tim Noakes was all about carbs.

"Athletes whose training involves prolonged high-intensity daily exercise must eat high-carbohydrates diets," Noakes made it clear. "Performance during prolonged exercise can potentially be enhanced by increasing the amount of carbohydrate stored before exercise," he went on, "and by maintaining a high rate of carbohydrate utilization, particularly when fatigued, via ingestion of carbohydrates in the appropriate amounts." It was all right there in chapter 3. And all those fifty-plus pages on "Energy Systems and Running Performance" could be nicely summed up in just seven words: *Stuff in carbs and keep on stuffing.*

And sorry—who was Phil Maffetone again? A ponytailed backcracker from suburban New York. Those were Stu's two options: the man who wrote The Book versus the man who probably hadn't read it. Ordinarily it would be an easy decision, but pain relief is the ultimate persuader. Stu decided to give the Maffetone Method a chance.

Okay, he told Phil. *How do we start?*

Simple, Phil began. To use fat as fuel, you need to do only two things: cut out sugar and lower your heart rate. "We store only a very limited amount of carbohydrate in our bodies," Phil explained. "Compare this with a relatively unlimited supply of fat." Carbs are a puddle; fat is the Pacific. At any time, your body has some 160,000 calories on tap: about 2,000 from sugar, 25,000 from protein, and nearly 140,000—*87 percent*—are fat. "Even an athlete with only 6 percent body fat will have enough fat to fuel exercise lasting for many hours," Phil explained. "When you use more fat, you generate more energy and your carbohydrate supply lasts longer. When you teach your body to rely on fat, your combustion of carbs goes down, and so does your craving for them."

But there's no pussyfooting around. Your body loves fat; it's a treasure your system would rather hoard than burn, so if it senses there's any other fuel at hand, it will use that first and convert the leftovers into more fat. To free himself from the sugar-burn cycle, Stu would have to go cold turkey: he could stuff himself silly all day, but only on meat, fish, eggs, avocados, vegetables, and nuts. No beans, no fruit, no grains. No soy, no wine, no beer. Whole dairy like sour cream and real cheese were in; low-fat milk was out.

That was Part 1. Part 2 was even more basic: *Slow down.* When you sprint, Phil explained, you jack up your heart rate. Your body interprets a hammering heart as *EMERGENCY!* so it goes looking for those gas-soaked rags. It wants the fastest-burning fuel it can find, and that means sugar. But once you've conditioned your body to rely on fat, you'll be able to run as fast as ever—and much faster. For Stu to keep his heart rate in his fat-burning zone, Phil had an easy formula: just subtract your age from 180. Stu was thirty-two years old, so Phil gave him a heart-rate monitor and set it for 153 beats per minute (148 plus five bonus beats because Stu was a highly conditioned athlete). Anytime the monitor beeped, it meant Stu had to slow to a walk until his pulse eased back down.

For three weeks, Stu was a perfect disciple. Come the six-day race in France, however, he'd had enough. It was humiliating enough when all the other runners shot off around the track while he trailed them at a walk ("*Yech!*" Stu grimaced), but to watch them snacking on cookies and candy at the aid stations while he had nothing but almonds . . . well, that just bordered on human-rights abuse. Unfortunately, Phil Maffetone had come to France with him, so Stu had to sneak cookies off the aid station table and hide them at the far end of the track, where he could munch later when Phil wasn't looking.

But before digging into his stash, Stu noticed something. For once, he could actually *see* what was going on. Usually during a race he was huffing along with his chin on his chest, but this time he was head high and breathing easy. Come to think of it, he'd felt that way during every run for the past three weeks. For most runners, enjoying the view is a rare sensation; as soon as fatigue kicks in, your eyes drop to the pavement and your vision tunnels. You're no longer in the present; you're locked on to how far you've come and how far you've got to go. Stu always assumed pain was the price of gain, but since he'd been on the Maffetone Method, his runs had actually been a pleasure.

"Each energy-producing state has specific and real sensory-based references," he'd learned. "Your body knows this by the way the world 'looks,' 'sounds,' and 'feels.' When you move in a comfortable fat-burning state, the visual information is distinct, expansive, and three dimensional with a peripheral vastness and expansiveness that is unique and identifiable. It's as though you are in a 3-D surround vision movie theatre."

You're seeing with the eyes of a hunter. But when your heart rate climbs, you become the hunted. "As soon as you shift into a more challenging sugar-burning state, visual information tends to collapse inward, the peripheral fringes tend to disappear and your attention gets drawn into a much narrower field of vision. Visual images tend to flatten out, become two-dimensional, and you begin to feel as though you are running through a tunnel with the world painted on the inside walls."

So that's how hunter-gatherers run antelopes to death. They don't act like the animal they're trying to kill; instead they're silent and graceful, moving easily with their eyesight sharp, their breathing controlled, their bottomless body-fat energy on tap. Much the way Stu was moving now, in fact, as he smoothly and stealthily pursued the runners who'd dropped him at the start. Three weeks earlier, Stu had been so hobbled by injury he couldn't compete; now, he was chasing down the best ultradistance runners in the world and getting faster by the day. Stu felt so good that for the entire six days, he never dug into his cookie stash. He set a new American record of 571 miles, crushing the old one by more than a half-marathon and finishing in second behind only the Beast himself, 24-Hour World Record holder Jean-Gilles Boussiquet of France.

That did it; Stu was now a fat-as-fuel true believer. For the next ten years he whirlwinded through the record books with such strength and style, it looked more like art than effort. In a display of "virtually flawless footracing," as one journalist put it, Stu defeated the reigning world champion in a thousand-mile showdown and not only shattered the old mark by sixteen hours, but even ran his second five hundred miles faster than his first. He handled the back half of his life the same way; instead of slowing down in his forties, he got stronger, running more than fifty miles a day as he set a new speed record from Los Angeles to New York City. "No other American ultrarunner, male or female, has exhibited national class excellence at such a wide range of racing distances," his American Ultrarunning Hall of Fame induction proclaimed.

But the funny thing is, Stu wasn't even Phil's best student. Compared with Mark Allen, Stu was . . . well, there's really no comparing anyone to Mark Allen. When Mark came to Phil in the late eighties, he was in his twenties but already feeling old. Triathlons were beating him up and not paying off; Mark was always hurt in training and blowing up in races, either fading toward the finish or dropping out altogether. Like Stu, his broken body gave him an open mind. "I was warned that his methods were probably going to sound crazy," Mark would recall. Not to mention embarrassing: Phil made Mark pedal far behind the pack during group rides and plod along at half speed during runs. Mark's training partners were convinced he was washed up . . . until four months later, when Mark went flying past. "I had become an aerobic machine!"

"I was now able to burn fat for fuel efficiently enough to hold a pace that a year before was red-lining my effort," Mark explained. "I was no longer feeling like I was ready for an injury the next run I went on, and I was feeling fresh after my workouts instead of being totally wasted." Mark soon tore off an insane streak: for two years, he didn't lose a race anywhere, at any distance. He won Ironman six times, including a stunning comeback victory at age thirty-seven, but what's more intriguing is what happened after he retired. Bikes got lighter, wetsuits got sleeker, training and nutrition became more lab-tested and sophisticated—yet no one could touch Mark's times. It was nearly *two decades* before another Ironman could match him.

"Mark Allen was well ahead of us scientists," agrees Dr. Asker Jeukendrup, a human metabolism expert at England's University of Birmingham and an accomplished Ironman himself. Jeukendrup is among the top ranks of endurance specialists, yet even he's a little foggy about the role played by the quiet guy with the ponytail. So was Mike Pigg, who only tracked Phil down at Mark Allen's urging. "Phil Maffetone is not crazy," Pigg insists, which suggests he wasn't always sure himself. "I feel very fortunate to have met him when I did." After switching to the Maffetone Method, Pigg won four USA Triathlon National Championships and remained resilient enough to compete for nearly a quarter-century. Dr. George Sheehan—the cardiologist, best-selling author, and "philosopher king of the marathon"—also put his legs in Dr. Phil's hands.

But oddly, Phil eventually began seeing more rock stars than Ironmen. An athlete has to be supremely confident or borderline desperate to gamble on a system that flips everything she's been told and guarantees she's heading straight to the back of the pack, possibly for an entire season. But rock stars don't have to deal with doubtful coaches and corporate sponsors; they just have to be strong enough to endure months of onstage musical marathons. "Musicians are all searching for the same two things," Maffetone learned. "How do I get more energy and how can I become more creative?"

James Taylor was an early Maffetone adopter ("I feel great!" he'd rave), and the Red Hot Chili Peppers brought Phil on board as tour doctor (years later, at age fifty, Peppers bassist Flea could still crank out a sub-four-hour marathon in a driving rainstorm). Rick Rubin, the great bearded sage of the sound studio, tracked down Phil in

2003 when Johnny Cash was on his deathbed. Phil got Johnny back on his feet, helped restore his eyesight, and began weaning him off his astonishingly high pill count of some forty different medications. Cash was so grateful, he gave Phil one of his guitars. But ultimately, Cash couldn't recover from the loss of his wife and the aftereffects of the chemical barrage. Phil had his hand on Cash's shoulder one afternoon when Cash turned and looked him in the eye.

"It's time," Cash said.

No one saw Dr. Phil at Ironman after that. No one saw much of him anywhere, unless you were Rick Rubin. Rubin owned Shangri-La, the secluded Malibu bungalow where Bob Dylan and the Band used to camp out and jam with Eric Clapton and Van Morrison (and where, for a time, TV horse Mr. Ed was stabled). Every once in a while, Phil would roll up at Shangri-La and play Rubin some songs he'd written. Then he'd climb back into his car and disappear into the Arizona desert. Phil was so out of touch, it was some time before he learned that after thirty years, he'd won both an argument and a convert:

Dr. Tim Noakes, the "High Priest of Carbo-Loading," was making a confession.

CHAPTER 33

I was quite wrong. Sorry, everyone.

—DR. TIMOTHY NOAKES

I WAS FAMISHED by the time I met Dr. Noakes in the lobby of his Washington, D.C., hotel and figured we'd head straight out to eat. It was pushing 1 P.M., and Noakes had been stuck in a conference all morning discussing, among other things, his biggest professional mistake. We just had time for a hearty lunch before his flight back home to South Africa. But Noakes had other ideas.

"I won't eat until tomorrow," he said. "Or the next day."

"You go two days without food?"

"Or more. Sometimes I've got to stop and think to remember my last meal."

Looking at him, it's hard to believe. At sixty-four, Noakes is tall and fit as a lumberjack, with the rangy look of the college rower he once was and the barely contained energy of a man whose mind is a constantly expanding to-do list. Everything about him seemed to demand constant refueling—his locked-in focus when listening, his Christmas-morning grin when amused, the unruly brown hair barely touched by time or a comb. It would all make sense, Noakes promised, when I heard his story. He suggested we grab coffee and get right to it. He had a lot to get off his chest.

"It's really funny when you think how chance events occur," he begins. In 2010, Noakes was finally reaching the end of a grim crusade. Back in 1981, he suspected joggers were being tricked into drinking themselves to death. Companies like Gatorade were pushing the idea that runners needed lots of fluids to avoid dehydration, and the race directors and running magazines who depend on sponsorship and advertising were quick to join the chorus. Suddenly, you could barely run a mile in a race without someone handing you a cup. Runners were told, "Drink until your eyeballs float," and "Don't just rely on thirst."

But hang on; when did thirst suddenly become unreliable? For millions of years, it's been fantastically effective. In fact, it's one of the most important aspects of our evolutionary development: humans lived or died by their ability to lope long on hot days, and the reason we survived is that our bodies told us when and how much to drink. It was precisely *because* we're resistant to dehydration that we could run other animals to death. "Humans evolved to be extremely adept long-distance runners with an unmatched ability to regulate their body temperatures when exercising in the heat," Noakes knew. "And our brains developed the ability to delay the need to drink—a crucial adaptation if we were to chase after our potential meals in the midday heat when there was little water available and no time to stop the hunt to search for fluid."

Noakes began checking the habits of runners from the pre-Gatorade era and discovered that old-school marathoners had no trouble going dry. "I only chew gum. I take no drink at all," Matthew Maloney said after he set the marathon world record in 1908. Mike Gratton won the London Marathon in 1983 without a single sip, and Arthur Newton, the legendary ultrarunner and five-time Comrades champion, believed, "Even in the warmest English weather, a 26-mile run ought to be manageable with no more than a single drink or, at most, two." To this day, the San people of the Kalahari can run up to seven hours in heat of 108° Fahrenheit on just a few swallows.

So now all of a sudden the American College of Sports Medicine, with major funding by its first platinum sponsor—Gatorade—was declaring, "Thirst may be an unreliable index of fluids needed during exercise"? Something else was fishy: the fifty-six-mile Comrades race never had a problem with dehydration and heat illness before it set up regular aid stations. "This paradox did not escape me," Noakes points out. "How could 'dehydration and heat illness' have become a significant problem in marathon and ultramarathon running *after* frequent drinking had become the accepted norm?"

Nothing added up—least of all the corpses. When Noakes researched postrace body weights, he found something peculiar: elite runners pump out more sweat than the midpack plodders. If dehydration were truly a danger, how did the elites even make it to the finish line? Logically, the faster runners should be knocked off their feet. Instead, they're stronger than everyone else in the field. And when Noakes went looking for all those marathoners who supposedly keeled over from too little to drink, he found . . .

None.

Not one. *Ever.* "There is not a single report in the medical literature of dehydration being a proven, direct cause of death in a marathon runner," Noakes discovered.

But if you look at runners who had plenty to drink, that's a different story. That's where the bodies turn up. In the United States, three marathoners died on days that weren't extraordinarily warm. In the UK, a fitness instructor in excellent shape and known for advising his own clients about hydration was dead soon after running the London Marathon. In the same race, a sports scientist with expertise in endurance conditioning became so delusional that she kept running in place while lying on a stretcher. Eight trekkers dropped into comas and never recovered while hiking the Kokoda Trail, a popular route for Australians on Papua New Guinea. For all of them, fluids weren't just available—they were *unavoidable*, just as they were at the Houston Marathon in 2000 when dozens were rushed to the medical tent, even though drinks were handed out every single mile.

None of these people were fleeing for their lives. None of them were pursuing food across the savanna. So if they were slowly dying of thirst, why on earth didn't they just pick up a cup? How could they be so blind to their own doom? Shipwreck victims survive on life rafts for weeks; how did these athletes die within a few hours?

Noakes was baffled. And then it hit him: they were drowning. Instead of too little to drink, they were dying from too much. They'd gulped so much fluid, they'd diluted their blood sodium concentration and caused their brains to swell. Water poisoning! Suddenly it all made sense. The Sports Drink Giants had been fantastically successful at tricking people into believing that, unlike every other creature on Earth, humans were too stupid to know when to drink. Cows and puppies and infants have it covered, but not you—no, you need to be told. The terrible irony was that by inventing a fake health scare, the Drink Giants had created a real one. They'd scared people into believing they were drinking too little, and fooled them into drinking too much. It was death by marketing.

Noakes found twelve confirmed deaths by water poisoning in sports events and thousands of close calls. "The 'Science of Hydration' is propaganda conceived by marketers who wished to turn a collection of kitchen chemicals into a multi-billion dollar industry," Noakes declared. "To their credit, they succeeded. To their unending shame, they cost the lives of some of those they were pretending to protect."

The scam was so outrageous, Noakes was sure it would explode as soon as it was revealed. Instead, he found himself battling the "Mafia of Science," as he calls it: doctors and researchers funded by corporate war chests. The more Noakes insisted the Drink Giants were a lethal menace, the more the Drink Giants and their paid Ph.D.'s blasted the message that humans were frail creatures who couldn't trust their own bodies. "Drink before you're thirsty or you'll just be playing catch-up," the Gatorade camp insisted. "Drink before, during and after exercise." When Asker Jeukendrup published a study that showed sports drinks are basically placebos—you can swish and spit and get the same benefit as if you'd swallowed—Gatorade knew just what to do: it hired him. As for Noakes—well, the Mafia of Science regretted that such a respected scientist was now just a mouthy crank. True, Noakes was possibly the world's top authority on distance-running physiology, but his warnings about excess hydration were just "one man's opinion," as the director of the Gatorade Sports Science Institute sniffed, and "not representative of the comprehensive research that is available on the topic of hydration during exercise."

Noakes persisted, gathering evidence from around the world for *Waterlogged*, his four-hundred-plus-page indictment of the sports-drink industry. On the night he wrote the last sentence, in December 2010, he went to bed thinking, *Tomorrow, you've got to start running again.* He'd been absorbed in work for too long. He hadn't run a marathon in four years. He'd put on thirty pounds. And he was about to wake up to a sickening discovery:

His own advice about carbs was killing him.

•   •   •

It was that first run that opened his eyes. Noakes got up as planned and huffed out a few miles, hating every step. He felt fat and slow, as if he'd never run a step before. His father and brother had both died from diabetes, and Noakes knew from his thickening waist and increasing sluggishness that he was heading in the same direction. He'd always persuaded himself that running would keep his weight under control, but now the misery of starting all over again made him face the truth: it wasn't going to work. It had *never* worked.

"In forty-one years of running I have learnt that the numerous benefits of exercise do not include any sustained effects on weight loss," Noakes realized. Even during his peak of nearly twenty miles a day, back in the seventies, he'd lost only a few pounds and yo-yoed them right back on again. His medical training told him that exercise and calorie control should do the trick, but after four decades as a conscientious eater and athlete, he was living proof that his medical training was wrong. With his book out of the way and his genetic time bomb ticking, Noakes set out to find out what was going on.

He began digging into nutrition science with the same intensity with which he'd gone after drinks, examining the primary research behind the dietary guidelines. What he found made Noakes angry, then heartsick. He'd been duped. Even worse: the whole time he'd been so self-righteous during his holy war with the Drink Giants, he'd been the instrument of something even deadlier. The food industry had pulled the same trick as the Drink Giants, and Noakes hadn't only missed it; he'd *endorsed* it. For decades, he'd advocated a carbohydrate-rich diet. He was so influential, he'd been dubbed the High Priest of Carbo-Loading—and processed carbs, he now understood, were toxic.

"Skillful marketing has made carbohydrate consumption a religion among athletes," he'd fume. "They believe that you cannot get energy from anywhere but carbs." The same foods Noakes had assured people would make them stronger and faster were a slow-acting poison making them fatter, weaker, and more prone to heart attacks, strokes, diabetes, and dementia.

Privately, Noakes was anguished for another reason. It wasn't well known, but Noakes's father had made his fortune as a tobacco broker. In medical school autopsies, Noakes had seen firsthand the kind of horror his father's profession wreaked on human bodies. He'd been troubled by Big Tobacco's stealth efforts to increase addiction and market to minors, and it gnawed at him that every time his father cut a check to pay his school fees, it was at the cost of "the ill-health of those who smoked cigarettes containing the tobacco he exported." In the end, Noakes's father begged him to make amends. "Tim, I did not help enough people in my life," his father told him. "You had better do so."

Now Noakes discovered he'd been pushing something that was even more addictive and shopped even more shamelessly, especially to children. If he'd been more careful, if he'd been more skeptical about the mass production and marketing of processed carbs, he could have saved so many people—starting with his own brother and father. He wished he'd been aware of these four key pieces of evidence:

HUMAN HISTORY

It's an inconvenient truth, but a truth nevertheless: animal fat made us who we are. When our ancestors first strayed from the African savanna, they weren't following the harvest. They were following the herds. They went in search of meat, and wherever they found it, no matter how harsh the environment, they stayed. For over two million years, we lived on the meats and chewy roots we could hunt and gather. Eggs, fatty flesh, and cheeses were prized because they were rich in energy, easy to preserve, and such a steadily burning nutrient that a few ounces could sustain someone all day. When the ancient Greeks offered the fattiest cut of meat to the gods, it was a *sacrifice*; they gave up what they wanted most. Only very recently did we switch to farm-raised grains, and since then we've seen a decrease in average human height and a spike in obesity and nutrition-deficiency diseases. The worst explosion began in the 1980s, after the United States embarked on a disastrous experiment. From 1960 to 1980, obesity remained constant. But in 1977, the United States separated itself from every other government in history by vilifying meat and pushing grains, which were traditionally used to fatten cattle. Soon after, America's obesity rate shot up and hasn't stopped.

PLUMBING THEORY

America's shift from proteins to grains was sparked by Ancel Keys, a biochemist from the University of Minnesota who made his name during World War II by inventing K-rations, the ready-to-eat meal for combat troops. Later, Keys was reading his local newspaper's obituary column when he noticed an unusual number of rich Minnesotans were dropping dead of heart disease. One thing America had after the war that other nations lacked was plenty of red meat, so Keys developed a plausible-sounding theory: If you pour bacon grease down your sink, it will thicken inside your pipes and eventually clog them. Our arteries must work the same way, Keys assumed.

"Keys hypothesized that heart disease was mostly a nutritional disorder linked directly to the amount of fat in the diet," one journalist explained. "High-fat foods raised cholesterol levels in the blood, which, in turn, increased the risk of clogged arteries and heart disease." That also sounded right to Senator George McGovern, who'd experimented with the low-fat Pritikin Diet. McGovern very quickly gave up on low-fat himself, but just because *he* didn't want to eat that way didn't mean other people shouldn't. McGovern would go on to become an extraordinarily influential voice in nutrition, serving as the United Nations' first global envoy on world hunger and teaming with Senator Bob Dole to create a worldwide school lunch program.

So largely on the whim of one powerful senator, the fat-is-fatal theory was rammed through U.S. health agencies in 1977 and propelled along by governmental "food faddists who hold the public in thrall," as *Science* magazine put it. Later, journalist Gary Taubes would reveal that Ancel Keys had built his argument on his "Seven Countries Study," ignoring data from three times as many other countries that weakened his theory. Dead people were also a problem; if Keys was right, the new U.S. dietary recommendations should have caused heart disease to plummet. Instead it's skyrocketed: in the twenty years after the fat warnings went into effect, medical procedures for heart disease *quintupled* from 1.2 million to 5.4 million a year.

INSULIN IS OZ

Whether you become fatter or skinnier, stronger or weaker, more alert or lethargic is largely influenced by insulin, the hormone that acts as your body's warehouse foreman. When sugars and carbohydrates are converted to glucose and enter your bloodstream, your pancreas deploys insulin to figure out where to store it. Glucose is great when your body needs it; it fuels brain and muscle cells, and is converted into fat for future use. It also acts as tinder so your body can burn fat as fuel.

But here's the catch: insulin evolved to handle complex carbs created by nature, like leafy greens, not simple carbs created by us, like cereal and bread. Simple carbs are absorbed too fast; your cells get their fill and the rest is turned into fat before your insulin has a chance to dissipate. The still-active insulin in your bloodstream goes looking for more sugar, which makes you feel hungry. So you chow another donut, starting the whole process all over again. Enough years of this abuse and your cells can become insulin resistant; they're tired of being asked to absorb all this glucose, so they just stop responding. What then happens to all that glucose? It goes straight to fat.

That's what killed Noakes's father and brother: their system needed fuel it wasn't getting, while storing fat it didn't need.

FAT AS FUEL

But there's a way out, Noakes discovered. Once you kick the carbohydrate habit, you can convert your body back into a fat burner. "If you're fat-adapted," Noakes posited, "then theoretically you should be able to source all your energy from fat metabolism, especially during very prolonged exercise, when the intensity of the activity is somewhat lower, so that there should not be any need to burn carbohydrates."

Bruce Fordyce, the legendary South African ultramarathon champ, put it to the test. Like Noakes, Fordyce had packed on the pounds since his glory days. But once he stopped eating grains and sugars and adopted a high-fat, low-carb diet, Fordyce underwent a running renaissance. At age fifty-six, he beat his best-ever Comrades time by *two hours* and chopped five minutes off his 5K, improving from 7:20 a mile to 5:40—a tremendous achievement for any experienced athlete, let alone one pushing sixty.

Still, Fordyce's self-experimentation is decades away from catching up with Dr. Fred Kummerow, a University of Illinois scientist who, since the 1950s, has taken the position that hardening of the arteries isn't caused by LDL, the so-called bad cholesterol found in eggs, red meat, and cheese. If LDL were deadly, Kummerow asks, then how come half of all heart disease patients have normal or low LDL levels? Something else must have killed them, and Kummerow believes it's exactly the food pushed by the U.S. government—polyunsaturated vegetable oils like soybean, corn, and sunflower.

"Cholesterol has nothing to do with heart disease, except if it's oxidized," Dr. Kummerow told the *New York Times*. And because soybean and corn oils are inherently unstable, they're quick to oxidize under the high heat of frying or even normal digestion. Kummerow put his own body on the firing line; he eats LDL food daily, including red meat, eggs scrambled in butter, and a glass of whole milk every day. He's one hundred years old, takes no meds, and runs his own university lab. Yes, you read that age correctly: one hundred.

When I met up with Noakes in D.C., he'd flown all the way from Cape Town for a one-day conference on "Innovations in Diabetes." That morning, he'd tucked away a farmhand's breakfast of eggs, sausage, and bacon. A meal like that will leave him satisfied all day, often longer. "I just don't get hungry anymore," he shrugged. "Sometimes I'll feel my energy waning and realize I haven't eaten in forty-eight hours."

"So basically, we're talking about Paleo?" I ask. The Paleo Diet is based on the premise that humans are healthiest when they follow the example of our Stone Age ancestors and eat grass-fed meats, wild-caught fish, vegetables, nuts, and seeds and stay away from rice, bread, pasta, and other grain-based foods from the agricultural age.

"Basically, yes," Noakes replies, although for the sake of precision, he'd replace "Paleo" with "Banting": Noakes can't be scientifically certain about what early humans ate, but he knows exactly what was on the menu of an overweight London embalmer named William Banting. Back in the 1860s, Banting was England's undertaker to the stars and so sought after that he was given the honor of building the coffin for the Duke of Wellington, one of Britain's most beloved heroes. Banting's success, however, was pushing him toward his own grave; he attended so many lavish funeral dinners that by age sixty-six he was "nearly spherical." He was only five foot five, yet weighed over two hundred pounds and was so belly heavy he had to walk downstairs backwards and couldn't tie his own shoes. Banting's doctors prescribed every known treatment for obesity—diets, Turkish baths, heavy exercise, spa retreats, even systematic vomiting—but every pound he took off boomeranged right back on again. Oddly, Banting made a breakthrough only when he began going deaf. He went to see a hearing specialist named William Harvey, who decided Banting's problem wasn't his ears, but his waistline. Poor circulation was damaging his auditory canal, so in August, Banting began following Dr. Harvey's eating instructions:

BREAKFAST: Five or six ounces of beef, mutton, kidneys, broiled fish, bacon, or cold meat of any kind, except pork. One small biscuit or one ounce of dry toast. A large cup of tea without milk or sugar.

LUNCH: Five or six ounces of any fish except salmon, any meat except pork, and any vegetable except potato. Any kind of poultry or game. One ounce of dry toast. Two or three classes of good claret, sherry, or Madeira.

DINNER: Three or four ounces of meat or fish, as for lunch. A glass of claret or two. Nightcap, if required.

So morning, noon, and night, Banting was feasting on roasts and fatty steaks with sides of buttery broccoli and washing it down with tasty wines, plus a snort of gin before bed. He was packing in the calories, too; Banting's meals amounted to nearly three thousand calories a day, *triple* what most weight-loss diets allow. Yet even in his midsixties, when weight loss is most difficult, Banting trimmed off twenty pounds in the first five months. Within a year he'd reduced his weight by fifty pounds and his waist by twelve inches, and he remained trim the rest of his life.

"The Banting plan was the foundation of the Atkins diet in the 1970s," Noakes explains. "We keep rediscovering these same fundamental principals of nutrition, then we forget them and start all over again."

In 2012, the Los Angeles Lakers began following in Banting's footsteps after a nutritionist consulting for the team became concerned about Dwight Howard, the superstar center nicknamed Superman for his Adonis abs and cannonball biceps. Howard was only twenty-seven years old and looked fantastic, with only 6 percent body fat, but there was something a little off about his hands. "It looked like he was wearing oven mitts," the nutritionist would recall. "It reminded me of patients who have pre-diabetes and neurological problems because of how sugar impacts the nervous system." A blood screening revealed Howard's glucose level was "through the roof," and a nutritional assessment found he was basically living on sugar: between candy, soda, and starches, he was downing the equivalent of twenty-four chocolate bars a day.

So the entire Lakers squad, including franchise player Kobe Bryant and seasoned veteran Steve Nash, joined Howard in a Banting-style meal makeover. "Not only are the Lakers unafraid of healthy fats, they practically freebase them," one journalist noted. "The pre-game beverage of choice is something the players call 'bullet-proof coffee'—coffee seasoned with two teaspoons of pastured butter and heavy, grass-fed cream."

"I've seen great results from it from when I started doing it last year—watching your sugar intake, making sure you're eating healthy fats," Kobe Bryant was quoted. "You've got to find a balance in that system. It's worked well for me." Lakers forward Shawne Williams showed up twenty pounds overweight for training camp; by doubling his fat intake and cutting out sugar, he took off twenty-five. Now most Lakers meals are built around grass-fed beef, humanely raised pork, raw nuts, squeezepacks of hazelnut butter, kale chips, and grass-fed beef jerky. Dwight Howard even remained faithful after he was traded; when he arrived in Houston, Howard persuaded Rockets management to start Banting. "We had to make that change," Rockets general manager Daryl Morey told a reporter, "and I should've pushed harder earlier."

For Dr. Noakes, it's been a three-year journey of scientific awakening and personal transformation. He's back down to 175 pounds—same as he was in his twenties—and feels like an athlete again. Eight weeks after he stopped eating sugar and processed carbs, Noakes was in Stockholm for a conference. It was dark when he arrived and twenty-five degrees below freezing, but Noakes went on a five-mile run anyway. He slept a few hours, then got up and ran ten more. "A few weeks earlier, I could barely finish 5K," he recalls. "I thought it was aging. But it was really carbohydrate intolerance. In two months, I lost eleven kilos. I turned it all around."

We've been brainwashed into being repulsed by the mention of the word *fat*, Noakes says, but the real heart danger is sugar. It's a corrosive that damages arterial walls, creating grooves that allow plaque to adhere. Which means the only real solution for cardiovascular disease and global obesity, Noakes feels, is pure scorched earth. "Ten companies produce 80 percent of processed foods in the world, and they're creating billions and billions of dollars in profits by poisoning people," he says. "I'd tax them out of existence. If you don't take addictive foods out of the environment, you'll never cure the addiction."

Some of Noakes's fellow scientists think he's going too far. The Heart Association was quick to urge caution; the same day Noakes began advocating saturated fats, the Heart Association issued a warning that "the 'Noakes Diet' is dangerous." It was an impressive performance, Noakes felt; cramming three mistakes into four words in one day isn't easy. It's not *his*, he argues, since it's been the basis of human nutrition for more than two million years. It's not a *diet*, because there are no portion or calorie restrictions. And how can it possibly be *dangerous* when humans have thrived on those very foods for most of our existence? If it were dangerous, we'd be extinct.

Rather than going too far, Noakes is furious with himself for starting so late. Back when he first began to suspect he'd been wrong about carbs, Noakes dug into the data on Ironman legend Mark Allen. Allen's eating habits were well-documented. Noakes could find almost no starches or processed carbs in the mix. So how could Allen possibly scorch out a marathon in two hours and forty minutes, immediately after swimming nearly two and a half miles and biking one hundred and twelve? There was only one explanation. "I knew that he had to start the race without any sugar or glycogen in his muscles," Noakes would say. "So he must've just been burning fat."

"Phil Maffetone knew this years ago," Noakes concluded. "Fat as fuel. It's exactly what he was saying all the way back in the eighties. Imagine the difference if we'd just listened to him."

Or knew where he was.

CHAPTER 34

Then they cut slices from the thighs, wrapped them
in layers of fat, and laid raw meat on top . . . while the young
men stood by, five-pronged forks in their hands.

—HOMER, the *Iliad*

FOR A MAN who'd spent years on the speed dial of athletes and rock
stars, Phil Maffetone knows how to make himself scarce. The only
online presence for a person by that name when I went looking for him
was a bare-bones Web page, a placeholder for some singer-songwriter
that provided no contact info or any mention of medical or athletic
work. But in an old paperback, long out of print, I came across a lead.

Back in the eighties, Maffetone published a slim manual called *In
Fitness and in Health.* Inside, I spotted a name I recognized: Hal Wal-
ter, a pro burro racer I'd met in Colorado during an annual ultramarathon in which athletes run up and down a mountain alongside a
pack burro. Prize money on the burro-racing circuit is pretty lean,
so in the off-season Hal was a freelance editor and outdoors writer.
That's how he met Phil Maffetone; in exchange for edits, Hal got fat-
as-fuel training. Whatever tips Maffetone gave him must have been
gold: Hal won his *seventh* world championship in fifteen years, at age
fifty-three, and could still average seven minutes per mile for thirty

miles, at thirteen thousand feet. During races that can last five or more hours, he only sips water.

I contacted Hal, who agreed to pass my message along to Maffetone. A week or so later, I received an e-mail from "pm." No name, just the two lowercase letters. If I was interested in talking, pm said, I should come to Oracle, Arizona.

> *Our home isn't that easy to find. Call when you get close and I'll talk you in. If your cell phone works. Don't count on it.*

So I was off to Oracle, a lonely desert outpost best known for UFO sightings and the occasional underground meth lab. Not far away is Biosphere 2, a self-contained environmental experiment constructed there deliberately to avoid being noticed by, basically, anyone. Edward Abbey had the same idea: decades ago, the irascible writer and eco-warrior began using Oracle as his mailing address so no one would know where he was. Geographically and psychologically, Oracle is out there.

I followed pm's directions, crossing an old railroad track and rumbling down a dusty, red-dirt road until I pulled up at a pleasant little cottage ringed by an artful garden of desert plants. Chickens scratched in the side yard, then scattered behind the cacti when the door opened and a lean, handsome man with a snow-white ponytail stepped out.

"Was I really that hard to find?" Maffetone asked.

"You mean the drive? Not so bad. But the rest—"

Maffetone shrugged and led me inside to meet his wife, Dr. Coralee Thompson, a physician who for fifteen years was medical director at Philadelphia's Institutes for the Achievement of Human Potential. "People seem to think I just went up in smoke like a genie."

In Maffetone's eyes, his sudden transformation from Dr. Ironman into InvisiPhil was a logical step. Fat-as-fuel was an intellectual challenge, and once he'd solved it—neatly, effectively, solid as a mathematical proof—it was on to the next endeavor. "I've had original music in my head since I was three years old," he says. "It was time to do something about it." So he shuttered his practice, referred his clients, rented his New York home, and rambled across the country until he found a place where he wouldn't be disturbed or tempted back into endurance sports.

Which, he's too polite to say, is exactly what I'm doing. The whole reason he settled out here, alone with coyote howls and Coralee and the guitar Johnny Cash gave him, was specifically to avoid people like me. But when he saw my message, he was intrigued; once Maffetone understood what I was up to, he spotted a connection I'd missed. I'd been wondering whether Paddy and Xan and their Cretan accomplices could have survived their long adventures through the mountains because they'd learned to tap into fat as fuel, but Maffetone realized something else.

"Do you know the healthiest diet in the world?" he asked.

"The Mediterranean?"

"Right. Do you know where it's from?

"Greece?"

"Close," he said. "Crete."

Crete was both the strangest and most enduring result of Ancel Keys's Seven Countries Study. Keys's goal was to pin down the lifestyle causes of heart attacks and strokes, so for twelve years—from 1958 to 1970—his team gathered biological markers from men aged forty to fifty-nine, in Italy, Japan, Yugoslavia, Finland, Holland, America, and Greece. It really was a noble experiment; in his own way, Keys was trying to save millions of lives by demonstrating that cardiovascular disease was an active choice, not an Act of God. No one disputes the data Keys collected; they just argued that he should have included regions that didn't necessarily fall in line with his saturated-fat-is-fatal theory.

For Greece, Keys took most of his subjects from Crete. It was a rare opportunity to travel back in time, because life in those mountain villages hadn't changed in three hundred years. Cretan farmers were still living like their ancestors; they used the same rough tools, ate the same foods, slept in the same huts, and raised sheep descended from the same family flock. If Keys was right, and heart attacks were the result of a decadent modern lifestyle, then these Middle Age throwbacks should be fantastically healthy. And they were—except for one weird twist. The Cretans had the lowest rate of heart disease in the entire study, yet their serum cholesterol was high and they ate a *ton* of fat, more than any other country in the study. Nearly half of the calories that went down a Cretan's throat came from fat. Going by Keys's model, heart disease should have been all over those mountains. Instead, the Cretans lived long and stayed strong.

So why were Cretans more heart healthy than everyone else, including the Japanese, who consumed only a quarter as much fat? The secret was partly what they ate—meat, butter, fish, olive oil, wild greens, and walnuts—but mostly what they didn't: sugar and starch. Unlike the rest of the industrialized world, Crete wasn't jolted by World War II into a new way of eating. Much of postwar Europe and Asia desperately needed aid, so cattle and dairy farms were repurposed to raise grain; in a pinch, bread and porridge could fill more bellies and wouldn't spoil in transit. Twenty years before Keys showed up with his research team, Finland had already begun converting grazing pasture into wheat fields and rows of sugar beets, which were processed into an all-purpose additive akin to high-fructose corn syrup. "During the Great Depression of the 1930s," a Finnish economic analysis noted, the government "encouraged farmers to shift from exportable animal products to basic grains, a policy that kept farm incomes from falling as rapidly as they did elsewhere and enabled the country to feed itself better." One result: more Finns died of heart disease than anyone else in the Seven Countries study.

Prosperity was its own peril in the United States. Giant factories constructed to feed the troops were now turning their attention to the family home, using wartime technologies to churn out canned soups, easy-grab snacks, and packaged bread. Orange juice, an exotic treat before the war, was suddenly *everywhere*; military contractors had figured out how to make frozen concentrate, and as soon as growers realized it could be sold as a "health" food, orange juice production skyrocketed from barely a quarter-million gallons a year to more than 115 million. Three out of every four Americans soon had OJ in the freezer, right next to another new sensation: frozen TV dinners, prepackaged with plenty of sugar, salt, and hydrogenated vegetable oil. In 1951, Kellogg's rolled out its twin juggernauts—Sugar Frosted Flakes and Sugar Pops—then removed even the need for milk by inventing Pop-Tarts. The Great American Breakfast of bacon and eggs was becoming a dinosaur, along with home-cooked dinners, locally baked bread, and backyard gardens. Sucrose, fructose, corn syrup, and bleached white flour—the difference between dinner and dessert had disappeared.

But up in the mountains of Crete, nothing had changed. Most villages were self-sustaining and barely reachable by road, so they remained untouched by the flood of starch and sugars engulfing the rest of the world. The Cretans kept foraging for wild plants, baking rough millet into loaves as chewy as jerky, frying free-range eggs in home-pressed olive oil, and eating every part of the sheep but the *baa*. Potatoes were rare in the rocky highlands; rice was unheard of; pastries were an occasional indulgence and nearly as jawbreaking as the bread. The Cretans, in other words, were eating the same high-performance food as their Olympic-athlete ancestors.

"Like this," Phil Maffetone said as we sat down with Coralee for lunch. They'd prepared steak—sliced thin and blood rare—alongside a jumbled salad of torn greens, tomatoes, cucumbers, and homemade goat-milk feta glistening with olive oil and sprinkled with fresh aromatic herbs. Break it down to raw components and it's the same food that Paddy and Xan survived on during their time in the caves: all slow-burn, all the time. "Those Resistance fighters couldn't have gotten their calories from starch and sugar, because it just wasn't available," Maffetone explains. "If they could only eat on the run, they needed food that would provide steady caloric energy all day." Greek battlefields didn't have Gatorade stations. Fugitives couldn't detour in search of snacks. Survival depended on two things: choosing slow-burn food and adapting your body to use it.

Maffetone was very late figuring this out, of course, at least compared with Pythagoras. The pioneering mathematician also had a side interest in sports science, and after he settled in Croton in the sixth century B.C., the city suddenly began churning out champions. At one Games, Croton swept the top seven places in the two-hundred-yard stadium race while winning both the boxing and wrestling crowns. Pythagoras's son-in-law, Milo of Croton, became ferocious enough in hand-to-hand combat to lead the annihilation of the kingdom of Sybaris and skillful enough in wrestling to rack up more victories than any other Olympian, a total of thirty-one victories over a twenty-four-year career.

And what contributed to their success?

"Pythagoras experimented with a special meat diet," it's reported, which was so effective that historians have battled for centuries over who deserves credit. Pausanias says it was Dromeus ("the Runner") who "proved true to his name" and dominated the distance events at four Games after he "conceived the idea of a flesh diet." A rival school says Pythagoras got there first; his student Milo "was famous for his meat consumption half a century before Dromeus is supposed to have discovered its efficacy in building up champion athletes." Ancient Greek trainers became so sophisticated in the nuances of slow-burn fueling that they could split hairs over "the relative merits of deep-sea versus in-shore fish based on what type of seaweed they would likely have eaten." On pork, there was no dissent; they all agreed you wanted to steer clear of pigs who'd foraged for crabs along the riverbanks and stick to the ones who fed on acorns and cornel berries.

But here's where the story gets strange: Milo retired, Pythagoras got into a political jam and moved away, and just like that, Croton was finished. No more sprinting laurels. No more titanic fighters. Whatever Croton was doing right, it wasn't doing it anymore. There's no record of Croton ever winning another title at the Games. The city didn't suddenly run out of strong young men or acorn-fattened ham, but whatever the magic was, it was gone.

"Food is only half the equation," Maffetone explains. "You can have the finest fuel in the world, but it's useless without the proper engine. It's two systems. It's input—what you eat—and output—how it's converted. But here's the funny part: it's really, *really*, simple."

"For anyone, or just seasoned athletes?"

"Anyone."

"How long does it take to learn?"

"Two weeks. Two weeks and you can master it. Two weeks and you'll be running on fat like your Resistance fighters."

I pushed my notebook toward him across the table.

Maffetone began scrawling notes. To give him time, I got up to help clear the table. Maybe I'd take a walk with Coralee until—

"Here you are." He couldn't have written more than a dozen sentences. I sat back down and started to read. *Really? It's that easy?*

Phil picked up the guitar and played me some of his songs. When it started getting late, Coralee packed me some of her special fat-as-fuel snacks for the road. Then I was heading home to see what the Maffetone Method could really do.

STEP 1: THE 2-WEEK TEST

Maffetone underlined "Test" in my notebook to make sure I got the point: this is emphatically Not a Diet. Diets, he believes, are a joke. They're based on a stupid, shame-based notion that losing weight is a matter of willpower and sacrifice, that you're heavy only because you're too lazy to starve yourself down to size. "It's baffling anyone still believes that, but they do," Maffetone told me. "Even when it's so clearly, *visibly*, unnatural." Humans are hunter-gatherers; we're born to search for food all day, every day, and scarf it down once we find it. Going hungry is the opposite of everything we've evolved to do.

So eat all you want, Maffetone urges. Just reboot your belly so it craves the food we've always hunted and gathered, not the fake stuff we've come to rely on. Once you've detoxed from the starch cycle and brought your body back to its natural metabolism, he says, you'll be free of hunger pangs and afternoon sugar crashes and midnight munchies. It only takes fourteen days, as long as you follow one rule of thumb: nothing high-glycemic. Nothing that jacks your blood sugar, in other words, and causes insulin to start storing fat.

By the end of two weeks I should be a fresh slate, glycemically speaking, and no longer cycling from sugar surge to sugar surge. Then, once the test is over, I can gradually add processed carbs back to my meals and see what happens. If I eat a slice of bread and feel fine, okay. But if it makes me feel bloated, sluggish, or sleepy, I'll know it's too much starch for my body to metabolize efficiently. That's what the 2-Week Test is all about; it's designed to reactivate your natural diagnostic panel, so that instead of relying on some diet book to tell you what to eat, you'll get instant, accurate feedback from your own body. "You'll actually know what it feels like to have normal insulin levels and optimal blood sugar," Maffetone explains.

So when I get home, I go shopping. I fill the cart with steak, fish, broccoli, avocados, canned squid, tuna, tomato juice, romaine lettuce, sour cream, and cashews—*tubs* of cashews, because they'll be my go-to temptation snuffer. Also on the "yes" list: eggs, cheese, whole cream, dry white wine, Scotch, and salsa.

But no fruit, breads, rice, potatoes, pasta, or honey. No beans, which means no tofu or soy of any stripe. No chips, no beer, no milk or yogurt. No deli ham or roast beef, either, since they're often cured in sugar. Turkey was fine if you cooked it yourself, but even then you have to be careful. I thought I'd hit the perfect multi-meal solution when I came across a stack of small Butterballs in the frozen food section, and only as an afterthought did I check the label and discover they were sugar-injected.

"Garbanzos are pretty moderate glycemically," I emailed Maffetone after I'd done a little research on my own. "So I'd like to lobby for hummus."

"Rule #1 of Step #1," he replied. "No lobbying."

The trick, I soon discovered, is solving one meal at a time. Breakfast was easy: by some whim I discovered that those $1.98 cans of squid from the Mexican food aisle are great in an omelette, so I'd fry up one of those, douse it with salsa, and be a happy man the rest of the morning. I kept cashews and spicy meat-sticks on hand throughout the day as snacks, and learned to add a splash of whole cream to my coffee instead of half-and-half. Lunch and dinner were only borderline crises when I got distracted and let myself get ravenous before planning what to eat.

By the end of Day 2, I felt like I had things under control—and then I stepped outside.

STEP 2: THE 180 FORMULA

I was barely a half-mile into an easy run and *whoa!* Why was my head spinning? I walked it off and began trotting again, but after another half-mile, I was bone-weary and panting. I wasn't tired, exactly; whenever I stopped running, I felt strong and rested and ready to go. But as soon as I began to push a little, my energy drained and that damn beeping started all over again.

For Step 2, Maffetone had me wearing a runner's heart rate monitor, a basic model with a chest strap and wristwatch console. The alarm was set to go off just before I hit my fat-burning threshold, which I'd calculated according to Maffetone's quick-and-easy equation. To figure out your fat-burning zone, you subtract your age from 180 and then fine-tune by this scale:

(a) If you've been sidelined for a while with injury or illness, subtract another 5.
(b) If you've been sidelined a *long* time (like recovering from a heart attack), subtract 10.
(c) If you've been training at least four times a week for two years, add 0.
(d) If you've trained hard for two years and are progressing in competition, add 5.

In my case, it works like this:

I'm fifty years old, so 180 − 50 = 130.
I run regularly and haven't been injured, putting me in
     category C: no additional points.
So: My fat-burning threshold is 130 heartbeats per minute.

That means I can work out as long, as fast, and as strenuously as I please, but whenever my heart rate hits 130 and my wrist alarm starts beeping, I have to ease off until my pulse drops back below the threshold. Maffetone believes your body is content to burn fat as long as it's not being pushed into oxygen debt. When you need more air, your heart begins to hammer; when your heart is pounding fast, it demands fast-burn fuel. So to wean yourself off sugar, you have to change both supply and demand: you cut the sugar from your diet and keep your pulse within your fat-burning zone.

Maffetone hit on the formula because of a happy accident. Heart rates "can be as low as 30 to 40 in those with great aerobic function to as high as 220 or higher in young athletes during all-out efforts," Maffetone explained. Using those numbers as his range, he originally put clients through extensive physiological tests to determine precisely when their metabolism kicked over from fat to sugar. After a few years of playing with the numbers, he realized he could just subtract their age from 180 and get the same results as if he'd done the testing. Why the math works, Maffetone can't say. It just does.

"One-eighty minus age itself is not a meaningful number," he explained. "It is not associated with VO2 max, lactate threshold, or other traditional measurements." It's just a shortcut to the end number: your maximum aerobic heart rate. Maffetone was delighted, because the magic equation allowed him to stop being the middleman between the athletes and their bodies. Maffetone believes the more you understand your own internal signals and stop listening to other people—even to him—the healthier you'll be. That was the beauty of the 180; it was so simple, anyone willing to invest fifty bucks in a heart-rate monitor could be their own sports-science lab.

Maffetone has tested it on hundreds of athletes, including triathlon legends like Mike Pigg and Mark Allen, and they've consistently come back with the same results: they recover faster from workouts, blow past their old records in competition, and leave chronic injuries behind. One reason they rarely get hurt is that they're no longer gritting through fatigue. When you go into oxygen debt, your form crumbles. Your head drops, your feet thump, your knees go cockeyed. You get sloppy, and you pay for it. "It was obvious that training at various intensities affected both posture and gait," Maffetone explained. "The more anaerobic, the more distortion of the body's mechanics."

"But if you're always going slow," I'd asked, "how do you ever get fast?"

"You work your way up a few heartbeats at a time."

You adapt. The more workouts you do in the fat-burning zone, the easier they get; the easier they get, the faster you can go. Maffetone predicted my workouts would feel ridiculously slow for the first few weeks. If you're used to running eight minutes a mile, he said, you might have to throttle back to ten and walk the hills to stop your heart-rate alarm from beeping. But you'll become so good at running ten-minute miles, he promised, you'll eventually be able to trot up any hill without breaking the 130-beat barrier. Before long, I should be able to run faster—and farther—than ever without hitting my heart-rate threshold or running low on fuel.

"Oh, and another thing," Maffetone added. "Don't be surprised if you feel a little bit, um . . . awful." When your body is denied its sugar supply, it can get grouchy.

Ugh. I saw what he meant about four minutes into the first run. Fatigue kept washing in and out like waves; I'd be clipping along easily, then suddenly feel like I coming down with the flu. It would pass after a few minutes of woozy walking, only to come roaring back shortly after I started running again. It was the eeriest sensation, like being yanked back and forth by a tug-of-war inside my own digestive system.

WE NEED SUGAR!

Shut your pie-hole, we're fine. Onward.

Maffetone had warned me to expect this, though, so I trudged on home and braced for a rough few days ahead.

Instead, I was greeted on the next morning's run by a pleasant surprise: instead of head spins, I got beeping. My heart-rate monitor began to chirp while I was a few hundred yards up an easy climb, and it dawned on me that I hadn't gotten dizzy yet. The storm had passed;

it was as if my body had given up the fight and surrendered the secret fuel stash it was hoarding. Now my challenge was keeping the damn wrist alarm quiet. Every time I got into a groove and started to leg it out a little—*beep beep beep*. Hills were the worst. I tried taking long, deep belly-breaths in hopes of Zen-mastering my pulse down a few blips, but it didn't help much. I spent that whole day—and the next, and the next—creaking along like a cyclist in granny gear.

At least Dutch skaters were going through the same thing. Back in the early '90s, the Dutch national speed skating team also began experimenting with low heart-rate training. It was a valiant quest, because as much as the Dutch love their skating, they were still up against ever more daunting powerhouses like the United States, Norway, and Canada. But despite the stiffening competition, the Dutch eased back; they replaced hard workouts with easier ones. In the seventies, 80 percent of their workouts were high-intensity; that total dwindled to 50 percent in 1992 and just 30 percent by 2010. It wasn't as if they were putting in more ice time, either. "We first hypothesized that the total amount of training hours would have been increased over the years. Our analyses showed that this was not the case," a research team concluded in 2014, after analyzing thirty-eight years of Dutch training logs. "Surprisingly, there was no increase in net training hours," the researchers added, "while performance increased considerably."

Considerably. Now that's a gentle way to put it. The Dutch *destroyed*. At the 2014 Winter Olympics, Dutch skaters crushed the field so relentlessly, on-air commentators complained it was bad for the sport. Together, Dutch men and women came home with twenty-three of thirty-six possible medals. Never in the history of the Games has one nation won so many gold medals in a single event. "The domination of their speed skating athletes has been total, with traditional rivals such as the USA, Canada and Norway utterly humiliated," the British *Guardian* summed it up.

The Dutch secret was as old as the Games themselves. The key to going fast, the Greeks believed, was a long time going slow. They called it "fatigue work," and until an ancient Greek athlete was twenty years old, he did little else. Fatigue work was raw, *Rocky IV*–style stuff: hiking mountains, carrying a heavy rock up and down a hill, climbing a rope slung over a tree branch, and the Ecplethrisma—running back and forth across the hundred-foot *plethron*, taking one step less every lap until you reached zero. The godfather of fatigue work, of course, was Milo of Croton; he came up with the idea of hoisting a newborn calf over his shoulders and carrying it around the stadium every day, gradually getting stronger as the heifer got bigger.

On the last day of my 2-Week Test, I tried a Milo of Croton experiment of my own. It was time to tally the results of my Maffetone immersion, which for me really boiled down to one question: was fat-as-fuel for real? Was it easy, sustainable, and effective? If by now I couldn't do more on less food—and find that food easily and eat it on the fly—then Maffetone's approach didn't explain how Paddy and Xan and their Cretan brothers-in-arms got stronger as life got harder.

Already I knew that in two out of three categories, Maffetone was scoring high. I'd lost eleven pounds in those two weeks, trimming me back to the same weight I'd been as a college rower nearly thirty years ago. I felt more like that teenage athlete again, too; not just skinnier but springier, more revved and rested. One afternoon I was about to head out for a run and suddenly remembered I'd done an hourlong Erwan-style workout that morning. I'd recovered so thoroughly, I felt fresh enough already to do it all over again. So I did. Even more surprising was the change that came over food: good old standbys like pizza, cheesesteaks, and doughnuts now seemed untempting and kind of gross. Soon I'd be allowed to ease them back into my meals, but it was hard to imagine why I'd want to.

The final exam, though, was out there on the Hill, the same place that made me woozy the first day and kept my heart-rate monitor beeping the next five. Since then, I'd stayed away. It was too aggravating. Even when I thought I'd adapted enough to glide to the top, the alarm always buzzkilled me down to a walk before I made it halfway. On this last day, though, I hit it just right. I warmed up on the approach and then backed off, easing into the climb. When I sensed I was passing the spot where I'd maxed out the first day, I didn't even turn my head to check. I kept eyes straight and everything else loose, trying to roll up and over this thing with my pulse slow-thumping in the fat-burning zone. Over and over in my mind, I looped the words of a wise old friend: "First focus on *easy*," Micah True used to say. "Because if that's all you get, that ain't so bad."

Halfway came and went without a beep, and I knew I had it. Why not? If Milo could work his way up to a thousand-pound bull, I should be able to handle a half-mile hill. The top was just steps away. I just had to remember to—

BEEP BEEP BEEP.

Breathe. Breathe, you idiot! *So close*, and I blew it by getting anxious and holding my breath. Still, if I could get that far on just fourteen days of adapting to fat-as-fuel, there was no telling how far I could get after a few months. Probably up and over the tallest mountain on Crete.

CHAPTER 35

If you really attack a fire, you put it out. But if you attack it
cautiously and fearfully, you get burned.

—GREEK PHILOSOPHER DIO CHRYSOSTOM,
the "Golden-Tongued"

I WASN'T counting on snow, though.

It was early May, the same time of year that Paddy was on the run,
when Chris White and I began tracking his escape route. Springtime
on Crete is like high summer anywhere else, so we'd spent the first
few days sweating under a blazing sun. It was so hot as we crossed the
Lasithi range that when we stumbled across a natural spring trickling
into a stone sheep trough, we tore off our clothes and plunged in for
a naked soak. For the rest of the day, we kept one eye on the trail and
the other scanning for more heaven-sent plunge pools.

Mount Ida was a different story. At daybreak, we stood at its base
and realized that high overhead, the gorge leading to the peak was
still choked with snow. There was no getting around it: the only way
Chris and I could cross the mountain would be to drop into that gully
and hope the snowpack was solid enough to hold our weight as we
crunched our way up to the top. If we were going to try, we had to
go now; the higher the sun rose, the deeper we'd sink if we crashed
through the crust.

"How high are we looking?" I asked Chris.

"High," he said. "Nearly three thousand meters." Chris glanced over his shoulder at the sun cresting the peaks behind us. We were starting at nearly sea level, so we had a long vertical ascent ahead before sunset. "Shall we?"

We shouldered our packs and began climbing, sidestepping through a long wash of crumbly scree as we traversed in an uphill diagonal toward the gorge. We were still on stone when the pitch suddenly veered upward, steepening so aggressively that I had to press my chest into the rock and climb with my hands to keep my pack from pulling me over backwards. The footing was so thin and crumbly, it was a relief two hours later to finally reach that long finger of snow-pack. We dropped into the gorge and were delighted—*It's frozen! Easy walking!*—until we crashed through and sank up to our hips.

The only way out was belly first. We clawed with our hands until we pulled ourselves far enough out to free our legs a little. Then, lying flat on the snow, we kicked and swam until we got ourselves back out and up on our feet—only to drop back in a few steps later. We foundered along, mastodons in a tar pit, until we hit a steep stretch frozen into a glassy sheet. This was even trickier; if we lost our footing, we'd slide backwards and rocket all the way down the slope until we crashed to a stop on the rocks. I was glad to have a few months of Erwan training under my belt to fall back on, but as usual, Chris knew what to do instinctively. He dropped to all fours and I copied him, kicking in with my toes and gripping as best I could with my hands as we inched along.

"Now," Chris panted. "Try this in the dark."

When Paddy and Billy eyed Mount Ida from the mouth of their cave, the sun worried them more than the snow. There was no way they could get the general across the mountain in a single night, which meant that no matter what time they started, at some point dawn would break and they'd be stuck out there in full daylight. The worst place was high above tree line—"the shaved scalp," as Billy called it— where they'd have nowhere to hide from planes and nowhere to run from pursuers.

So they dashed for it. After a recon plane passed in midafternoon,

Paddy and his band slipped out of the cave and went on the move. They'd attack the lower slope immediately, then duck for cover before the planes circled back at dusk. They'd wait for the high roar of the engines to fade away, then set off again, crossing the snow in the dark before making the last hard push off the mountain before dawn. It was a gamble, especially because the general would be on his own two feet.

"The steepness and irregularity of the track were too much for the mule," Paddy observed. "Back it had to go and the General, to his despair and ours, had to continue on foot up a slippery and collapsing staircase of loose boulders and shale and scree." But if they'd timed it right, it was their best chance to stay alive.

Waiting for Paddy at the foot of the mountain were the Five Georges: five shepherds, all named George, who'd been sent by the local rebel leader as guides and bodyguards. The Georges quickly fanned out, some taking point while others trailed behind to keep an eye on the prisoner. They led Paddy's band along spidery goat paths, zigzagging them up the steep stone until, just before dark, they reached snow line. "The last stunted mountain cedar vanished, leaving us in a stricken world where nothing grew and a freezing wind threatened to blow us off our feet. Then deep snow turned every step into torment," Paddy would say. "Mist surrounded us and rain began to fall. We stumbled on, bent almost double against the blast; no breath or energy was left even for objurgation."

Frozen and soaked to the skin, they fought through the snow at eight thousand feet, desperate for a warm sun but doomed if it came up. Paddy's plan, they all knew, had failed. They'd never make it off that mountain before dawn. So shortly before sunrise, the Five Georges improvised a Plan B.

The Georges led the band to an old shepherd's hut, a tumbled-down stone ruin with a collapsed roof that would give them a little shelter from the wind but not enough to draw attention. From the air, it would look like a pile of rubble and conceal them enough to wait for night to fall again. Paddy and Billy slunk back outside on a quick forage, hunting among the icy rocks until they spotted those familiar gray-leafed weeds. "Mountain dandelions," explained Billy, who'd grown to savor their "pleasant, bitter taste."

The two Brits brought breakfast back to the hut, where they found the Five Georges muttering and glaring at the general. "I think he must have sensed the atmosphere of antagonism," Billy observed, "for he kept very quiet and sat by himself in a corner, not speaking."

You've got a pistol, the Georges told Paddy. *Use it.*

The general was dragging his heels on purpose, they suspected. He knew they were vulnerable on the mountain, so he was playing a waiting game, dawdling along to keep them up there as long as he could. The Georges weren't going to be captured because Paddy was a nice guy. It was time to put a gun to the general's head and give him a choice: *Move or die.*

You're right, Paddy agreed. *But that will only work once. We need to reserve it as a last resort.*

Which, it turned out, was just a few hours away.

At nightfall, the band slipped out of the hut and began their descent. Going down, Billy soon discovered, was scarier than going up. The moon faded behind clouds, forcing them to grope their way blindly. If any one of them fell, he could tenpin the rest of the group and send them on a long slide into the teeth of a boulder field. "It took us two hours to reach the bottom of the snow belt," Billy said. And then it got worse.

"The mountain steepened to the tilt of a ladder," Paddy would recall. "It was channelled and slippery with rain and each footfall unloosed a landslide of shifting stones. We were descending, hand over hand, through what seemed, in the dark and the wind, to be a jungle of hindering branches, spiked leaves, and vindictive twigs." Every step was an act of faith; if the Georges accidentally led them off a dead drop, Paddy and Billy wouldn't know until they were falling through the air. Below, the rebels were supposed to signal all's-clear by lighting fires. Paddy and his band strained their eyes, searching the distance for pinpoints of flame, as Billy had to ask himself the only question that really mattered:

Why?

Why were they still pushing toward the coast, when the only ones who knew they were heading that way were the Germans? Did the British even know they were alive? How could they, when the one man they were counting on to coordinate their escape was still missing?

There was still no word about Tom Dunbabin's mysterious disappearance, and Paddy's attempts to improvise backup communication to Cairo were becoming deadly: a Cretan runner carrying a message to a wireless operator on the far side of the mountain was intercepted by Germans and shot to death, while two others barely got away. "They brought us ugly news," the rebel fighter Scuttle George would recall. "The Germans were hunting along the coast and up all the valleys. It was hopeless to go there. They also said it would be impossible for the English ship we were waiting for to approach the shore."

What was the point, then? Why cross this mountain when they had no idea if a boat could ever meet them on the other side?

But if the Five Georges felt any doubt, it wasn't slowing them down. They flowed down the back side of Mount Ida, sure-stepping along crumbling trails no wider than their feet and pivoting around boulders that suddenly loomed ahead in the dark. Keeping Billy and Paddy alive was the test of a true *hērōs*—a true protector—and there was only one way to pull it off: the Cretan way. They'd been raised to run farther, adapt faster, and survive on less than the men trying to kill them. All they had to do was find a donkey for the general, and they could stay on the move and fade back into the wilderness.

But first they had to get off that mountain.

From the top of Mount Ida, Chris White and I looked down and considered our options.

Off-trail, there was a skinny snake of a route that was somehow free of snow, but parts of it were too steep to walk and the rest was a crazy obstacle course of boulders and scree patches and sudden mini-cliffs where rocks had sheared from the mountain face. Or we could stick to the wandering thread of switchbacks, except they were so crosshatched by snowpack that we'd constantly be sidestepping on a forty-five-degree angle across frozen sliding boards.

"I've got an idea," I called over to Chris. "But you might hate it."

"I hate *this*," he said, kicking at the ice. "What've you got?"

I told him about Parkour, and my apprenticeship in drugstore parking lots and London housing projects. I filled him in on the way Shirley bounded over walls, and the fact that the Yamakasi believed elastic recoil was the secret of effortless movement in the new urban jungle. I'd even asked Dan Edwardes specifically about Crete, and he wasn't surprised that newcomers like Xan and Paddy and Billy Moss could learn to adapt. "The same thing we do in the city, they do in mountain terrain," Dan had said. "That 'Cretan Bounce' you were asking about? That comes from precision. When you hit a rock and bounce off, it's because you hit it square. You can't brake or doubt. You have to trust your body and go."

"So," I asked Chris White. "Do you want to try?"

"What, running down the mountain?"

"More like bouncing."

Chris toed the snowpack, then cinched his backpack tight. "After you."

I yanked in my waist strap and glanced down to check my boot laces. *Strip away conditioning and return to an innate, effortless way of moving that utilizes the entire body,* I recalled one Parkour disciple urging. *The elusive "flow state."* I jumped into the scree, sliding sideways down the steepest part of the slope until I got my balance and began to run, my feet stutter-stepping faster than my brain could process. I ran right off the edge of a mini-cliff, landing in a crouch so deep my butt almost hit the ground, and surged right back into a careening sprint.

"YES!" Chris was shouting behind me. "IT REALLY—"

My feet went out and I crashed, missing the rest.

CHAPTER 36

THE BUTCHER, DAY 8 OF THE ABDUCTION:

Cretans, beware! The edge of the German sword will
strike down every one of the guilty men and all the bandits
and all the henchmen and hirelings of the English.

CRETAN SHEPHERD TO PADDY:

He'd better look out or we'll capture him too.

I RUMBLED OVER ROCKS, sliding out of control, until I was able to
brake to a stop with my heels. I was still trying to figure out what
happened and how badly banged up I was when footsteps thundered
past close to my head.

"YOU OKAY?" Chris White shouted as he galloped by.

"Yeah," I called.

"GOOD! CAN'T STOP!"

Chris looked like a nervous kid at his first ice rink, with his back all
stiff and his arms wide and slightly flappy as he braced for the wipe-
out he knew was coming. *Loosen up*, I was about to shout, but decided
to keep my mouth shut. I didn't want to distract him, plus the guy
sprawled in the dirt wasn't really the one to be giving out pointers.
And as awkward as Chris seemed to me, it was working. He'd prob-

ably look just fine to Dr. Schleip, the fascia research specialist who demonstrated human elastic recoil by clipping his keys to a spring and letting them *sproing* up and down. Your body works the same way: as long as your movement is rhythmic and your center is stacked—head over shoulders over hips over knees, as erect as a boxer in the ring or a girl on a pogo stick—you can bounce along indefinitely. But when you break tempo or fall off-balance, you short out all that free energy from your rubbery tendons and connective tissue. That's what happened to me; I'd gotten a little fancypants with my tiny bit of Parkour and my Erwan jungle training and began adding quick-cuts and leaps. I was forcing it; Chris was flowing.

He's a marvel, I thought, then realized I was wrong: he's exactly what I should have expected. Chris is the natural born hero I've been looking for, the one that Georges Hébert and Teddy Roosevelt and the Heavenly Twins were certain was lurking in all of us. That's why Chris was mastering this stuff while I kept bumbling. I'd tried to data-dump it all into my system over the course of three years, but in his own instinctive way, Chris had been absorbing the art of the hero for six decades. As with all true heroes, his starting points were compassion and curiosity. He became his own Camp Half-Blood: instead of searching for instructors in London housing projects and lonely Arizona outposts, he's hiked and sailed and wandered about on his own, getting in over his head and finding a way back out again. His backyard cabin was full of maps and memoirs, making it a window into the minds of the people he was trying to understand. As a psychologist, he listened for a living, and on his adventures he'd turn that same encouraging attention on an old farmer telling a story in a language that Chris doesn't speak, and before he knew it he was being served a tasty dish he'd never heard of or being led to a cave that no other historian could find. In his own natural way, Chris had become the bond that united Erwan and Plutarch, Phil Maffetone and Paddy, Norina Bentzel and the Heavenly Twins: wherever Chris went, he was useful.

I was struggling to get there myself. I'd made a lot of right steps: instead of half-assing around with weights for a strength workout, I now climbed the twenty-five-foot rope I hung from a tree limb in my backyard. I practiced Steve Maxwell's personal invention, the "Traveling Maxercist," a functional fitness drill that takes three minutes and challenges just about every conceivable body movement. I followed Erwan and Shirley Darlington's lead and turned many of my afternoon runs into trouble-quests: I focused less on speed and distance and more on challenges, like scrambling up hills on all fours, sprinting from tree to tree, rolling under fences and vaulting over guardrails. Useful stuff.

But the key, as Chris was demonstrating in his mad contortions down the mountain, was forgetting about everything except the mountain. The reason I crashed, I had to admit, was because I'd been thinking about getting to the bottom first and staying ahead of Chris. I was trying to win, instead of trying to learn. Chris didn't care what he looked like; much the way Mark Allen only conquered Ironman after he stopped looking at every workout as a competition and instead submitted to Phil Maffetone's agonizingly slow fat-as-fuel method, Chris had absorbed enough of the heroic ideal to understand that the payoff comes after you stop grabbing for it. Learn the skills, and when the time comes, you'll be ready.

Watching him now as he learned on the fly how to Cretan Bounce down an Alpine descent was like watching Paddy and Xan Fielding and John Pendlebury in action. Chris was an unqualified man on an improbable mission, and so far he was succeeding brilliantly. He'd gotten us nearly as far as Paddy had gotten himself, and even though we'd started at eight thousand feet, Chris looked like he'd run out of mountain before he ran out of wind.

I hustled to my feet before he dropped out of sight. As I began to run, a tiny cluster of rooftops appeared below: the village of Nivathris.

"What are you doing here, boys?" Andoni Zoidakis exclaimed when Paddy and his band arrived at the bottom of Mount Ida near Nivathris. "You ought all to be dead!" Andoni touched his fingers to his forehead and belly, over and over, in the sign of the cross.

Then he paused, puzzled. But why did you ignore my warning?

After helping Paddy with the abduction and then killing the general's driver, Andoni had crossed Mount Ida ahead of the band to scout an escape route. What he found was terrifying. Troops were already linked in an unbroken chain and marching up the slope in a total comb-out. Columns of dust were heading toward Mount Ida from all directions with reinforcements, while observation planes were blanketing the southern villages with leaflets offering a choice between cash rewards and blood revenge.

Andoni scrawled an urgent message to Paddy and put it in the hands of a runner who knew where the band was hiding. In the darkness of a slit cave, Paddy flicked on his flashlight just long enough to read:

"In God's name come tonight!"

Tonight? Why on earth would Andoni tell them to leave the cave when Germans were all around them? They were in an excellent hideout, deep and dark, with only the thinnest crack of an entrance shrouded by thick brambles. You could pass within inches and never see a thing—and that was exactly what the Butcher's men were doing. Outside, shouts and stomping boots were everywhere. "I personally think that the airplane spotted us on the treeless expanse," Scuttle George would surmise. "The search parties were hunting the valleys inch by inch, firing off flares—and bullets too—and shouting, 'KREIPE! SPEAK UP! DON'T BE AFRAID!'"

The general grew smug as he heard his troops approaching. "Perhaps," he told Paddy, "you and your company will soon be *my* prisoners."

Scuttle George watched Paddy stare the general down. Paddy spoke, slowly and deliberately, and Scuttle George finally saw the leader he'd been counting on. "You will *never* escape these men," Paddy told the general. "They're ready to kill you right now. No matter how close your troops get, don't even dream of opening your mouth."

The general went silent. And long after dark, Paddy decided to swallow his doubts and trust Andoni's judgment. Leaving the cave seemed foolish, but Paddy and Manoli had both been struck by how "urgent and precise" the message had been. Andoni didn't suggest they come at once; he all but promised they were dead if they didn't. As the band crept out of the cave, it began to rain, then sleet. Warily, they felt their way through the dark and icy trees. Somehow, they arrived at Andoni's meeting place—a little clump of oaks with the watering trough cut from a fallen log—but Andoni wasn't there.

For two hours they shivered in the dark, growing more nervous as the sky lightened. Finally, they couldn't wait anymore. The Cretans led Paddy and Billy down the slope to the edge of Andoni's home village, where they crawled into a gully covered by a thick bed of thyme and myrtle. *Poor Andoni,* Paddy thought. First Tom Dunbabin disappeared, now him. Only a bullet would have stopped Andoni, Paddy knew. Only a bullet or . . .

Paddy dug out the slip of paper. He and Manoli pulled a coat over their heads to hide the flashlight beam, and with their heads pressed together they read the message again:

"In God's name come tonight!" Right. Exactly as they'd—

Wait a second. After "name," the paper was creased and a little soggy. Paddy spread the note flat, and as he smoothed out the wrinkle, two letters emerged: *bu*. Somehow they'd missed the single most important word in the entire message:

"In God's name *don't* come tonight!"

Good Lord. Andoni must have seen the troops moving out and realized they were marching shoulder-to-shoulder straight toward Paddy's cave. He'd implored Paddy to lie low until the Germans passed, but instead the band set off on a collision course straight at them—and passed through to the other side. "God exists!" Andoni exclaimed in amazement later that morning, after one of the Georges retrieved him from the village and brought him to the band's hiding place. "You ought all to build churches. What churches—cathedrals! How did you get through? The whole place was full of them. *Hundreds*, especially where you came down."

In a flash, Paddy understood what happened. "The Germans nearly always stuck to the main paths; when they wandered away from them, they usually got lost," he'd learned. "Everything ahead was a looming wilderness of peaks and canyons, and in the rougher bits it would be impossible for a large party to keep formation, or even contact, except at a slow crawl which could be heard and seen for miles." On a dark night over icy ground, the Butcher's men would have instinctively bunched together near the trail and not strayed off alone toward a deadly enemy in the dark, leaving narrow corridors for Paddy's band to slip through.

Where were the Germans now? Paddy asked.

"All gone up Mount Ida, after you and the General," Andoni exulted.

Paddy was ecstatic, but not for long. Andoni had more to say. Remember those two secret coves you were counting on as escape points? Both were blown. The Butcher had troops guarding them around the clock. Even the Preveli monastery, on the extreme edge of the island, was under surveillance, and the monks were being questioned by the Gestapo. "Our way of escape from the island was blocked," Paddy realized. "We had to begin all over again." They had outrun the Butcher, but they'd run out of island.

One hope remained: Paddy's favorite outlaw, the unstoppable George Psychoundakis, was on his way. George suspected that Paddy would need his help, so he raced across the northern mountains and found his way to the hideout. Beside him was "a great tough, free-booting giant," as Paddy put it, who'd slash the throat of anyone who even looked at the Clown crossways. Paddy knew why; this was the father of the little girls George had saved by carrying them to safety on his back. Yanni Katsias was a sheep thief and murderer with a price on his head and twenty corpses to his credit, but he became bonded for life to the little sprite by his side on the day George risked his life to save Yanni's children from a German attack.

With George and his arch-criminal blood brother there to help, Paddy began brainstorming a fresh plan. Paddy had stashed his Cretan costume in a village about five hours away. Could George retrieve it and come right back?

"Don't worry," George replied.

Good. Then Paddy would go full undercover, disguising himself as a goatherd and joining the Clown to scout the coastline. Somewhere along that rocky smugglers' shoreline, there had to be *some* forgotten nook where a British boat could slip in. Billy would stay behind and keep the general hidden, despite the handicap of speaking no Greek or German and barely knowing where he was. But nearby was a wild maze of a ravine where Billy and the general could go underground, and in the neighboring village of Patsos was a good man who could bring them a donkey and join them on the run. Yiorgos Pattakos was a young country boy, but among the guerrillas he was already known as "a determined and fearless *palikari*"—a true hero.

"Mr. Yiorgos Pattakos?" the voice said. "You are looking for Yiorgos Pattakos?"

Chris White and I had trudged into Patsos and shucked our sweat-soaked packs on the front porch of the village café—and by "village," I mean a handful of homes packed so tightly together at the bottom of a grotto, it seemed its most fervent civic wish was to never be noticed. The fog helps; as we were hiking toward Patsos across an endless boggy moor, we got lost in a fog that rolled so creamily off the sluggish horseshoe of a river, it felt like we were high in the Andes. We had to keep circling and backtracking, mucking through our own bootprints, until finally the sun cut through and we caught a glint of windows in the distance.

At the café, Chris showed his paper to the elderly woman behind the counter. She held up a finger: Wait. She dialed the wall phone, then handed Chris the receiver.

"You are interested in Mr. Yiorgos?" the crackly voice asked.

"Yes, we're hoping to—"

"I'm two hours away. I'll be there in ninety minutes."

Chris and I sat down to eat, tucking into giant Greek salads and a plateful of cheese. Before we'd finished, a black SUV roared down the thin slash of road and screeched to a stop in front of us. A bruiser of a man stepped out, big-armed and thick-chested with a jaw that looked like it could crack walnuts. He pulled off his wrap-arounds and scowled up at the café, pivoting his head like a tank turret from table to table until he locked in on us. His face split in a grin.

"Chreestopher!"

"So good to see you, Vasilios."

"A man of his word. You came back. I couldn't hear you on the phone."

Chris met Vasilios the previous year when he and Pete had gone in search of—and ultimately discovered—one of the more vexing of the kidnappers' hideouts, a narrow gash beneath a cliff which Billy Moss had described as being close to a shrouded waterfall that was so enticing, even the general stripped down to bathe. After being led to the falls by a shepherd, Chris and Pete trekked on to Patsos, where they got to know Vasilios, a Greek Special Forces combat diver and paratrooper whose mother owns the café. Vasilios liked the White brothers immediately and enjoyed telling them what he knew about his little village's commitment to the Resistance. Chris had promised to return, but it was evident from Vasilios's reaction that few visitors to Patsos ever found their way back.

"Mr. Yiorgos," Chris said. "Is he still alive?"

"Alive?" Vasilios asked, perplexed. "He's right here."

We turned and for the first time noticed an old gentleman in a gray beret sitting against the wall, his hands and chin on his walk-ing stick as he gazed out at the hills. Vasilios squatted beside him and spoke quietly, then beckoned us over. We pulled our chairs close as this remarkable survivor began to speak, bringing us back to the nightmare he endured and the day he was asked to choose between his family and his country.

"There was only one mule in the village," Vasilios translated. "And it belonged to the Kourkoulas family. . . ."

When the Hunters first appeared in the sky above Crete, Yiorgos was still a teenager. Somehow, he and the Kourkoulases' four-legged livelihood both survived the bombings and the burnings, the mass executions and the body-snatching raids by German troops hunting slave labor for their work crews. In a mountain village like Patsos, a mule is a life-support system, the only emergency-response vehicle that can carry a hurt child to the doctor and haul food across the peaks to the stranded and starving. The entire village depended on that one animal, so when a whisper arrived from the hills that a Brit-ish soldier was hurt and needed a mule to outrun a German manhunt, the only smart response was to keep your mouth shut and head down.

Instead, the mule's owner grabbed a harness and turned the mule over to Yiorgos. "They told us the officer was British," Yiorgos explained, "because they knew we'd never give the mule to a Ger-man." Yiorgos made his way down to the hiding place, accompanied by his sister with a basket of food. Ten guerrillas were waiting, along with a portly older man in a dark overcoat. "My sister passed around a bottle of raki and gave everyone some cheese," Yiorgos said. "One said, 'Don't forget our cousin, the policeman.' That was their nick-name for the general, because of his long coat. When the general took it off to piss, a boy who came with us saw the medals on his chest and was so scared, he ran away. Until we saw it with our eyes, we couldn't believe they really captured a German general."

When it was time to move out, Yiorgos helped the general mount. "We led the party right this way," Yiorgos told us, pointing to the lane in front of the café. "Everyone in Patsos saw him, and no one in Patsos told a soul."

"We never betray a secret!" Vasilios thundered, slapping the table.

"Never," Yiorgos agreed. "That's why the Germans never burned us. No betrayers, so they never knew."

Once past the village, the band started up a rocky slope into the mountains. "In a flash," Yiorgos said, "the mule jumped and threw the general, injuring his shoulder." Yiorgos helped the general back up, but the mule threw him again, this time so badly the general needed a sling for his arm. "He didn't like Germans," Yiorgos shrugged. To this day, the Midnight Payback of the Patsos Mule is commemorated on Crete by the expression *Tou stratigá to perasma*—"A general can fall into your lap," meaning "Even big shots get cut down to size."

For the next three days, Yiorgos was the general's personal escort as the band scrambled just out of reach of the search parties. The same night the kidnappers left Patsos, the Butcher's men surrounded the village. "They searched it, and though they found nothing, they took 40 villagers hostage," Yiorgos's cousin, George Harokopos, would recall. "Fortunately, they were all released five weeks later after exhaustive but fruitless interrogation." The Germans were getting dangerously close, but even more worrying, they were getting dangerously smart. Since the beginning of the war, Cretan men had been sleeping in the woods at night to avoid being surrounded in their villages before dawn. The ploy had been nearly foolproof—until the Germans, desperate to find the general, grew more cunning.

"The raiders used a new system," Harokopos explained. "They hid at key points among the trees, in the cornfields and up trees. They even let the unsuspecting villagers leave with their animals in the morning to work in the fields and the village. When they approached, the Germans leaped out at them." Every time the band thought it had a little breathing space, a scout arrived with a fresh warning. One night, the kidnappers were just tucking into a thickly wooded hollow when a shepherd burst from the trees.

"My friends, get up quickly!" he panted.

More than a hundred troops were heading right at them, storming down the dirt road from the mountains in trucks. Yiorgos and George Harokopos grabbed Billy Moss and the general and hurried them into a slit cave in the side of a ravine. The rest of the band scattered into the trees. Within minutes, machine-gun fire and grenades were exploding just west of their hiding place. Yiorgos and his cousin readied their weapons, but instead of drawing closer, the shooting drifted away. Local Resistance fighters had been shadowing the kidnap gang as an invisible escort, and as the troop convoy approached, they opened fire, creating a diversion and drawing the Germans in the wrong direction.

"*Yasou*," Yiorgos said not long after they emerged from hiding. "Farewell." He'd reached the limit of the countryside he knew, so it was time for a fresh mount and guide to take over. "Yiorgos Pattakos left to return east with the Kourkoulases' wonderful mule, which had made our journey so much faster in spite of the General's accident," recalled his cousin, who remained on with the kidnappers. Within a few days Yiorgos had retraced his stealthy steps back through the German patrols and arrived home.

"If I can ask a question," I said. "Would you do it again? Now that you're ninety-one years old, looking back—the Germans were murdering entire villages. Was it wise to put your family at risk?"

Vasilios began translating, but erupted before he finished. "Everyone from this village was a patriot!" he simmered, outraged I'd suggest otherwise. But Yiorgos quietly raised a hand.

"It's a good question," Yiorgos said, and then gave an answer which stayed with me for a long time and, the more I thought about it, kept extending further and further—from the four of us around the table to the ends of that tiny village, all the way across this embattled island and back to my own home and family. "When you live in a place like this—small, by itself—you're brought up to give help, not wait for it," Yiorgos began. When your neighbor needs something, he needs *you*. The person he knows. Not the army. Not the police. You. And if you're not there, someday you'll have to look him in the face and explain.

Vasilios was listening so intently, Chris had to prompt him to translate. "The Germans didn't know us, and they believed they could not lose," Yiorgos continued. "They believed they'd never have to look anyone in the face and explain. They'd never have to pay for what they did. And I believe that is why we defeated them." *Because we have to answer to one another, and they did not.*

Even Kreipe, who barely escaped the Russian front with his life and was now a prisoner in the wilderness, was still convinced Hitler would come out of this a winner. Kreipe told his captors exactly that: when Yiorgos's cousin joked that Kreipe was the last general they'd have to kidnap, since the Allies were on their way to victory, Kreipe responded—quite sincerely—that Germany was unbeatable. "The 'Wall of the Atlantic' was unbreakable," Kreipe said. "If the Allies tried to land in France or the Low Countries, they would be crushed." Germany might get pushed back, but eventually the Allies would wear out and negotiate for peace—just the way the Butcher, at that moment, was wearing out Paddy and his kidnap band.

Certainly, Paddy and his Cretan friends had their moment of glory—"This *Husarenstück*," as Kreipe called it, a "show-off's prank"— but playtime was coming to an end. Every day, the Butcher's men were getting closer. German soldiers were streaming down the mountains, they were lying in wait along the coastline, they had just missed rescuing Kreipe twice in the past few days alone. Kreipe could see Paddy was breaking down, and Paddy knew it himself. ("My right arm felt stranger and stranger; it was quite painless, but I found I could neither straighten it nor raise it very high," Paddy discovered). The kidnappers were outgunned and outmanned, and it was only a matter of time until they were out of options. This little heroic fantasy, Kreipe knew, was about to come to its painful and inevitable finale.

It was around that time, Yiorgos said—around the very day we were talking, in fact, May 10—that Paddy returned from his undercover recon mission. Yiorgos's cousin was there, and he could tell at a glance that something was up. "Late at night, Leigh Fermor himself arrived, astonishingly lively despite the distance of over 100 kilometers he had to cover in the last three days," George Harokopos would recall. Paddy always knew how to make an entrance, and this time he had a reason.

Yasou, koumbaroi. We're back, god brothers. And we may have something.

CHAPTER 37

If the Russian Peoples succeeded in raising their tired bodies
in front of the gates of Moscow to set back the German
torrent, they owe it to the Greek people. . . . The gigantomachy
of Crete was the climax of the Greek contribution.

—SOVIET GENERAL GEORGY ZHUKOV

Gigantomachy: the struggle between the gods of Olympus
and the demons of underworld

CHRIS AND I heaved our backpacks over the wire fence, then belly-crawled after them and into the final chapter of the chase.

Gunfire was crackling a few miles from this olive grove when Paddy and Billy's band got here. In one direction, Paddy could hear so many villages being dynamited that "it sounded like a naval battle." In another, Gestapo interrogators were going house to house in search of the man that, sooner or later, they always found: the one who said more than he meant to. A German garrison was less than an hour away over the hills, and the weird semi-paralysis in Paddy's arm was spreading down his right side, making him wonder, privately, how much farther he could go.

During his undercover recon, Paddy found trouble in every direction. The Butcher had studied the chessboard and realized the kidnappers had only one move left; they had to be running along the southern coast, hurrying from east to west in search of a safe beach. Unfortunately, British command helped confirm the Butcher's suspicions. Cairo had sent a rescue boat one night in the blind hope that Paddy was waiting near a drop spot the Brits had used before. When the captain flashed a cautious signal toward shore, machine-gun fire answered. Immediately after, two neighboring villages were destroyed. "They have burnt the place down and lots of Huns have been snooping round there," Paddy was told. "There was a lot of going and coming of Germans all along the coast. It was very sinister." Now that he was sure where the bandits were headed, the Butcher could do more than give chase; he could head them off. German troops began splashing ashore, securing the western shoreline. "Not only had the garrison at Preveli been doubled, but a strong German contingent had been landed by sea," Paddy learned.

The dragnet was looped together, and the Butcher was pulling it tight. Paddy and Billy had to face facts: it was time to stop running from the Germans.

And start running toward them. Crazy as it seemed, Paddy had enough close shaves under his belt by then to know that when it came to battling the Butcher, the worst strategy usually worked best. When Xan Fielding walked into the Chania mayor's office, he expected to find German officers, but they never expected to find him, allowing him to saunter in and out without attracting a glance. Paddy nearly got pinched when he was high in the remote mountains, yet he found it relatively easy to operate in the Butcher's backyard, where he pilfered documents from a staff sergeant's bedroom, whisked an Italian general out of the capital, staged a crackerjack of an ambush on the island's busiest road, and drove a kidnapped general at parade pace past the front door of Gestapo headquarters. The trick was getting so close, the enemy looked right past you.

So, in this olive grove below the village of Photeinou, Paddy and Billy knew their worst, best chance was right here—in the shadow of a German stronghold, on a stretch of beach that was suicidally exposed. It was awfully risky, which might just make it perfect. Paddy sent a message off by runner to the radio operator, and then the band climbed into Photeinou to prepare for the final showdown.

· · ·

Chris White and I were driving our knees down with our hands as we made the final push up the donkey trail that winds from the grove toward Photeinou. When Chris arrived here the previous year, he and his brother showed their paper to the first person they saw, an old woman passing by the village fountain. She had read it, then pointed to herself. Despina Perros had met the kidnappers as a young bride and made such an impression on them that Billy never forgot her.

Despina was in the midst of the wildest week of her life even before Paddy and Billy slunk into the grove. Her family had an ancient blood feud with a rival clan, and, after an eighty-year lull, it had erupted again when Despina's father killed a member of the Perros clan. Seven people were killed in the back-and-forth revenge attacks before someone dreamed up a way to stop the bloodshed: marry the kids. Despina was promised to Andoni, the youngest of the Perros boys. She sewed herself a wedding dress from salvaged German parachute silk, and peace between the families was restored.

"The time-lapse between their engagement and wedding had broken all speed-records in Crete," an amused Billy Moss observed, "but it seems to me that they are very fond of each other despite the stormy overture to their betrothal." The clans were staunch Resistance fighters when not battling each other, so they hurried down to the olive grove as soon as they got word that Paddy's band was approaching. The Perros boys set themselves around the perimeter on guard duty, while Despina cooked chickpeas and lentils. Paddy and Billy were famished and dug right in, but something about the armed-to-the-teeth Perros family made the general suspicious.

"The general thought they were going to poison him, so my father brought him boiled eggs," Stephanos Perros, Despina's nephew, told Chris and me after we made our way up to Photeinou. The village is even tinier than Patsos, with fewer than ten homes and no café. Stephanos lives only a few steps from the fountain where the White brothers first met Despina, who was away this time. "Kreipe wouldn't touch the eggs, either, so my father said, 'You have to eat something, general.' "

"I used to be a general," Kreipe replied. "Now I'm shit."

Stephanos invited us into his backyard garden, and there, over homemade wine and plates of nuts and olives, he told us about the last time anyone on Crete saw the General alive. As he spoke, we looked down at where it all unfolded, at those green hills tumbling from Photeinou straight to the twinkling blue sea—the Greek sea that was so close, so tempting, so skilled at luring men to their deaths.

Paddy knew that if they kept fleeing west, they'd be snared by the Germans who'd landed by boat. If they pushed back into the mountains, they'd run into the search parties coming down. So he sent word to Cairo that this would be the place: from here, they'd gamble that the Butcher was too preoccupied with distant beaches to worry about one right under his nose, just one mile from a German outpost.

Whether Cairo would agree, Paddy had good reason to doubt; in all likelihood, they wouldn't sign on for such a high-wire scheme from a military school reject they believed "requires firm handling." Still, Paddy was already fantasizing about what kind of booze a rescue boat might carry—"Pink Gin? Whisky? Brandy? *Champagne* perhaps . . . ?"—when he heard "a sudden, hysterical shriek," as Billy put it, ending in a heavy thud.

Some twenty feet below, a limp figure lay on the ground. The band had just set off from Photeinou toward a fresh hideout when the general slipped off a cliff and tumbled over the rocks. Billy couldn't believe it. For more than half a month, they'd fought and starved and scrambled to keep the general alive, and *now*, just before their last throw of the dice, he accidentally kills himself? The kidnappers slid down in a panic and found the general had landed on a thick bed of rotten leaves. He was uninjured, but furious and screeching curses. "The poor man must have lost whatever nerve he had been able to retain over the period of the past seventeen days," Billy acknowledged. They quieted him down and moved on.

The band made its way to a snug cave to wait for Cairo's reply—which, astonishingly, arrived almost immediately. Cairo finally had a communication link with the kidnappers, and it wasn't going to waste the opportunity. Every British wireless on Crete was soon buzzing with variations of these instructions:

Affirmative. Pickup vessel to approach location on May 14 at 22:00 hours. Code signals are S.B.

"Ten o'clock tomorrow night!" Paddy was stunned when he got the message. "We would only just be able to manage it." Quickly, Paddy split the band in two. He sent Billy off as a decoy with the Clown's outlaw companions—"Yanni Katsias and his two wild boys," Billy called them—since the four of them had the best hope of shooting their way out of an ambush. Then Paddy and Manoli pulled the general off the donkey and went the long way on foot, feeling their way by moonlight over the "limestone sickles and daggers," as Paddy put it, of boot-shredding Krioneritis mountains.

"Not one of the highest ranges of Crete," Paddy knew, "but they are among the steepest and are certainly the worst going." They were facing a long night, but not long enough: both bands had to be under cover by sunrise, yet close enough to the shore to reach the boat by dark. Billy's outlaw escorts faced this kind of challenge all the time with contraband deliveries, so they knew exactly what to do. "At times we almost ran, our route taking us up and down steep gradients like a madman's switchbacks," Billy marveled. "I don't think I have ever walked so fast in my life; and this was largely due to the cat-like maneuvers of the two sheep thieves."

By dawn, they'd reached an overlook above the beach. Billy pulled out his binoculars and saw gray-green uniforms everywhere. "Just below us, within full view, is a German coastal post," he noted. "There are a further forty Germans stationed less than one mile to the west, and since these positions are linked by telephone we have been careful to keep out of sight behind the rocks." At the moment, though, one of Billy's biggest worries was his partner. "Paddy is walking very stiffly and his cramp seems to be getting much worse," Billy realized. "He doesn't know what is wrong with him, and says he has never had anything like this before."

But soon after, Billy and the bandits were delighted to see Paddy and the general creep into camp. "It had taken them less than thirteen hours," Billy marveled. "Only five hours slower than our own break-neck rush." Somehow, the playboy poet who'd barely survived officer training and had a life expectancy of about three weeks when he first ventured behind enemy lines was now strong and adaptable enough—even with his right arm seizing up—to march a prisoner over the mountains all night through razor-sharp rocks. Paddy and Billy might never make it across that last bit of sand to safety, but it wouldn't be from any lack of hero schooling from the Cretan underground.

It was their own army training, in fact, that let them down in the end.

"How do you spell *S.B.* in dots and dashes?" Billy whispered on the beach that night.

"Haven't a clue," Paddy whispered back. "I thought you knew how to do it."

"Not I."

"Sure?"

"I know how to do *SOS.*"

"God forbid!"

Through the deep fog hanging over the sea, the muffled throb of engines approached. Billy and Paddy knew at least one letter, so maybe they could fake the other. They flashed three crisp dots for *S*, then a few hopeful blinks before starting over with three more dots. The boat engines came closer, slowed—and then began fading away. Paddy and Billy were staring into the mist, heartsick and helpless, when someone called their names from the rocks. Dennis Ciclitira, a British agent filling in for Xan Fielding, had just arrived over the mountain with a German deserter and two prisoners he wanted to ship out with the general.

"Do you know the Morse code?" Paddy and Billy hissed.

Dennis grabbed the flashlight and began blinking.

S . . . B . . .
S . . . B . . .
S . . . B . . .

Dennis kept flashing, hoping the light would cut through the fog to the departing boat yet remain invisible to the Germans down the beach. After half an hour, the only reply was hissing surf. Billy was trying so hard to *will* the boat back, he could hear his heartbeat thudding in his ears—and then he realized the thudding was approaching through the waves. A black shadow detached from the dark and drifted toward shore.

Billy's outlaws hugged him hard and scraped his cheeks with good-bye kisses. In return, Billy and Paddy yanked off their tattered boots and presented them to the sheep thieves and shepherds, the Clowns and the killers, who were staying behind to carry on the fight. Billy and Paddy helped the general into the dinghy, then pulled themselves aboard. Soon they were gliding into the darkness. Paddy kept staring at the beach, watching as the men who transformed him slowly disappeared.

"Crete is always difficult to leave," Paddy sighed. "It was especially so now."

All at once I heard shouts and music and cheers,
and realizing the entry had begun, I ran toward the shouting
as fast as my legs would carry me.

—GEORGE PSYCHOUNDAKIS, on the day Crete was liberated

BILLY MOSS enjoyed kidnapping generals so much, he went back for another one.

Six weeks after delivering General Kreipe to Cairo, Billy returned to Crete to snatch Kreipe's replacement. This time, the plan was a little messier. There was no chance of another roadside abduction, since all German officers were now traveling with heavily armed escorts—so Billy's scheme was to creep right into the general's bedroom and pull him out by force. Billy and a small band of Cretans managed to sneak up to the edges of Ano Arkhanais, a remote village that the new general had fortified into his stronghold, but at the last moment they received a warning that eight hundred troops were speeding their way. The local Communists, unhappy with Britain's influence in Greece, had tipped off the enemy to Billy's plot.

Billy escaped and decided to give up bedeviling generals in order to focus his attention on, basically, every other German he could find. He masterminded ambushes across the island, at one point crawling through the middle of a firefight to blow up a tank by chucking a grenade down the hatch. Billy returned to Egypt at the end of the war to enjoy what should have been a hero's reward: he married Countess Sophie Tarnowska, the beautiful Polish refugee who ran the Cairo party house, and wrote two popular memoirs of his adventures on Crete. But danger and adventure continued to tempt him, and it wasn't long before Billy abandoned his family to party and sail the Pacific. Drinking heavily, he died in Jamaica at just forty-four years old.

The mystery of Tom Dunbabin's disappearance was solved only after Paddy and Billy arrived in Cairo with General Kreipe. A severe relapse of malaria, it turned out, had flattened Tom just when Paddy and Billy were moving into position by the side of the road in their German uniforms. It was a dire situation: Tom was growing too weak to escape a German manhunt, and he knew the names, locations, and support network of every British operative on the island. So rather than jeopardize the entire Resistance, Tom had to vanish. He dispatched his radio operator to help Paddy and then dragged himself off to a secret hiding place. He didn't let anyone know where he was, or even what happened, for fear of being discovered.

Tom later recovered and returned to the fight. While trekking across the mountains, he and Paddy's loyal and extraordinarily courageous sidekick Andoni Zoidakis were locked in a gun battle with a German patrol. Tom shot his way out, but Andoni fell wounded. The Germans chained him by the feet, alive, to the back of a truck and gunned it, dragging him for miles across the rocky roads. His mangled corpse was dumped on the outskirts of a village as a Dark Ages warning to other rebels.

"I tried to persuade Andoni to come with us; he wavered a moment and then decided against it," a heartsick Paddy lamented. "I wish he had."

George Psychoundakis also remained on Crete and was rewarded for his years of danger and self-sacrifice by being chucked in jail.

George was awarded the British Empire Medal for gallantry, but in a cruel bit of irony, his work with clandestine forces meant the Greeks had no record of his military service. George was arrested as a deserter and "locked up in cells," as he'd later tell Paddy, "with brigands and Communists and all the dregs of the mainland." George began jotting down his recollections of the war while he was in prison and kept at it after his release, working by day as a road laborer and writing by candlelight at night in the cave where he slept. When Paddy returned to Crete years later, George had filled five student notebooks. Paddy was astonished to discover that this poor mountain shepherd who'd barely attended grade school had composed one of the finest accounts of the Resistance ever written. Paddy translated it himself, then persuaded his publisher to bring it out in English as *The Cretan Runner*.

George was at home in Asi Gonia, sitting with his wife beneath the grape trellis, when he received a message from Paddy about the publication. He ran inside, grabbed his gun, and began firing joyfully into the air. Then he buckled back down to his next work: translating the *Iliad* and the *Odyssey* into Cretan rhyming couplets. "It was a brilliant and almost unbelievable achievement," Paddy marveled.

George shrugged and said he mostly had a feel for the Cyclopes. "I am a shepherd, too, like Polyphemus, so I knew all about it."

Xan Fielding hated missing out on the kidnapping, but he had other things to deal with—namely, a firing squad.

Instead of returning to Crete, Xan was parachuted into France in 1944 on a sabotage mission ahead of the Allied invasion of Normandy. On his first drive through enemy-occupied countryside, he and two seasoned Resistance operators were stopped by the Gestapo at a roadblock. Xan wasn't all that worried: his French was excellent, his fake identity card was impeccable, and he was with Francis Cammaerts, the legendary master of mayhem who was already famous in Britain for seemingly impossible escapes. Xan also had a nifty cover story; he was searching for a new home for his elderly parents, and the other two gents were strangers who'd picked him up hitchhiking.

"You say you don't know these men?" the Gestapo agent asked.

"I've never seen them before in my life," Xan replied.

"Then can you explain how these bank notes, which each of you was carrying individually, happen to be all in the same series?"

Xan and Cammaerts had been lucky for too long and they'd gotten sloppy. They'd made the rookie mistake of divvying up one stack of cash for pocket money, all of it in sequential numbers. No amount of slick talking could convince the Gestapo that a straight run of serial numbers in the wallets of three complete strangers was a coincidence. Xan and his two fellow spies were hauled off to Digne prison and slated for execution. On the day they were to die, the three men were led into the prison courtyard—and out the other side. A staff car was waiting, and the three were ordered inside. The doors slammed shut and the car roared off. Christine Glanville, the Polish countess turned freedom fighter, had gotten word of the pending execution and raced to the rescue. Through some exquisite combination of tearful pleading and gentle bribery, she persuaded the Vichy guards who were keeping an eye on the prisoners that the Gestapo was about to make a horrible mistake. She got the spies out the door three hours before they were to be shot.

"Characteristically, Christine never told us exactly what methods she used to secure our release," a still bewildered Xan would say. But one thing was certain: "She had voluntarily risked her life in the hope of saving ours." Xan went on to further clandestine adventures in Cambodia before settling down to write. He found a kindred spirit in Pierre Boulle, the French secret agent who'd survived a hard-labor camp in Vietnam, and translated two of Boulle's most famous works into English—*The Bridge over the River Kwai* and *Planet of the Apes*. Like Billy Moss, Xan remained close to Paddy until the end of his life and penned two stirring accounts of his time on Crete. When Xan died, in 1991, Paddy summed him up with four words: "He was altogether outstanding."

The Butcher also got to tell his side of the story. General Friedrich-Wilhelm Müller was transferred late in the war to the Russian front and there was taken prisoner by the Soviets. He and one of his fellow Crete commanders, General Bruno Bräuer, were remanded to Greece to stand trial for war atrocities. Paddy visited the Butcher in prison and found him in a surprisingly receptive mood; when Paddy revealed that he was the one who'd kidnapped Kreipe, Müller laughed.

"*Mich hätten Sie nicht so leicht geschnappt!*" the Butcher retorted. "You wouldn't have captured me so easily!" Soon after, he and Bräuer were taken out and shot.

• • •

For a long, *long* time, Paddy kept Crete to himself.

By the time he arrived in Egypt after the kidnapping, Paddy was burning with fever, and the paralysis that had locked his right arm had spread into his legs. "Within a week I was in hospital stiff as a plank," he'd recall. Doctors were baffled. Was it polio? Rheumatic fever? Or post-traumatic stress, as one doctor speculated? "One is more anxious than one realizes," he told Paddy, "and somehow, when the subconscious anxiety relaxes a bit, nature steps in indignantly." Paddy spent three months in the hospital, sipping Moët & Chandon champagne from an ice bucket by his unfrozen left arm, until the ailment finally disappeared as mysteriously as it had arrived.

Back on his feet and with the war over, Paddy drifted in and out of romances and sponged off friends while trying to establish himself as a writer. He wangled an invitation to visit Somerset Maugham, who promptly kicked Paddy out of the house and called him "that middle-class gigolo for upper-class women." Like Billy, Paddy struggled to find his bearings in a world that seemed so peculiarly normal; but unlike Billy, he refused to write about his two greatest adventures. No one else had ever kidnapped a general *and* witnessed Hitler's rise while walking from the Netherlands to Constantinople, taking time out along the way to woo countesses, befriend gypsies, and sip old brandy with even older archdukes. Paddy was a truly magical story-teller, but the two stories he refused to tell were the ones everyone wanted to read.

But how could he? How could Paddy make himself out to be a hero after Crete taught him what a hero really is? Paddy was supposed to be a protector, a true companion whose *arete* and *paideia*—strength and skill—never outstripped his *xenía:* his humility and humanity. Villages were burned after the general was kidnapped. Women and children were murdered. Paddy's own good friend Yanni Tsangarakis died at the point of Paddy's gun. An accident, yes—but it's hard to feel peace in your heart when the dead man's nephew has sworn for thirty years to avenge his uncle's death by putting a bullet in your head, and once even staked Paddy out with binoculars and a hunting rifle. Had Paddy truly been a protector on Crete, or just an adventurer? Heroes, after all, aren't measured by the stories they tell—they're measured by the stories told about them.

So Paddy wrote a forgettable novel and a few respectable travel books, all the while struggling to turn the magic that flowed from his mouth into something that would stick to the page. He found and married his soul mate, and together they built a home on a lonely stretch of the Greek coast. And it was there, in the land of the heroes, that he was struck by a magnificent idea. Godlike skill comes only with a human connection. A hero, in other words, needs a sidekick. . . .

Paddy typed two words—"Dear Xan"—and memories came flooding back. Gypsies and boatmen. Hoofbeats and violins. Snatches of poems in forgotten languages. A beautiful girl at a Budapest ball, singing a song about birds so haunting that for the rest of his life Paddy would make it his signature: little scrawled wings of freedom and fantasy. He wasn't behind a typewriter; he was back in a cave on Crete, sharing his adventures with a friend. Paddy shaped this letter to Xan into a literary marvel, a two-book series of adventure, history, and scholarship called *A Time of Gifts* and *Between the Woods and the Water*.

But for forty years, Crete remained a dark spot in his heart. Then at age sixty, Paddy received an urgent phone message from George Psychoundakis: *Get here. Fast!*

For decades, George had been pleading with Yorgo Tsangarakis to call off the vendetta and forgive Paddy for his uncle's death. Yorgo finally gave his answer: *My daughter needs a godfather,* he told George. *Paddy will be my god brother and choose her name.* Paddy rushed to the airport, and soon after, was holding up baby Ioanna—named in honor of long-dead Yanni and Paddy's wife, Joan. Amid the wild dancing and embracing that night, Yorgo pulled Paddy aside to make peace, Cretan style.

I still have the binoculars and rifle, Yorgo said. *Who do you want killed?*

"It was the end of a miserable saga." Paddy glowed. "All wartime Crete rejoiced."

In 2011, at age ninety-six, Paddy returned to England to die. At a memorial, his final words were read: "Love to all and kindness to all friends, and thank you all for a life of great happiness."

Chris White, of course, was there.

ACKNOWLEDGMENTS

I couldn't choose between two different book ideas—one about Natural Movement, the other about a crazy wartime adventure on Crete—when conversations with my daughters about Rick Riordan's magnificent Percy Jackson series suddenly made me realize the two concepts were the same thing: the art of the hero *is* the art of natural movement. So thank you, Sophie and Maya; without you, this book would have been weaker at least by half. While I was beginning research, I made one lucky decision: after I repeatedly wrote to Patrick Leigh Fermor and never heard back, I was going to show up at his door and barge in for an interview. Instead, I first visited his lifelong friends, the husband and wife historians Artemis Cooper and Antony Beevor. Paddy was dying of cancer, so disturbing him would have been an awful mistake, but Artemis and Antony were warm and welcoming and astonishingly generous with their personal insights and unrivaled expertise (not to mention wine and pasta). I'm not the only one who feels that way; every Paddy enthusiast I've ever met has been overwhelmed by their graciousness. Chief among my Paddy guides, of course, are Chris and Pete White; I still don't know why the wonderful White Brothers allowed me to bumble along in their footsteps, but man, am I glad they did. Alun Davies and Christopher Paul were kind enough not only to share their stories about Paddy but treat me to drinks in Paddy's favorite club in London and show me, in its place of pride over the fireplace, Paddy's hand-drawn map of his Great Walk, complete with his signature flying-birds doodle. Alun was even kinder not to complain when I stuck him with the dinner bill because I'd forgotten to change money; four years later, I'm still cringing. Anything that's amiss in this book is probably something my editor, Edward Kastenmeier, tried mightily to get me to change. Why someone as patient as Edward is saddled with someone as stubborn as me is a mystery I'm sure he's pondered often. Luckily, he's assisted by fellow editor Emily Giglierano, whose deft touch brightened many passages. Normally I try to avoid any outside voices when I'm putting work together, which is why I'm so grateful for the dead-on comments from the one person I gave an advance look: Deb Newmyer, my friend and the head of Outlaw Productions. If this book becomes the next *Guns of Navarone*, we'll be thanking Deb. Last time around, I was busy ruining an early draft of *Born to Run* when Maria Panaritis sped to my home and helped get me back on course by stuffing me with those two Greek cure-alls: food and confidence. It worked. What a hero.

A NOTE ON SOURCES

For a man who became famous for his amazing recall, Patrick Leigh
Fermor could be oddly inaccurate at the most unexpected times.
Sometimes he fudged on purpose—claiming to be galloping on
horseback, for instance, to spice up a story about endless trudging—
and sometimes he simply flubbed, losing track of details as adventures
suddenly rose up and carried him along. That makes sense; you can't
live a life like Paddy's and still be a slave to facts and plans and daily
diary entries. And that's why, of all the accounts of Paddy's time
on Crete, his own is the most poetic and perplexing. Decades later,
Paddy could tell you exactly where he and George Psychoundakis
were hiding at precise moments of the Kreipe kidnapping (Day 10:
"The goat-fold of Zourbobasili"), yet he occasionally couldn't keep
straight if the island's biggest mountain was ahead of him or behind,
or whether the Butcher had been hot on his heels and leading the
chase or already transferred off the island. But that was Paddy's
genius, and the reason he became the only man in modern history to
successfully kidnap a commanding general. Paddy created excitement
by always being open to it, instantly veering the second he sniffed
something a bit more enticing than whatever he was supposed to
be doing. It led him to bizarre plots, like his attempts to infiltrate
a Haitian voodoo cult and his fortunately derailed scheme to break
into a notorious German prison camp, and it set him apart even from
fellow adventurers: in the midst of a grueling mountain expedition, as
Artemis Cooper notes, "everyone began to dread the familiar sight of
a solitary shepherd. Paddy would invariably hail the man and engage
him in a long conversation, which left everyone else hanging about,

kicking stones, for a good twenty minutes." He surged along through the years without a compass, which meant facts and his journals were occasionally lost in the tumult. Luckily, there are reliable outside resources that can reorient Paddy's memories. First and foremost are Paddy's biographer, Artemis Cooper, and her husband, the military historian Antony Beevor. No one was closer to Paddy during the last decades of his life, and I'd be amazed if even Paddy could tell his stories any better than they can. When I first contacted Artemis and Antony, they immediately invited me out to their country home, answering every question I had and prompting many I hadn't thought of. They were equally generous with their address book, putting me in touch with one of the last surviving members of Paddy's circle, Xan Fielding's ex-wife, Magouche. They told me tales that were beyond the body of this book but helped inform its spirit, like the way Paddy in his late eighties could still down twenty-six glasses of champagne without slurring a syllable, and the time Xan ran into a German officer years after the war and informed him they'd actually met before—the pretty girl the German had danced with in a Cretan tavern during the Occupation was actually Xan in disguise.

When Artemis was working through Paddy's long-withheld account of the kidnapping, she was aided by Chris White, whose boots-on-the-ground research uncovered elements that even Paddy didn't know. Chris and his brother, Pete, tracked down the most obscure references, like the young Cretan bride who delivered food one night to the general and his abductors. Paddy and Billy Moss didn't mention her name, only that she'd been forced into marriage to settle a blood feud between two rival clans. Chris found her and showed her a copy of Billy Moss's book, *Ill Met By Moonlight*. "She insisted that we mark the paragraph that features her and that we write her name—Despina Perros—next to it," Chris was later able to pencil into Paddy's account. "She was clearly very attached to her husband and mourning him as he is now deceased—so an arranged but happy marriage we assume!"

Tim Todd, Chris Paul, and Alun Davies likewise shared their discoveries from retracing Paddy's steps, and Alun in particular opened my eyes to details of the invasion and subsequent Resistance that only a military man would understand. They steered me toward so many written references that my backyard office finally looked like Chris White's, with faded maps pinned to the walls and rows of out-of-print books squeezed together in tight rows covering every flat surface. Some of the most useful were the following:

Chapter 1 (On the run)

Ill Met By Moonlight, by W. Stanley Moss. London: George G. Harrap & Co., 1950.

The best version of Billy Moss's epic is the limited 2010 edition published in Philadelphia by Paul Dry Books, because it contains a brief afterword by Paddy with his first print comments on the abduction.

Abducting a General: The Kreipe Operation and SOE in Crete, by Patrick Leigh Fermor. London: John Murray, 2014.

I only had access to the prepublication manuscript with embedded comments by Chris White. Since then, the book has been published with an excellent foreword by military historian and Resistance expert Roderick Bailey.

The Abduction of General Kreipe, by George Harokopos. Heraklion, Crete: V. Kouvidis–V. Manouros, 1973.

George Harokopos was one of the Cretan Resistance fighters who joined Paddy in spiriting General Kreipe toward the coast after descending the southern flank of Mt. Ida.

Patrick Leigh Fermor: An Adventure, by Artemis Cooper. London: John Murray, 2012.

Artemis's account of Paddy's life is a remarkable mixture of both painstakingly accurate detail and personal affection.

Chapter 2 (Occupied Crete)

The Fortress Crete, 1941–1944, by George Harokopos. Athens: B. Giannikos & Co., 1971.

Inside Hitler's Greece: The Experience of Occupation, 1941–1944, by Mark Mazower. New Haven and London: Yale University Press, 1993.

Mazower's study of archived German military orders offer a unique look at the Occupation from the perspective of the occupiers, especially the command that German soldiers were to view any Greek resistance as the work of "subhuman criminals who refused to recognize the legitimate authority in their country."

Crete: The Battle and the Resistance, by Antony Beevor. London: John Murray, 1991.

On the Run: Anzac Escape and Evasion in Enemy-occupied Crete, by Seán Damer and Ian Frazer. New Zealand: Penguin Group (NZ), 2006.

Dare to be Free: One of greatest true stories of World War II, by W. B. "Sandy" Thomas. London: Allen Wingate, 1951.

Chapter 3 (Art of the hero)

Justice at Nuremberg, by Robert E. Conot. New York: HarperCollins, 1983.

The Nuremberg Trial, by Ann Tusa and John Tusa. New York: Scribner, 1984.

The Cretan Runner, by George Psychoundakis. Translated by Patrick Leigh Fermor. London: John Murray, 1955.

Escape to Live, by Wing Commander Edward Howell, OBE, DFC. London: Grosvenor Books, 1947.

Greek Gods, Human Lives: What We Can Learn from Myths, by Mary Lefkowitz. New Haven: Yale University Press, 2003.

The World of Odysseus, by M. I. Finley. New York: Viking Press, 1954.

Chapter 4 (Churchill's scheme)

Franklin and Winston: An Intimate Portrait of an Epic Friendship, by Jon Meacham. New York: Random House, 2003.

Churchill: A Life, by Martin Gilbert. New York: Henry Holt and Co., 1991.

The Last Lion: Winston Spencer Churchill: Visions of Glory, 1874–1932, by William Manchester. New York: Bantam Doubleday, 1983.

Inferno: The World at War, 1939–1945, by Max Hastings. New York: Alfred A. Knopf, 2011.

Adolf Hitler, by John Toland. New York: Anchor Books, 1976.

Undercover: The Men and Women of the S.O.E., by Patrick Howarth. London: Arrow Books, 1980.

SOE: The Special Operations Executive 1940–46, by M. R. D. Foot. London: British Broadcasting Corporation, 1984.

A Prince of Our Disorder: The Life of T. E. Lawrence, by John E. Mack. Cambridge: Harvard University Press, 1976.

Chapter 5 (Norina Bentzel and the mystery of the hero)

Apart from news reports of the attack and subsequent trial, I conducted personal interviews with Norina Bentzel, as well as with responding officers and Norina's school colleagues.

Chapters 6–9 (Invasion and resistance)

Hide and Seek: The Story of a Wartime Agent, by Xan Fielding. London: Martin Secker & Warburg Ltd., 1954.

Ten Days to Destiny: The Battle for Crete, 1941, by G. C. Kiriakopoulos. New York: Avon Books, 1985.

Greece and Crete, 1941, by Christopher Buckley. Athens: Efstathiadis Group S.A., 1977.

Hunters from the Sky: The German Parachute Corps 1940–1945, by Charles Whiting. New York: Stein and Day, 1974.

Greek Women in Resistance: Journals, Oral Histories, by Eleni Fourtoni. New Haven: Thelphini Press, 1978.

Fourtoni's collection of first-person accounts by Greek women who fought in the Resistance is a rare glimpse into the lives of some of the most courageous and determined opponents the German army ever faced.

Crete, 1941: Eyewitnesses, by Costas N. Hadjipateras and Maria S. Fafalios (with a foreword by the British special agent, C. M. Woodhouse). Athens: Efstathiadis Group S.A., 1989.

Chapters 10–12 (Wobble power)

Forgotten Voices of the Secret War: An Inside History of Special Operations During the Second World War, by Roderick Bailey. London: Ebury Press, 2008.

S.O.E. Assignment: The Story of the Special Operations Executive by Its Second-in-Command, by Donald Hamilton-Hill. London: William Kimbler and Co. Ltd, 1973.

Secret War Heroes: Men of the Special Operations Executive, by Marcus Binney. London: Hodder & Stoughton, 2006.

How to Be a Spy: The World War II SOE Training Manual. Toronto: Dundurn Group, 2001.
This is the actual training syllabus and method guidelines developed by Fairbairn and Sykes and other instructors for use by wartime SOE agents.

"The Art of Guerrilla Warfare," a twenty-three-page training booklet by Colin Gubbins, architect of Churchill's special operations directive.

Shooting to Live with the One-Hand Gun, by W. E. Fairbairn and E. A. Sykes. Boulder, Colorado: Paladin Press reprint, 2008.

Get Tough! How to Win in Hand-to-Hand Fighting, as Taught to the British Commandos, and the U.S. Armed Forces, by W. E. Fairbairn. Boulder, Colorado: Paladin Press, 1974.

The Close-Combat Files of Colonel Rex Applegate, by Rex Applegate and Chuck Melson. Boulder, Colorado: Paladin Press, 1998.

Wing Chun Kung Fu: Traditional Chinese Kung Fu for Self-Defense and Health, by Grandmaster Ip Chun, with Michael Tse. New York: St. Martin's Griffin, 1998.

Chapter 13–17 (Xan Fielding and John Pendlebury)

Inside Hitler's Greece: The Experience of Occupation, 1941–1944, by Mark Mazower. New Haven and London: Yale University Press, 1993.

Auden and Isherwood: The Berlin Years, by Norman Page. Palgrave Macmillan, 1998.
Page digs into the strange, tragic saga of Xan's first and perhaps most important mentor: Francis Turville-Petre, "Der Fronny."

The Stronghold: An Account of Four Seasons in the White Mountains of Crete, by Xan Fielding. London: Secker & Warburg, 1953.

Xan returned to Crete after the war to hike its breadth and width. The result is a deep, sometimes tart, reflection on himself, the island, and the war.

Something Ventured: The Autobiography of C. M. Woodhouse. London: Granada Publishing Ltd. 1982.

Monty went on to distinguish himself as a member of Parliament and secretary under two prime ministers. His perspective on the clandestine work on Crete is even more stark than Xan's and Paddy's; as a diplomat, he was less impressed by his own derring-do and more concerned about lasting consequences.

Classical Spies: American Archeologists with the OSS in World War II Greece, by Susan Heuck Allen. Ann Arbor: University of Michigan Press, 2011.

The Bull of Minos, by Leonard Cottrell. London: Evans Brothers Ltd, 1953.

Cottrell provides a magnificent account of the stranger-than-fiction saga of Arthur Evans and Heinrich Schliemann as they both began lifelong quests to solve the "Homeric Problem": how could the *Iliad* and the *Odyssey* be so detailed and realistic if they were just make-believe?

The Will of Zeus: A History of Greece from the Origins of Hellenic Culture to the Death of Alexander, by Stringfellow Barr. New York: Barnes & Noble, Inc., 1961.

The Civilization of Ancient Crete, by R. F. Willets. New York: Barnes & Noble, Inc., 1976.

Willets provides an indispensable study of how the heroic ideal took root on Crete, rising from Minoan culture and creating the notion that each Cretan citizen is a *dromeus*—a runner who needs strength, skill, and compassion to care for his fellow citizens. Willets also fills in many details about John Pendlebury's exploration of the island.

The Villa Ariadne, by Dilys Powell. London: RC&C, 1973.

Powell's husband once mentored young Pendlebury, and her memoir is a breathtaking account of what it was like to roam the Cretan mountains with them.

The Archeology of Crete, by J. D. S. Pendlebury. London: Methuen, 1939.

There's no better look at the imagination, scholarship, and daring of Pendlebury as archeologist.

The Rash Adventurer: A Life of John Pendlebury, by Imogen Grundon. With a foreword by Patrick Leigh Fermor. London: Libri Publications, 2007.

Grundon created a thrilling and remarkably thorough biography (including the choice detail of the shared love Pendlebury and T. E. Lawrence had for the awful *Richard Yea-and-Nay*). She also provided an opportunity for Paddy Leigh Fermor, shortly before his death, to look back on the magnificent figure who dazzled him when he first arrived on Crete.

The Secret of Crete, Hans George Wunderlich. New York: Macmillan Publishing, 1974.

Chapters 18–22 (Xan and Paddy)

Hide and Seek: A Story of a Wartime Agent, by Xan Fielding. London: Martin Secker & Warburg Ltd., 1954.

The Nearest Way Home, by Daphne Fielding. London: Eyre & Spottiswoode, 1970.

Xenia: A Memoir. Greece 1919–1949, by Mary Henderson. London: Weidenfield and Nicholson, 1988.

Paddy makes a colorful appearance in this recollection of life in Greece before and during the German occupation.

A Time of Gifts, by Patrick Leigh Fermor. London: John Murray, 1977.

Between the Woods and the Water, by Patrick Leigh Fermor. London: John Murray, 1986.

A Time to Keep Silence, by Patrick Leigh Fermor. London: John Murray, 1957.

Roumeli: Travels in Northern Greece, by Patrick Leigh Fermor. London: John Murray, 1966.

Mani: Travels in the Southern Peloponnese, by Patrick Leigh Fermor. London: John Murray, 1958.

Vasili, the Lion of Crete: the Heroic Story of a New Zealand Special Agent Behind Enemy Lines During World War II, by Murray Elliott. Auckland: Century Hutchinson, 1987.

Botany, Ballet, & Dinner from Scratch: A Memoir with Recipes, by Leda Meredith. New York: Heliotrope Books LLC, 2008.

Jump Westminster: Parkour in Schools. A documentary film by Julie Angel. May 2007.

Ciné Parkour: A Cinematic and Theoretical Contribution to the Understanding of the Practice of Parkour, by Julie Angel, Ph.D. Self-published doctoral dissertation, 2011.

The Cretan Runner, by George Psychoundakis. Translated by Patrick Leigh Fermor. London: John Murray, 1955.

Chapters 23–31 (Escape by natural method)

"Eagles of Mount Ida," an unpublished manuscript by George Phrangoulitakis, aka "Scuttle George." Translated by Patrick Leigh Fermor. Stored in the Sir Patrick Leigh Fermor archive in the National Library of Scotland.

The Nazi Occupation of Crete, 1941–1945, by G. C. Kiriakopoulos. Westport, Connecticut: Praeger, 1995.

The Cretan Resistance, 1941-1945. The official British report of 1945 together with comments by British officers who took part in the Resistance, compiled by N. A. Kokonas, M.D. Forewords by Jack Smith-Hughes, Patrick Leigh Fermor, and Ralph Stockbridge. Rethymnon: 1991.

Unpublished memoir by Tom Dunbabin, 1955. Manuscript saved by his son, John Dunbabin, after his father's death in 1955 and provided to Patrick Leigh Fermor.

The War Magician, by David Fisher. New York: Coward-McCann, 1983.

The Last Days of St. Pierre: the Volcanic Disaster that Claimed Thirty Thousand Lives, by Ernest Zebrowski, Jr. New Brunswick: Rutgers University Press, 2002.

The Violins of Saint-Jacques: A Tale of the Antilles, by Patrick Leigh Fermor. London: John Murray, 1953.

Natural Method of Physical Culture, by Paul C. Bragg, Ph.D., and Patricia Bragg, Ph.D. Santa Barbara: Health Science, 1975.

A Natural Method of Physical Training: making muscle and reducing flesh without dieting or apparatus, by Edwin Checkley. New York: W.C. Bryant & Co., 1892.

Building Strength: Alan Calvert, the Milo Bar-Bell Company, and the Modernization of American Weight Training, by Kimberly Ayn Beckwith. Ann Arbor: Proquest, 2006.

L'éducation physique, ou l'entrainement complet par la méthode naturelle, by Georges Hébert. Paris: Librairie Vuibert, 1912.

La Culture Virile et les Devoirs Physiques de L'Officier Combattant, by Georges Hébert. Paris: Librairie Vuilbert, 1913.

The Rise of Theodore Roosevelt, by Edmund Morris. New York: Coward, McCann & Geoghegan, 1979.

Ill Met By Moonlight, by W. Stanley Moss. London: George G. Harrap & Co., 1950.

Abducting a General: The Kreipe Operation and SOE in Crete, by Patrick Leigh Fermor. London: John Murray, 2014.

A War of Shadows, by W. Stanley Moss. New York: MacMillan, 1952.

The Abduction of General Kreipe, by George Harokopos. Heraklion, Crete: V. Kouvidis–V. Manouros, 1973.

Chapters 32–36 (Fueling an escape on fat and fascia)

Slow Burn, by Stu Mittleman. New York: Harper Collins, 2000.

Training for Endurance, by Phil Maffetone. Stamford, New York: David Barmore Productions, 1996.

In Fitness and In Health, Phil Maffetone. Stamford, New York: David Barmore Productions, 1997.

Cheng Hsin: the Principles of Effortless Power, by Peter Ralston. Berkeley: Blue Snake Books, 1989.

Why We Get Fat: And What to Do About It, by Gary Taubes. New York: Anchor Books, 2010.

The Lore of Running, by Tim Noakes, M.D. London: Oxford University Press, 1985.

Challenging Beliefs: Memoir of a Career, by Tim Noakes, M.D. Cape Town: Zebra Press, 2012.

The Real Meal Revolution, by Sally-Ann Creed, Tim Noakes, Jonno Proudfoot and David Grier. Cape Town: Quivertree Publications, 2014.

The Way They Ate: Origins of the Mediterranean Diet, by Dario Gugliano, Michael Sedge, and Joseph Sepe. Naples: Idelson-Gnocchi Publishers, 2001.

"Eagles of Mount Ida," an unpublished manuscript by George Phrangoulitakis, aka "Scuttle George." Translated by Patrick Leigh Fermor. Stored in the Sir Patrick Leigh Fermor archive in the National Library of Scotland.

Ill Met By Moonlight, by W. Stanley Moss. London: George G. Harrap & Co, 1950.

Abducting a General: The Kreipe Operation and SOE in Crete, by Patrick Leigh Fermor. London: John Murray, 2014.

A War of Shadows, by W. Stanley Moss. New York: MacMillan, 1952.

The Abduction of General Kreipe, by George Harokopos. Heraklion, Crete: V. Kouvidis–V. Manouros, 1973.

A NOTE ABOUT THE AUTHOR

Christopher McDougall is the author of *Born to Run: A Hidden Tribe, Superathletes, and the Greatest Race the World Has Never Seen.* He began his career as an overseas correspondent for the Associated Press, covering wars in Rwanda and Angola. He now lives and writes (and runs, swims, climbs, and bear-crawls) among the Amish farms around his home in rural Pennsylvania.

www.chrismcdougall.com

A NOTE ON THE TYPE

This book was set in Janson, a typeface long thought to have been made by the Dutchman Anton Janson, who was a practicing typefounder in Leipzig during the years 1668–1687. It has been conclusively demonstrated, however, that these types are actually the work of Nicholas Kis (1650–1702), a Hungarian, who most probably learned his trade from the master Dutch typefounder Dirk Voskens. The type is an excellent example of the influential and sturdy Dutch types that prevailed in England up to the time William Caslon (1692–1766) developed his own incomparable designs from them.

Typeset by Scribe, Philadelphia, Pennsylvania

Printed and bound by Berryville Graphics, Berryville, Virginia

Designed by Maggie Hinders